Medical Statistics
at a Glance

A companion website for this book is available at:

www.medstatsaag.com

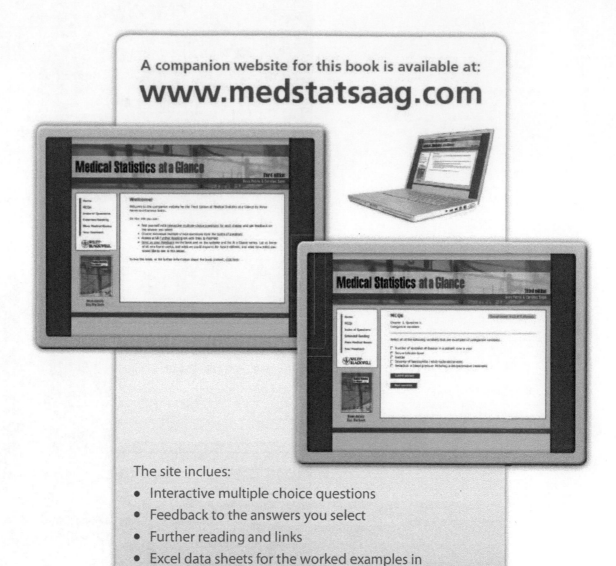

The site inclues:

- Interactive multiple choice questions
- Feedback to the answers you select
- Further reading and links
- Excel data sheets for the worked examples in the Workbook

This title is also available as an e-book.
For more details, please see
www.wiley.com/buy/9781119167815

Also available to buy!

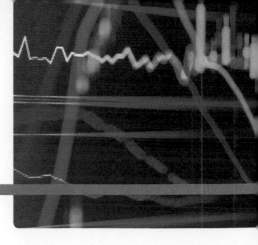

Medical Statistics at a Glance Workbook

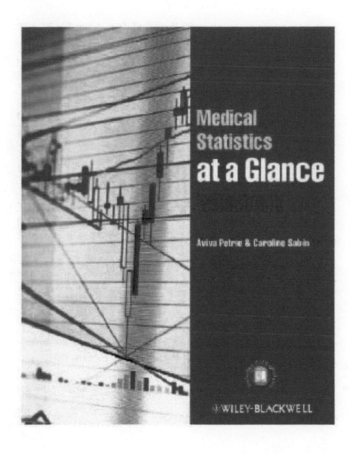

A comprehensive workbook containing a variety of examples and exercises, complete with model answers, designed to support your learning and revision.

Fully cross-referenced to *Medical Statistics at a Glance*, this workbook includes:

• Over 80 MCQs, each testing knowledge of a single statistical concept or aspect of study interpretation
• 29 structured questions to explore in greater depth several statistical techniques or principles

• Full appraisals of two published papers to demonstrate the use of templates for clinical trials and observational studies
• Detailed step-by-step analyses of two substantial data sets (also available at www.medstatsaag.com) to demonstrate the application of statistical procedures to real-life research

Medical Statistics at a Glance Workbook is *the* ideal resource to improve statistical knowledge together with your analytical and interpretational skills.

Medical Statistics at a Glance

Fourth Edition

Aviva Petrie

Honorary Associate Professor of Biostatistics
UCL Eastman Dental Institute
London, UK

Caroline Sabin

Professor of Medical Statistics and
Epidemiology
Institute for Global Health
UCL
London, UK

WILEY Blackwell

Registered Office(s)
John Wiley & Sons, Inc., 111 River Street, Hoboken, NJ 07030, USA
John Wiley & Sons Ltd, The Atrium, Southern Gate, Chichester, West Sussex, PO19 8SQ, UK

Editorial Office
9600 Garsington Road, Oxford, OX4 2DQ, UK
For details of our global editorial offices, customer services, and more information about Wiley products visit us at www.wiley.com.

Wiley also publishes its books in a variety of electronic formats and by print-on-demand. Some content that appears in standard print versions of this book may not be available in other formats.

Library of Congress Cataloging-in-Publication Data

Names: Petrie, Aviva, author. | Sabin, Caroline, author.
Title: Medical statistics at a glance / Aviva Petrie, Caroline Sabin.
Description: Fourth edition. | Hoboken, NJ : Wiley-Blackwell, 2020. |
   Includes bibliographical references and index. |
Identifiers: LCCN 2019008181 (print) | LCCN 2019008704 (ebook) | ISBN
   9781119167822 (Adobe PDF) | ISBN 9781119167839 (ePub) | ISBN 9781119167815
   (pbk.)
Subjects: | MESH: Statistics as Topic | Research Design
Classification: LCC R853.S7 (ebook) | LCC R853.S7 (print) | NLM WA 950 | DDC
   610.72/7—dc23
LC record available at https://lccn.loc.gov/2019008181

Cover Design: Wiley
Cover Image: © Somyot Techapuwapat/EyeEm/Getty Images
Set in Minion Pro 9.5/11.5 by Aptara
Printed and bound by CPI Group (UK) Ltd, Croydon, CR0 4YY

C9781119167815_260723

Contents

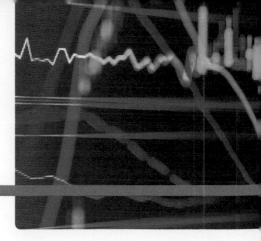

Categorical data

Regression and correlation

Important considerations

Additional chapters 115

Appendices 147

Preface

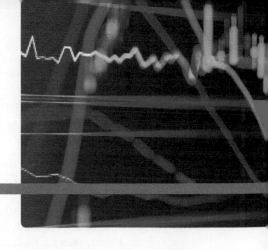

Medical Statistics at a Glance is directed at undergraduate medical students, medical researchers, postgraduates in the biomedical disciplines and at pharmaceutical industry personnel. All of these individuals will, at some time in their professional lives, be faced with quantitative results (their own or those of others) which will need to be critically evaluated and interpreted, and some, of course, will have to pass that dreaded statistics exam! A proper understanding of statistical concepts and methodology is invaluable for these needs. Much as we should like to fire the reader with an enthusiasm for the subject of statistics, we are pragmatic. Our aim in this new edition, as it was in the earlier editions, is to provide the student and the researcher, as well as the clinician encountering statistical concepts in the medical literature, with a book which is sound, easy to read, comprehensive, relevant, and of useful practical application.

We believe *Medical Statistics at a Glance* will be particularly helpful as an adjunct to statistics lectures and as a reference guide. The structure of this fourth edition is the same as that of the first three editions. In line with other books in the *At a Glance* series, we lead the reader through a number of self-contained two-, three- or occasionally four-page chapters, each covering a different aspect of medical statistics. There is extensive cross-referencing throughout the text to help the reader link the various procedures. We have learned from our own teaching experiences and have taken account of the difficulties that our students have encountered when studying medical statistics. For this reason, we have chosen to limit the theoretical content of the book to a level that is sufficient for understanding the procedures involved, yet which does not overshadow the practicalities of their execution.

Medical statistics is a wide-ranging subject covering a large number of topics. We have provided a basic introduction to the underlying concepts of medical statistics and a guide to the most commonly used statistical procedures. Epidemiology, concerned with the distribution and determinants of disease in specified populations, is closely allied to medical statistics. Hence some of the main issues in epidemiology, relating to study design and interpretation, are discussed. Also included are chapters that the reader may find useful only occasionally, but which are, nevertheless, fundamental to many areas of medical research; for example, evidence-based medicine, systematic reviews and meta-analysis, survival analysis, Bayesian methods and the development of prognostic scores. We have explained the principles underlying these topics so that the reader will be able to understand and interpret the results from them when they are presented in the literature.

A basic set of statistical tables is contained in Appendix A. Neave, H.R. (1995) *Elementary Statistical Tables*, Routledge: London, and Diem, K. Lenter, C. and Seldrup (1981) *Geigy Scientific Tables*, 8th rev. and enl. edition, Basle: Ciba-Geigy, amongst others, provide fuller versions if the reader requires more precise results for hand calculations. We have included a new appendix, Appendix D, in this fourth edition. This appendix contains guidelines for randomized controlled trials (the CONSORT checklist and flow chart) and observational studies (the STROBE checklist). The CONSORT and STROBE checklists are produced by the EQUATOR Network, initiated with the objectives of providing resources and training for the reporting of health research. Guidelines for the presentation of study results are now available for many other types of study and we provide website addresses in a table in Appendix D for some of these designs. Appendix D also contains templates that we hope you will find useful when you critically appraise or evaluate the evidence in randomized controlled trials and observational studies. The use of these templates to critically appraise two published papers is demonstrated in our *Medical Statistics at a Glance Workbook*. Due to the inclusion of the new Appendix D, the labeling of the final two appendices differs from that of the third edition: Appendix E now contains the Glossary of terms with readily accessible explanations of commonly used terminology, and Appendix F provides cross-referencing of multiple choice and structured questions from *Medical Statistics at a Glance Workbook*.

The chapter titles of this fourth edition are identical to those of the third edition. Some of the first 46 chapters remain unaltered in this new edition and some have relatively minor changes which accommodate recent advances, cross-referencing or re-organization of the new material. In particular, where appropriate, we have provided references to the relevant EQUATOR guidelines.

As in the third edition, we provide a set of learning objectives for each chapter. Each set provides a framework for evaluating understanding and progress. If you are able to complete all the bulleted tasks in a chapter satisfactorily, you will have mastered the concepts in that chapter.

Most of the statistical techniques described in the book are accompanied by examples illustrating their use. We have replaced many of the older examples that were in previous editions by those that are commensurate with current clinical research. We have generally obtained the data for our examples from collaborative studies in which we or colleagues have been involved; in some instances, we have used real data from published papers. Where possible, we have used the same data set in more than one chapter to reflect the reality of data analysis, which is rarely restricted to a single technique or approach. Although we believe that formulae should be provided and the logic of the approach explained as an aid to understanding, we have avoided showing the details of complex calculations – most readers will have access to computers and are unlikely to perform any but the simplest calculations by hand.

We consider that it is particularly important for the reader to be able to interpret output from a computer package. We have therefore chosen, where applicable, to show results using extracts from computer output. In some instances, where we believe individuals may have difficulty with its interpretation, we have included (Appendix C) and annotated the complete computer output from an analysis of a data set. There are many statistical packages in common use; to give the reader an indication of how output can vary, we have not restricted the output to a particular package and have, instead, used four well-known ones – SAS, SPSS, Stata and R.

We know that one of the greatest difficulties facing non-statisticians is choosing the appropriate technique. We have therefore produced two flow charts which can be used both to aid the decision as to what method to use in a given situation and to locate a particular technique in the book easily. These flow charts are displayed prominently on the inside back cover for easy access.

The reader may find it helpful to assess his/her progress in self-directed learning by attempting the interactive exercises on our website (www.medstatsaag.com) or the multiple choice and structured questions, all with model answers, in our *Medical Statistics at a Glance Workbook*. The website also contains a full set of references (some of which are linked directly to Medline) to supplement the references quoted in the text and provide useful background information for the examples. For those readers who wish to gain a greater insight into particular areas of medical statistics, we can recommend the following books:

• Altman, D.G. (1991) *Practical Statistics for Medical Research*. London: Chapman and Hall/CRC.
• Armitage, P., Berry, G. and Matthews, J.F.N. (2001) *Statistical Methods in Medical Research*. 4th edition. Oxford: Blackwell Science.
• Kirkwood, B.R. and Sterne, J.A.C. (2003) *Essential Medical Statistics*. 2nd edition. Oxford: Blackwell Publishing.
• Pocock, S.J. (1983) *Clinical Trials: A Practical Approach*. Chichester: Wiley.

We are extremely grateful to Mark Gilthorpe and Jonathan Sterne who made invaluable comments and suggestions on aspects of the second edition, and to Richard Morris, Fiona Lampe, Shak Hajat and Abul Basar for their counsel on the first edition. We wish to thank everyone who has helped us by providing data for the examples. Naturally, we take full responsibility for any errors that remain in the text or examples. We should also like to thank Mike, Gerald, Nina, Andrew and Karen who tolerated, with equanimity, our preoccupation with the first three editions and for their unconditional support, patience and encouragement as we laboured to produce this fourth edition.

Aviva Petrie
Caroline Sabin
London

Handling data

Part 1

Chapters

1 Types of data

Learning objectives

By the end of this chapter, you should be able to:
- Distinguish between a sample and a population
- Distinguish between categorical and numerical data
- Describe different types of categorical and numerical data
- Explain the meaning of the terms: variable, percentage, ratio, quotient, rate, score
- Explain what is meant by censored data

Relevant Workbook questions: MCQs 1, 2 and 16; and SQ 1 available online

Data and statistics

The purpose of most studies is to collect **data** to obtain information about a particular area of research. Our data comprise **observations** on one or more variables; any quantity that varies is termed a **variable**. For example, we may collect basic clinical and demographic information on patients with a particular illness. The variables of interest may include the sex, age and height of the patients.

Our data are usually obtained from a **sample** of individuals that represents the **population** of interest. Our aim is to condense these data in a meaningful way and extract useful information from them. **Statistics** encompasses the methods of collecting, summarizing, analysing and drawing conclusions from the data: we use statistical techniques to achieve our aim.

Data may take many different forms. We need to know what form every variable takes before we can make a decision regarding the most appropriate statistical methods to use. Each variable and the resulting data will be one of two types: **categorical** or **numerical** (Fig. 1.1).

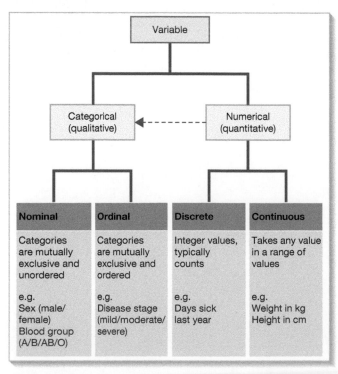

Figure 1.1 Diagram showing the different types of variable.

Categorical (qualitative) data

These occur when each individual can only belong to one of a number of distinct categories of the variable.
- **Nominal data** – the categories are not ordered but simply have names. Examples include blood group (A, B, AB and O) and marital status (married/widowed/single, etc.). In this case, there is no reason to suspect that being married is any better (or worse) than being single!
- **Ordinal data** – the categories are ordered in some way. Examples include disease staging systems (advanced, moderate, mild, none) and degree of pain (severe, moderate, mild, none).

A categorical variable is **binary** or **dichotomous** when there are only two possible categories. Examples include 'Yes/No', 'Dead/Alive' or 'Patient has disease/Patient does not have disease'.

Numerical (quantitative) data

These occur when the variable takes some numerical value. We can subdivide numerical data into two types.
- **Discrete data** – occur when the variable can only take certain whole numerical values. These are often counts of numbers of events, such as the number of visits to a GP in a particular year or the number of episodes of illness in an individual over the last 5 years.
- **Continuous data** – occur when there is no limitation on the values that the variable can take, e.g. weight or height, other than that which restricts us when we make the measurement.

Distinguishing between data types

We often use very different statistical methods depending on whether the data are categorical or numerical. Although the distinction between categorical and numerical data is usually clear, in some situations it may become blurred. For example, when we have a variable with a large number of ordered categories (e.g. a pain scale with seven categories), it may be difficult to distinguish it from a discrete numerical variable. The distinction between discrete and continuous numerical data may be even less clear, although in general this will have little impact on the results of most analyses. Age is an example of a variable that is often treated as discrete even though it is truly continuous. We usually refer to 'age at last birthday' rather than 'age', and therefore, a woman who reports being 30 may have just had her 30th birthday, or may be just about to have her 31st birthday.

Do not be tempted to record numerical data as categorical at the outset (e.g. by recording only the range within which each patient's age falls rather than his/her actual age) as important information is often lost. It is simple to convert numerical data to categorical data once they have been collected.

Derived data

We may encounter a number of other types of data in the medical field. These include:
- **Percentages** – these may arise when considering improvements in patients following treatment, e.g. a patient's lung

function (forced expiratory volume in 1 second, FEV1) may increase by 24% following treatment with a new drug. In this case, it is the level of improvement, rather than the absolute value, which is of interest.

• **Ratios** or **quotients** – occasionally you may encounter the ratio or quotient of two variables. For example, body mass index (BMI), calculated as an individual's weight (kg) divided by her/ his height squared (m^2), is often used to assess whether s/he is over- or underweight.

• **Rates** – disease rates, in which the number of disease events occurring among individuals in a study is divided by the total number of years of follow-up of all individuals in that study (Chapter 31), are common in epidemiological studies (Chapter 12).

• **Scores** – we sometimes use an arbitrary value, such as a score, when we cannot measure a quantity. For example, a series of responses to questions on quality of life may be summed to give some overall quality of life score on each individual.

All these variables can be treated as numerical variables for most analyses. Where the variable is derived using more than one value (e.g. the numerator and denominator of a percentage), it is important to record all of the values used. For example, a 10% improvement in

a marker following treatment may have different clinical relevance depending on the level of the marker before treatment.

Censored data

We may come across **censored** data in situations illustrated by the following examples.

• If we measure laboratory values using a tool that can only detect levels above a certain cut-off value, then any values below this cut-off will not be detected, i.e. they are censored. For example, when measuring virus levels, those below the limit of detectability will often be reported as 'undetectable' or 'unquantifiable' even though there may be some virus in the sample. In this situation, if the lower cut-off of a tool is x, say, the results may be reported as '$<x$'. Similarly, some tools may only be able to reliably quantify levels below a certain cut-off value, say y; any measurements above that value will also be censored and the test result may be reported as '$>y$'.

• We may encounter censored data when following patients in a trial in which, for example, some patients withdraw from the trial before the trial has ended. This type of data is discussed in more detail in Chapter 44.

2 Data entry

Learning objectives

By the end of this chapter, you should be able to:
• Describe different formats for entering data on to a computer
• Outline the principles of questionnaire design
• Distinguish between single-coded and multi-coded variables
• Describe how to code missing values

Relevant Workbook questions: MCQs 1, 3 and 4; and SQ 1 available online

When you carry out any study you will almost always need to enter the data into a computer package. Computers are invaluable for improving the accuracy and speed of data collection and analysis, making it easy to check for errors, produce graphical summaries of the data and generate new variables. It is worth spending some time planning data entry – this may save considerable effort at later stages.

Formats for data entry

There are a number of ways in which data can be entered and stored on a computer. Most statistical packages allow you to enter data directly. However, the limitation of this approach is that often you cannot move the data to another package. A simple alternative is to store the data in either a spreadsheet or database package. Unfortunately, their statistical procedures are often limited, and it will usually be necessary to output the data into a specialist statistical package to carry out analyses.

A more flexible approach is to have your data available as an **ASCII** or **text** file. Once in an ASCII format, the data can be read by most packages. ASCII format simply consists of rows of text that you can view on a computer screen. Usually, each variable in the file is separated from the next by some **delimiter**, often a space or a comma. This is known as **free format**.

The simplest way of entering data in ASCII format is to type the data directly in this format using either a word processing or editing package. Alternatively, data stored in spreadsheet packages can be saved in ASCII format. Using either approach, it is customary for each row of data to correspond to a different individual in the study, and each column to correspond to a different variable, although it may be necessary to go on to subsequent rows if data from a large number of variables are collected on each individual.

Planning data entry

When collecting data in a study you will often need to use a form or questionnaire for recording the data. If these forms are designed carefully, they can reduce the amount of work that has to be done when entering the data. Generally, these forms/questionnaires include a series of boxes in which the data are recorded – it is usual to have a separate box for each possible digit of the response.

Categorical data

Some statistical packages have problems dealing with non-numerical data. Therefore, you may need to assign numerical codes to categorical data before entering the data into the computer. For example, you may choose to assign the codes of 1, 2, 3 and 4 to categories of 'no pain', 'mild pain', 'moderate pain' and 'severe pain', respectively. These codes can be added to the forms when collecting the data. For binary data, e.g. yes/no answers, it is often convenient to assign the codes 1 (e.g. for 'yes') and 0 (for 'no').

• **Single-coded** variables – there is only one possible answer to a question, e.g. 'Is the patient dead?' It is not possible to answer both 'yes' and 'no' to this question.

• **Multi-coded** variables – more than one answer is possible for each respondent. For example, 'What symptoms has this patient experienced?' In this case, an individual may have experienced any of a number of symptoms. There are two ways to deal with this type of data depending upon which of the two following situations applies.

▪ **There are only a few possible symptoms, and individuals may have experienced many of them.** A number of different binary variables can be created that correspond to whether the patient has answered yes or no to the presence of each possible symptom. For example, 'Did the patient have a cough?', 'Did the patient have a sore throat?'

▪ **There are a very large number of possible symptoms but each patient is expected to suffer from only a few of them.** A number of different nominal variables can be created; each successive variable allows you to name a symptom suffered by the patient. For example, 'What was the first symptom the patient suffered?', 'What was the second symptom?' You will need to decide in advance the maximum number of symptoms you think a patient is likely to have suffered.

Numerical data

Numerical data should be entered with the same precision as they are measured, and the unit of measurement should be consistent for all observations on a variable. For example, weight should be recorded in kilograms or in pounds, but not both interchangeably.

Multiple forms per patient

Sometimes, information is collected on the same patient on more than one occasion. It is important that there is some unique identifier (e.g. a serial number) relating to the individual that will enable you to link all of the data from an individual in the study.

Medical Statistics at a Glance, Fourth Edition. Aviva Petrie and Caroline Sabin. © 2020 Aviva Petrie and Caroline Sabin. Published 2020 by John Wiley & Sons Ltd.
Companion Website: www.medstatsaag.com

Problems with dates and times

Dates and times should be entered in a consistent manner, e.g. either as day/month/year or month/day/year, but not interchangeably. It is important to find out what format the statistical package can read.

Coding missing values

You should consider what you will do with missing values before you enter the data. In most cases you will need to use some symbol to represent a missing value. Statistical packages deal with missing values in different ways. Some use special characters (e.g. a full stop or asterisk) to indicate missing values, whereas others require you to define your own code for a missing value (commonly used values are 9, 999 or –99). The value that is chosen should be one that is not possible for that variable. For example, when entering a categorical variable with four categories (coded 1, 2, 3 and 4), you may choose the value 9 to represent missing values. However, if the variable is 'age of child' then a different code should be chosen. Missing data are discussed in more detail in Chapter 3.

Example

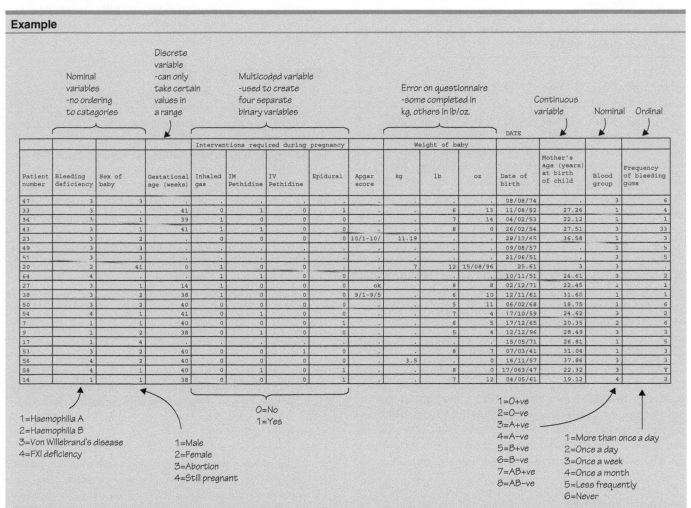

Figure 2.1 Portion of a spreadsheet showing data collected on a sample of 64 women with inherited bleeding disorders.

As part of a study on the effect of inherited bleeding disorders on pregnancy and childbirth, data were collected on a sample of 64 women registered at a single haemophilia centre in London. The women were asked questions relating to their bleeding disorder and their first pregnancy (or their current pregnancy if they were pregnant for the first time on the date of interview). Figure 2.1 shows the data from a small selection of the women after the data have been entered onto a spreadsheet, but before they have been checked for errors. The coding schemes for the categorical variables are shown at the bottom of Fig. 2.1. Each row of the spreadsheet represents a separate individual in the study; each column represents a different variable. Where the woman is still pregnant, the age of the woman at the time of birth has been calculated from the estimated date of the baby's delivery. Data relating to the live births are summarized in Table 37.1 in Chapter 37.

Data kindly provided by Dr R.A. Kadir, University Department of Obstetrics and Gynaecology, and Professor C.A. Lee, Haemophilia Centre and Haemostasis Unit, Royal Free Hospital, London.

3 Error checking and outliers

In any study there is always the potential for errors to occur in a data set, either at the outset when taking measurements, or when collecting, transcribing and entering the data into a computer. It is hard to eliminate all of these errors. However, you can reduce the number of typing and transcribing errors by checking the data carefully once they have been entered. Simply scanning the data by eye will often identify values that are obviously wrong. In this chapter we suggest a number of other approaches that you can use when checking data.

Typing errors

Typing mistakes are the most frequent source of errors when entering data. If the amount of data is small, then you can check the typed data set against the original forms/questionnaires to see whether there are any typing mistakes. However, this is time-consuming if the amount of data is large. It is possible to type the data in twice and compare the two data sets using a computer program. Any differences between the two data sets will reveal typing mistakes. Although this approach does not rule out the possibility that the same error has been incorrectly entered on both occasions, or that the value on the form/questionnaire is incorrect, it does at least minimize the number of errors. The disadvantage of this method is that it takes twice as long to enter the data, which may have major cost or time implications.

Error checking

- **Categorical data** – it is relatively easy to check categorical data, as the responses for each variable can only take one of a number of limited values. Therefore, values that are not allowable must be errors.
- **Numerical data** – numerical data are often difficult to check but are prone to errors. For example, it is simple to transpose digits or to misplace a decimal point when entering numerical data. Numerical data can be **range checked** – that is, upper and lower limits can be specified for each variable. If a value lies outside this range then it is flagged up for further investigation.
- **Dates** – it is often difficult to check the accuracy of dates, although sometimes you may know that dates must fall within certain time periods. Dates can be checked to make sure that

they are valid. For example, 30th February must be incorrect, as must any day of the month greater than 31, and any month greater than 12. Certain logical checks can also be applied. For example, a patient's date of birth should correspond to his/her age, and patients should usually have been born before entering the study (at least in most studies). In addition, patients who have died should not appear for subsequent follow-up visits!

With all error checks, a value should only be corrected if there is evidence that a mistake has been made. You should not change values simply because they look unusual.

Handling missing data

There is always a chance that some data will be missing. If a large proportion of the data is missing, then the results are unlikely to be reliable. The reasons why data are missing should always be investigated – if missing data tend to cluster on a particular variable and/or in a particular subgroup of individuals, then it may indicate that the variable is not applicable or has never been measured for that group of individuals. If this is the case, it may be necessary to exclude that variable or group of individuals from the analysis. There are different types of missing data[1]:

- **Missing completely at random (MCAR)** – the missing values are truly randomly distributed in the data set and the fact that they are missing is unrelated to any study variable. The resulting parameter estimates are unlikely to be biased (Chapter 34). An example is when a patient fails to attend a hospital appointment because he is in a car accident.
- **Missing at random (MAR)** – the missing values of a variable do not depend on that variable but can be completely explained by non-missing values of one or more of the other variables. For example, suppose that individuals are asked to keep a diet diary if their BMI is above 30 kg/m²: the missing diet diary data are MAR because missingness is completely determined by BMI (those with a BMI below the cut-off do not complete the diet diary).
- **Missing not at random (MNAR)** – the chance that data on a particular variable are missing is strongly related to that variable. In this situation, our results may be severely biased For example, suppose we are interested in a measurement that reflects the health status of patients and this information is missing for some patients because they were not well enough to attend their clinic appointments: we are likely to get an overly optimistic overall view of the patients' health if we take no account of the missing data in the analysis.

Provided the missing data are *not* MNAR, we may be able to estimate (**impute**) the missing data[2]. A simple approach is to replace a missing observation by the mean of the existing observations for that variable or, if the data are longitudinal, by the last observed value. These are examples of **single imputation**. In **multiple imputation**, we create a number (generally up to five) of imputed data sets from the original data set, with the missing values replaced by imputed values which are derived from an appropriate model that incorporates random variation. We then use standard statistical procedures on each complete imputed data set and finally combine the results from these analyses. Alternative statistical approaches to dealing with missing data are available[2], but the best option is to minimize the amount of missing data at the outset.

Outliers

What are outliers?

Outliers are observations that are distinct from the main body of the data, and are incompatible with the rest of the data. These values may be genuine observations from individuals with very extreme levels of the variable. However, they may also result from typing errors or the incorrect choice of units, and so any suspicious values should be checked. It is important to detect whether there are outliers in the data set, as they may have a considerable impact on the results from some types of analyses (Chapter 29).

For example, a woman who is 7 feet tall would probably appear as an outlier in most data sets. However, although this value is clearly very high, compared with the usual heights of women, it may be genuine and the woman may simply be very tall. In this case, you should investigate this value further, possibly checking other variables such as her age and weight, before making any decisions about the validity of the result. The value should only be changed if there really is evidence that it is incorrect.

Checking for outliers

A simple approach is to print the data and visually check them by eye. This is suitable if the number of observations is not too large and if the potential outlier is much lower or higher than the rest of the data. Range checking should also identify possible outliers. Alternatively, the data can be plotted in some way (Chapter 4) – outliers can be clearly identified on histograms and scatter plots (see also Chapter 29 for a discussion of outliers in regression analysis).

Handling outliers

It is important not to remove an individual from an analysis simply because his/her values are higher or lower than might be expected. However, the inclusion of outliers may affect the results when some statistical techniques are used. A simple approach is to repeat the analysis both including and excluding the value – this is a type of **sensitivity analysis** (Chapter 35). If the results are similar, then the outlier does not have a great influence on the result. However, if the results change drastically, it is important to use appropriate methods that are not affected by outliers to analyse the data. These include the use of transformations (Chapter 9) and non-parametric tests (Chapter 17).

References

1 Bland, M. (2015) *An Introduction to Medical Statistics*. 4th edition. Oxford University Press.
2 Horton, N.J. and Kleinman, K.P. (2007) Much ado about nothing: a comparison of missing data methods and software to fit incomplete data regression models. *American Statistician*, 61(1), 71–90.

Example

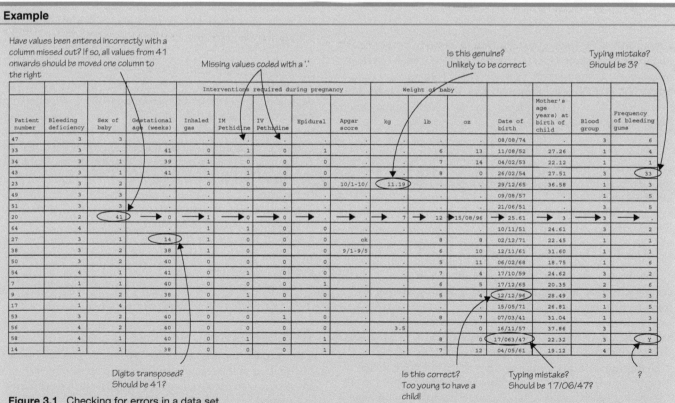

Figure 3.1 Checking for errors in a data set.

After entering the data described in Chapter 2, the data set is checked for errors (Fig. 3.1). Some of the inconsistencies highlighted are simple data entry errors. For example, the code of '41' in the 'Sex of baby' column is incorrect as a result of the sex information being missing for patient 20; the rest of the data for patient 20 had been entered in the incorrect columns. Others (e.g. unusual values in the gestational age and weight columns) are likely to be errors, but the notes should be checked before any decision is made, as these may reflect genuine outliers. In this case, the gestational age of patient number 27 was 41 weeks, and it was decided that a weight of 11.19 kg was incorrect. As it was not possible to find the correct weight for this baby, the value was entered as missing.

4 Displaying data diagrammatically

One of the first things that you may wish to do when you have entered your data into a computer is to summarize them in some way so that you can get a 'feel' for the data. This can be done by producing diagrams, tables or summary statistics (Chapters 5 and 6). Diagrams are often powerful tools for conveying information about the data, for providing simple summary pictures, and for spotting outliers and trends before any formal analyses are performed.

One variable

Frequency distributions

An **empirical frequency distribution** of a variable relates each possible observation, class of observations (i.e. range of values) or category, as appropriate, to its observed **frequency** of occurrence. If we replace each frequency by a **relative frequency** (the percentage of the total frequency), we can compare frequency distributions in two or more groups of individuals.

Displaying frequency distributions

Once the frequencies (or relative frequencies) have been obtained for *categorical* or some *discrete numerical* data, these can be displayed visually.
- **Bar or column chart** – a separate horizontal or vertical bar is drawn for each category, its length being proportional to the frequency in that category. The bars are separated by small gaps to indicate that the data are categorical or discrete (Fig. 4.1a).
- **Pie chart** – a circular 'pie' is split into sectors, one for each category, so that the area of each sector is proportional to the frequency in that category (Fig. 4.1b).

It is often more difficult to display *continuous numerical* data, as the data may need to be summarized before being drawn. Commonly used diagrams include the following:
- **Histogram** – this is similar to a bar chart, but there should be no gaps between the bars as the data are continuous (Fig. 4.1d). The width of each bar of the histogram relates to a range of values for the variable. For example, the baby's weight (Fig. 4.1d) may be categorized into 1.75–1.99 kg, 2.00–2.24 kg, …, 4.25–4.49 kg. The area of the bar is proportional to the frequency in that range. Therefore, if one of the groups covers a wider range than the others, its base will be wider and height shorter to compensate. Usually, between five and 20 groups are chosen; the ranges should be narrow enough to illustrate patterns in the data, but should not be so narrow that they are the raw data. The histogram should be labelled carefully to make it clear where the boundaries lie.
- **Dot plot** – each observation is represented by one dot on a horizontal (or vertical) line (Fig. 4.1e). This type of plot is very simple to draw, but can be cumbersome with large data sets. Often a summary measure of the data, such as the mean or median (Chapter 5), is shown on the diagram. This plot may also be used for discrete data.
- **Stem-and-leaf plot** – this is a mixture of a diagram and a table; it looks similar to a histogram turned on its side, and is effectively the data values written in increasing order of size. It is usually drawn with a vertical **stem**, consisting of the first few digits of the values, arranged in order. Protruding from this stem are the **leaves** – i.e. the final digit of each of the ordered values, which are written horizontally (Fig. 4.2) in increasing numerical order.
- **Box plot** (often called a **box-and-whisker plot**) – this is a vertical or horizontal rectangle, with the ends of the rectangle corresponding to the upper and lower quartiles of the data values (Chapter 6). A line drawn through the rectangle corresponds to the median value (Chapter 5). Whiskers, starting at the ends of the rectangle, usually indicate minimum and maximum values but sometimes relate to particular percentiles, e.g. the 5th and 95th percentiles (Fig. 6.1). Outliers may be marked.

The 'shape' of the frequency distribution

The choice of the most appropriate statistical method will often depend on the shape of the distribution. The distribution of the data is usually **unimodal** in that it has a single 'peak'. Sometimes the distribution is **bimodal** (two peaks) or **uniform** (each value is equally likely and there are no peaks). When the distribution is unimodal, the main aim is to see where the majority of the data values lie, relative to the maximum and minimum values. In particular, it is important to assess whether the distribution is:
- **symmetrical** – centred around some mid-point, with one side being a mirror-image of the other (Fig. 5.1);
- **skewed to the right (positively skewed)** – a long tail to the right with one or a few high values. Such data are common in medical research (Fig. 5.2);
- **skewed to the left (negatively skewed)** – a long tail to the left with one or a few low values (Fig. 4.1d).

Two variables

If one variable is categorical, then separate diagrams showing the distribution of the second variable can be drawn for each of the categories. Other plots suitable for such data include **clustered** or **segmented** bar or column charts (Fig. 4.1c).

If both of the variables are numerical or ordinal, then the relationship between the two can be illustrated using a **scatter diagram** (Fig. 4.1f). This plots one variable against the other in a two-way diagram. One variable is usually termed the *x* variable and is represented on the horizontal axis. The second variable, known as the *y* variable, is plotted on the vertical axis.

Medical Statistics at a Glance, Fourth Edition. Aviva Petrie and Caroline Sabin. © 2020 Aviva Petrie and Caroline Sabin. Published 2020 by John Wiley & Sons Ltd.
Companion Website: www.medstatsaag.com

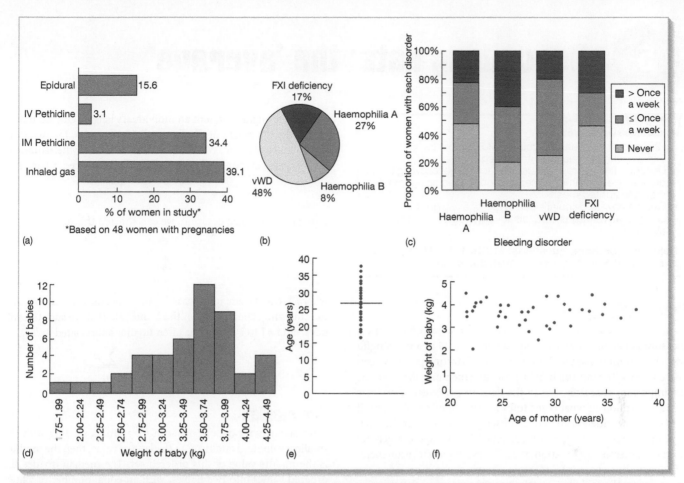

Figure 4.1 A selection of diagrammatic output which may be produced when summarizing the obstetric data in women with bleeding disorders (Chapter 2). (a) **Bar chart** showing the percentage of women in the study who required pain relief from any of the listed interventions during labour. (b) **Pie chart** showing the percentage of women in the study with each bleeding disorder. (c) **Segmented column chart** showing the frequency with which women with different bleeding disorders experience bleeding gums. (d) **Histogram** showing the weight of the baby at birth. (e) **Dot plot** showing the mother's age at the time of delivery, with the median age marked as a horizontal line. (f) **Scatter diagram** showing the relationship between the mother's age at delivery (on the horizontal or *x*-axis) and the weight of the baby (on the vertical or *y*-axis).

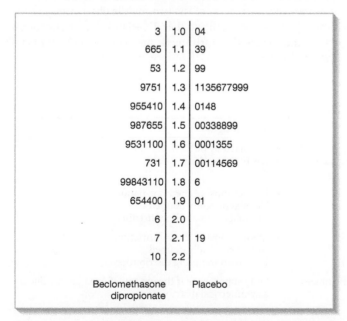

Figure 4.2 Stem-and-leaf plot showing the FEV1 (litres) in children receiving inhaled beclomethasone dipropionate or placebo (Chapter 21).

Identifying outliers using graphical methods

We can often use single-variable data displays to identify outliers. For example, a very long tail on one side of a histogram may indicate an outlying value. However, outliers may sometimes only become apparent when considering the relationship between two variables. For example, a weight of 55 kg would not be unusual for a woman who was 1.6 m tall, but would be unusually low if the woman's height was 1.9 m.

The use of connecting lines in diagrams

The use of connecting lines in scatter diagrams may be misleading. Connecting lines suggest that the values on the *x*-axis are ordered in some way – this might be the case if, for example, the *x*-axis reflects some measure of time or dose. Where this is not the case, the points should not be joined with a line. Conversely, if there is a dependency between different points (e.g. because they relate to results from the same individual at two different time points, such as before and after treatment), it is helpful to connect the relevant points by a straight line (Fig. 20.1) and important information may be lost if these lines are omitted.

⑤ Describing data: the 'average'

Summarizing data

It is very difficult to have any 'feeling' for a set of numerical measurements unless we can summarize the data in a meaningful way. A diagram (Chapter 4) is often a useful starting point. We can also condense the information by providing measures that describe the important characteristics of the data. In particular, if we have some perception of what constitutes a representative value, and if we know how widely scattered the observations are around it, then we can formulate an image of the data. The **average** is a general term for a measure of **location**; it describes a typical measurement. We devote this chapter to averages, the most common being the mean and median (Table 5.1). We introduce measures that describe the scatter or **spread** of the observations in Chapter 6.

The arithmetic mean

The **arithmetic mean**, often simply called the mean, of a set of values is calculated by adding up all the values and dividing this sum by the number of values in the set.

It is useful to be able to summarize this verbal description by an algebraic formula. Using mathematical notation, we write our set of n observations of a variable, x, as $x_1, x_2, x_3, …, x_n$. For example, x might represent an individual's height (cm), so that x_1 represents the height of the first individual, and x_i the height of the ith individual, etc. We can write the formula for the arithmetic mean of the observations, written $\bar{x}$ and pronounced 'x bar', as

$$\bar{x} = \frac{x_1 + x_2 + x_3 + … + x_n}{n}$$

Using mathematical notation, we can shorten this to

$$\bar{x} = \frac{\sum\limits_{i=1}^{n} x_i}{n}$$

where Σ (the Greek uppercase 'sigma') means 'the sum of', and the sub- and superscripts on the Σ indicate that we sum the values from $i = 1$ to $i = n$. This is often further abbreviated to

$$\bar{x} = \frac{\sum x_i}{n} \quad \text{or to} \quad \bar{x} = \frac{\sum x}{n}$$

The median

If we arrange our data in order of magnitude, starting with the smallest value and ending with the largest value, then the **median** is the middle value of this ordered set. The median divides the ordered values into two halves, with an equal number of values both above and below it.

It is easy to calculate the median if the number of observations, n, is **odd**. It is the $(n + 1)/2$th observation in the ordered set. So, for example, if $n = 11$, then the median is the $(11 + 1)/2 = 12/2 = 6$th observation in the ordered set. If n is **even** then, strictly, there is no median. However, we usually calculate it as the arithmetic mean of the two middle observations in the ordered set (i.e. the $n/2$th and the $(n/2 + 1)$th). So, for example, if $n = 20$, the median is the arithmetic mean of the $20/2 = 10$th and the $(20/2 + 1) = (10 + 1) = 11$th observations in the ordered set.

Table 5.1 Advantages and disadvantages of averages.

Type of average	Advantages	Disadvantages
Mean	• Uses all the data values • Algebraically defined and so mathematically manageable • Known sampling distribution (Chapter 9)	• Distorted by outliers • Distorted by skewed data
Median	• Not distorted by outliers • Not distorted by skewed data	• Ignores most of the information • Not algebraically defined • Complicated sampling distribution
Mode	• Easily determined for categorical data	• Ignores most of the information • Not algebraically defined • Unknown sampling distribution
Geometric mean	• Before back-transformation, it has the same advantages as the mean • Appropriate for right-skewed data	• Only appropriate if the log transformation produces a symmetrical distribution
Weighted mean	• Same advantages as the mean • Ascribes relative importance to each observation • Algebraically defined	• Weights must be known or estimated

Medical Statistics at a Glance, Fourth Edition. Aviva Petrie and Caroline Sabin. © 2020 Aviva Petrie and Caroline Sabin. Published 2020 by John Wiley & Sons Ltd.
Companion Website: www.medstatsaag.com

The median is similar to the mean if the data are symmetrical (Fig. 5.1), less than the mean if the data are skewed to the right (Fig. 5.2), and greater than the mean if the data are skewed to the left (Fig. 4.1d).

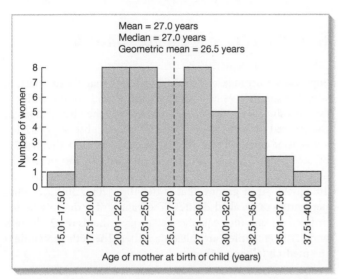

Figure 5.1 The mean, median and geometric mean age of the women in the study described in Chapter 2 at the time of the baby's birth. As the distribution of age appears reasonably symmetrical, the three measures of the 'average' all give similar values, as indicated by the dashed line.

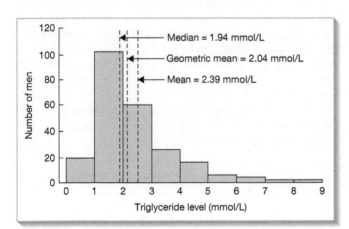

Figure 5.2 The mean, median and geometric mean triglyceride level in a sample of 232 men who developed heart disease (Chapter 19). As the distribution of triglyceride levels is skewed to the right, the mean gives a higher 'average' than either the median or geometric mean.

The mode

The **mode** is the value that occurs most frequently in a data set; if the data are continuous, we usually group the data and calculate the modal group. Some data sets do not have a mode because each value only occurs once. Sometimes, there is more than one mode; this is when two or more values occur the same number of times, and the frequency of occurrence of each of these values is greater than that of any other value. We rarely use the mode as a summary measure.

The geometric mean

The arithmetic mean is an inappropriate summary measure of location if our data are skewed. If the data are skewed to the right, we can produce a distribution that is more symmetrical if we take the logarithm (typically to base 10 or to base e) of each value of the variable in this data set (Chapter 9). The arithmetic mean of the log values is a measure of location for the transformed data. To obtain a measure that has the same units as the original observations, we have to back-transform (i.e. take the antilog of) the mean of the log data; we call this the **geometric mean**. Provided the distribution of the log data is approximately symmetrical, the geometric mean is similar to the median and less than the mean of the raw data (Fig. 5.2).

The weighted mean

We use a **weighted mean** when certain values of the variable of interest, x, are more important than others. We attach a weight, w_i, to each of the values, x_i, in our sample, to reflect this importance. If the values $x_1, x_2, x_3, ..., x_n$ have corresponding weights $w_1, w_2, w_3, ..., w_n$, the weighted arithmetic mean is

$$\frac{w_1 x_1 + w_2 x_2 + ... + w_n x_n}{w_1 + w_2 + ... + w_n} = \frac{\sum w_i x_i}{\sum w_i}$$

For example, suppose we are interested in determining the average length of stay of hospitalized patients in a district, and we know the average discharge time for patients in every hospital. To take account of the amount of information provided, one approach might be to take each weight as the number of patients in the associated hospital.

The weighted mean and the arithmetic mean are identical if each weight is equal to one.

6 Describing data: the 'spread'

Summarizing data

If we are able to provide two summary measures of a continuous variable, one that gives an indication of the 'average' value and the other that describes the 'spread' of the observations, then we have condensed the data in a meaningful way. We explained how to choose an appropriate average in Chapter 5. We devote this chapter to a discussion of the most common measures of **spread** (**dispersion** or **variability**) which are compared in Table 6.1.

The range

The **range** is the difference between the largest and smallest observations in the data set; you may find these two values quoted instead of their difference. Note that the range provides a misleading measure of spread if there are outliers (Chapter 3).

Ranges derived from percentiles

What are percentiles?

Suppose we arrange our data in order of magnitude, starting with the smallest value of the variable, x, and ending with the largest value. The value of x that has 1% of the observations in the ordered set lying below it (and 99% of the observations lying above it) is called the 1st **percentile**. The value of x that has 2% of the observations lying below it is called the 2nd percentile, and so on. The values of x that divide the ordered set into 10 equally sized groups, that is the 10th, 20th, 30th, …, 90th percentiles, are called **deciles**. The values of x that divide the ordered set into four equally sized groups, that is the 25th, 50th and 75th percentiles, are called **quartiles**. The 50th percentile is the **median** (Chapter 5).

Using percentiles

We can obtain a measure of spread that is not influenced by outliers by excluding the extreme values in the data set, and then determining the range of the remaining observations. The **interquartile range** is the difference between the 1st and the 3rd quartiles, i.e. between the 25th and 75th percentiles (Fig. 6.1). It contains the central 50% of the observations in the ordered set, with 25% of the observations lying below its lower limit, and 25% of them lying above its upper limit. The **interdecile range** contains the central 80% of the observations, i.e. those lying between the 10th and 90th percentiles. Often we use the range that contains the central 95% of the observations, i.e. it excludes 2.5% of the observations above its upper limit and 2.5% below its lower limit (Fig. 6.1). We may

Table 6.1 Advantages and disadvantages of measures of spread.

Measure of spread	Advantages	Disadvantages
Range	• Easily determined	• Uses only two observations • Distorted by outliers • Tends to increase with increasing sample size
Ranges based on percentiles	• Usually unaffected by outliers • Independent of sample size • Appropriate for skewed data	• Clumsy to calculate • Cannot be calculated for small samples • Uses only two observations • Not algebraically defined
Variance	• Uses every observation • Algebraically defined	• Units of measurement are the square of the units of the raw data • Sensitive to outliers • Inappropriate for skewed data
Standard deviation	• Same advantages as the variance • Units of measurement are the same as those of the raw data • Easily interpreted	• Sensitive to outliers • Inappropriate for skewed data

Medical Statistics at a Glance, Fourth Edition. Aviva Petrie and Caroline Sabin. © 2020 Aviva Petrie and Caroline Sabin. Published 2020 by John Wiley & Sons Ltd.
Companion Website: www.medstatsaag.com

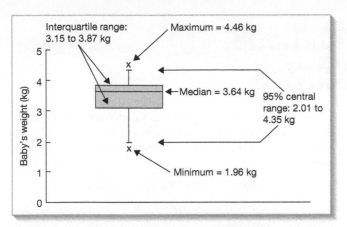

Figure 6.1 A box-and-whisker plot of the baby's weight at birth (Chapter 2). This figure illustrates the median, the interquartile range, the range that contains the central 95% of the observations and the maximum and minimum values.

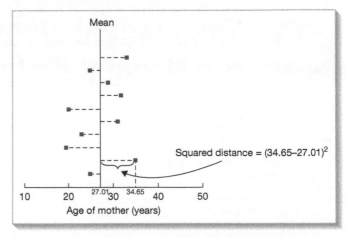

Figure 6.2 Diagram showing the spread of selected values of the mother's age at the time of the baby's birth (Chapter 2) around the mean value. The variance is calculated by adding up the squared distances between each point and the mean, and dividing by ($n-1$).

use this interval, provided it is calculated from enough values of the variable in healthy individuals, to diagnose disease. It is then called the **reference interval**, **reference range** or **normal range** (Chapter 38).

The variance

One way of measuring the spread of the data is to determine the extent to which each observation deviates from the arithmetic mean. Clearly, the larger the deviations, the greater the variability of the observations. However, we cannot use the mean of these deviations as a measure of spread because the positive differences exactly cancel out the negative differences. We overcome this problem by squaring each deviation, and finding the mean of these squared deviations (Fig. 6.2); we call this the **variance**. If we have a sample of n observations, $x_1, x_2, x_3, \ldots, x_n$, whose mean is $\bar{x} = \sum x_i / n$, we calculate the variance, usually denoted by s^2, of these observations as

$$s^2 = \frac{\sum (x_i - \bar{x})^2}{n-1}$$

We can see that this is not quite the same as the arithmetic mean of the squared deviations because we have divided by ($n-1$) instead of n. The reason for this is that we almost always rely on *sample* data in our investigations (Chapter 10). It can be shown theoretically that we obtain a better sample estimate of the population variance if we divide by ($n-1$).

The units of the variance are the square of the units of the original observations, e.g. if the variable is weight measured in kg, the units of the variance are kg².

The standard deviation

The **standard deviation** is the square root of the variance. In a sample of n observations, it is

$$s = \sqrt{\frac{\sum (x_i - \bar{x})^2}{n-1}}$$

We can think of the standard deviation as a sort of average of the deviations of the observations from the mean. It is evaluated in the same units as the raw data.

If we divide the standard deviation by the mean and express this quotient as a percentage, we obtain the **coefficient of variation**. It is a measure of spread that is independent of the unit of measurement, but it has theoretical disadvantages and thus is not favoured by statisticians.

Variation within- and between-subjects

If we take repeated measurements of a continuous variable on an individual, then we expect to observe some variation (**intra-** or **within-subject** variability) in the responses on that individual. This may be because a given individual does not always respond in exactly the same way and/or because of measurement error (Chapter 39). However, the variation within an individual is usually less than the variation obtained when we take a single measurement on every individual in a group (**inter-** or **between-subject** variability). For example, a 17-year-old boy has a lung vital capacity that ranges between 3.60 and 3.87 litres when the measurement is repeated 10 times; the values for single measurements on 10 boys of the same age lie between 2.98 and 4.33 litres. These concepts are important in study design (Chapter 13).

7 Theoretical distributions: the Normal distribution

In Chapter 4 we showed how to create an **empirical frequency distribution** of the observed data. This contrasts with a theoretical **probability distribution** which is described by a mathematical model. When our empirical distribution approximates a particular probability distribution, we can use our theoretical knowledge of that distribution to answer questions about the data. This often requires the evaluation of probabilities.

Understanding probability

Probability measures uncertainty; it lies at the heart of statistical theory. A probability measures the chance of a given event occurring. It is a number that takes a value from zero to one. If it is equal to zero, then the event *cannot* occur. If it is equal to one, then the event *must* occur. The probability of the **complementary** event (the event *not* occurring) is one minus the probability of the event occurring. We discuss **conditional probability**, the probability of an event, given that another event has occurred, in Chapter 45.

We can calculate a probability using various approaches.
- **Subjective** – our personal degree of belief that the event will occur (e.g. that the world will come to an end in the year 2050).
- **Frequentist** – the proportion of times the event would occur if we were to repeat the experiment a large number of times (e.g. the number of times we would get a 'head' if we tossed a fair coin 1000 times).
- **A priori** – this requires knowledge of the theoretical *model*, called the **probability distribution**, which describes the probabilities of all possible outcomes of the 'experiment'. For example, genetic theory allows us to describe the probability distribution for eye colour in a baby born to a blue-eyed woman and brown-eyed man by specifying all possible genotypes of eye colour in the baby and their probabilities.

The rules of probability

We can use the rules of probability to add and multiply probabilities.

- **The addition rule** – if two events, A and B, are *mutually exclusive* (i.e. each event precludes the other), then the probability that either one or the other occurs is equal to the sum of their probabilities.

$$\text{Prob}(A \ or \ B) = \text{Prob}(A) + \text{Prob}(B)$$

For example, if the probabilities that an adult patient in a particular dental practice has no missing teeth, some missing teeth or is edentulous (i.e. has no teeth) are 0.67, 0.24 and 0.09, respectively, then the probability that a patient has some teeth is $0.67 + 0.24 = 0.91$.

- **The multiplication rule** – if two events, A and B, are *independent* (i.e. the occurrence of one event is not contingent on the other), then the probability that both events occur is equal to the product of the probability of each.

$$\text{Prob}(A \ and \ B) = \text{Prob}(A) \times \text{Prob}(B)$$

For example, if two unrelated patients are waiting in the dentist's surgery, the probability that both of them have no missing teeth is $0.67 \times 0.67 = 0.45$.

Probability distributions: the theory

A **random variable** is a quantity that can take any one of a set of mutually exclusive values with a given probability. A **probability distribution** shows the probabilities of all possible values of the random variable. It is a theoretical distribution that is expressed mathematically, and has a mean and variance that are analogous to those of an empirical distribution. Each probability distribution is defined by certain **parameters** which are summary measures (e.g. mean, variance) characterizing that distribution (i.e. knowledge of them allows the distribution to be fully described). These parameters are estimated in the sample by relevant **statistics**. Depending on whether the random variable is discrete or continuous, the probability distribution can be either discrete or continuous.

- **Discrete** (e.g. Binomial and Poisson) – we can derive the probabilities corresponding to every possible value of the random variable. *The sum of all such probabilities is one*.
- **Continuous** (e.g. Normal, Chi-squared, *t* and *F*) – we can only derive the probability of the random variable, *x*, taking values in certain ranges (because there are infinitely many values of *x*). If the horizontal axis represents the values of *x*, we can draw a curve from the equation of the distribution (the **probability density function**); it resembles an empirical relative frequency distribution (Chapter 4). *The total area under the curve is one*; this area represents the probability of all possible events. The probability that *x* lies between two limits is equal to the area under the curve between these values (Fig. 7.1). For convenience, tables have been produced to enable us to evaluate probabilities of interest for commonly used continuous probability distributions (Appendix A). These are particularly useful

Medical Statistics at a Glance, Fourth Edition. Aviva Petrie and Caroline Sabin. © 2020 Aviva Petrie and Caroline Sabin. Published 2020 by John Wiley & Sons Ltd.
Companion Website: www.medstatsaag.com

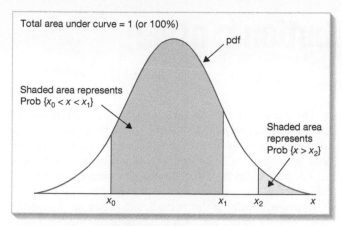

Figure 7.1 The probability density function, pdf, of x.

in the context of confidence intervals (Chapter 11) and hypothesis testing (Chapter 17).

The Normal (Gaussian) distribution

One of the most important distributions in statistics is the **Normal distribution**. Its probability density function (Fig. 7.2) is:
- completely described by two parameters, the *mean* (μ) and the *variance* (σ^2);
- bell-shaped (unimodal);
- symmetrical about its mean;
- shifted to the right if the mean is increased and to the left if the mean is decreased (assuming constant variance);
- flattened as the variance is increased but becomes more peaked as the variance is decreased (for a fixed mean).

Additional properties are that:
- the mean and median of a Normal distribution are equal;
- the probability (Fig. 7.3a) that a Normally distributed random variable, x, with mean, μ, and standard deviation, σ, lies between

$$(\mu - \sigma) \text{ and } (\mu + \sigma) \text{ is } 0.68$$
$$(\mu - 1.96\sigma) \text{ and } (\mu + 1.96\sigma) \text{ is } 0.95$$
$$(\mu - 2.58\sigma) \text{ and } (\mu + 2.58\sigma) \text{ is } 0.99$$

These intervals may be used to define **reference intervals** (Chapters 6 and 38).

We show how to assess Normality in Chapter 35.

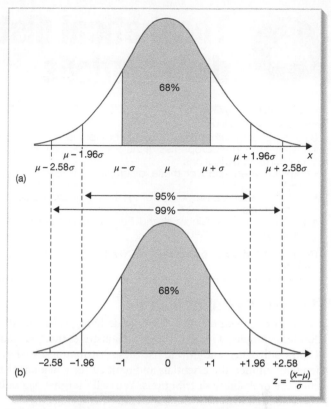

Figure 7.3 Areas (percentages of total probability) under the curve for (a) Normal distribution of x, with mean μ and variance σ^2, and (b) Standard Normal distribution of z.

The Standard Normal distribution

There are infinitely many Normal distributions depending on the values of μ and σ. The Standard Normal distribution (Fig. 7.3b) is a particular Normal distribution for which probabilities have been tabulated (Appendices A1 and A4).
- The Standard Normal distribution has a **mean of zero** and a **variance of one**.
- If the random variable x has a Normal distribution with mean μ and variance σ^2, then the **Standardized Normal Deviate** (SND), $z = \dfrac{x - \mu}{\sigma}$, is a random variable that has a Standard Normal distribution.

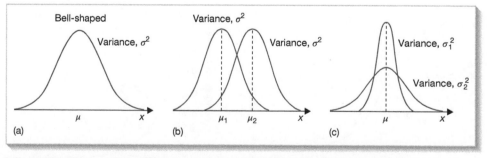

Figure 7.2 The probability density function of the Normal distribution of the variable x. (a) Symmetrical about mean = μ : variance = σ^2. (b) Effect of changing mean ($\mu_2 > \mu_1$). (c) Effect of changing variance ($\sigma_1^2 < \sigma_2^2$).

8 Theoretical distributions: other distributions

Some words of comfort

Do not worry if you find the theory underlying probability distributions complex. Our experience demonstrates that you want to know only when and how to use these distributions. We have therefore outlined the essentials and omitted the equations that define the probability distributions. You will find that you only need to be familiar with the basic ideas, the terminology and, perhaps (although infrequently in this computer age), know how to refer to the tables.

More continuous probability distributions

These distributions are based on continuous random variables. Often it is not a measurable variable that follows such a distribution but a statistic derived from the variable. The total area under the probability density function represents the probability of all possible outcomes, and is equal to one (Chapter 7). We discussed the Normal distribution in Chapter 7; other common distributions are described in this chapter.

The *t*-distribution (Appendix A2, Fig. 8.1)
- Derived by W.S. Gossett, who published under the pseudonym 'Student'; it is often called Student's *t*-distribution.

- The parameter that characterizes the *t*-distribution is the **degrees of freedom (*df*)**, so we can draw the probability density function if we know the equation of the *t*-distribution and its degrees of freedom. We discuss degrees of freedom in Chapter 11; note that they are often closely affiliated to sample size.
- Its shape is similar to that of the Standard Normal distribution, but it is more spread out, with longer tails. Its shape approaches Normality as the degrees of freedom increase.
- It is particularly useful for calculating confidence intervals for and testing hypotheses about one or two means (Chapters 19–21).

The Chi-squared (χ^2) distribution (Appendix A3, Fig. 8.2)
- It is a right-skewed distribution taking positive values.
- It is characterized by its **degrees of freedom** (Chapter 11).
- Its shape depends on the degrees of freedom; it becomes more symmetrical and approaches Normality as the degrees of freedom increase.
- It is particularly useful for analysing categorical data (Chapters 23–25).

The *F*-distribution (Appendix A5)
- It is skewed to the right.
- It is defined by a ratio. The distribution of a ratio of two estimated variances calculated from Normal data approximates the *F*-distribution.
- The two parameters that characterize it are the **degrees of freedom** (Chapter 11) of the numerator and the denominator of the ratio.
- The *F*-distribution is particularly useful for comparing two variances (Chapter 35), and more than two means using the analysis of variance (ANOVA) (Chapter 22).

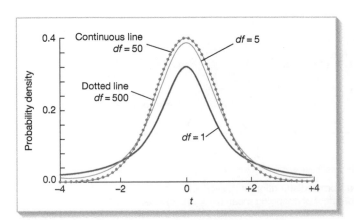

Figure 8.1 *t*-distributions with degrees of freedom (*df*) = 1, 5, 50 and 500.

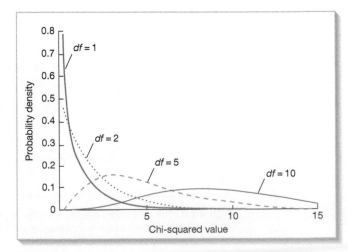

Figure 8.2 Chi-squared distributions with degrees of freedom (*df*) = 1, 2, 5 and 10.

Medical Statistics at a Glance, Fourth Edition. Aviva Petrie and Caroline Sabin. © 2020 Aviva Petrie and Caroline Sabin. Published 2020 by John Wiley & Sons Ltd.
Companion Website: www.medstatsaag.com

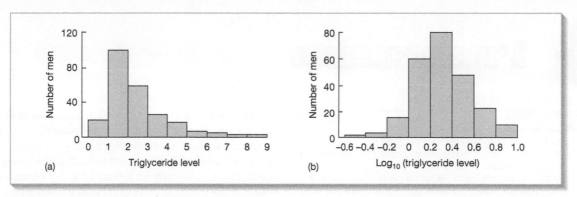

Figure 8.3 (a) The Lognormal distribution of triglyceride levels (mmol/L) in 232 men who developed heart disease (Chapter 19). (b) The approximately Normal distribution of $\log_{10}$ (triglyceride level) in $\log_{10}$ (mmol/L).

The Lognormal distribution

- It is the probability distribution of a random variable whose log (e.g. to base 10 or e) follows the Normal distribution.
- It is highly skewed to the right (Fig. 8.3a).
- If, when we take logs of our raw data that are skewed to the right, we produce an empirical distribution that is nearly Normal (Fig. 8.3b), our data approximate the Lognormal distribution.
- Many variables in medicine follow a Lognormal distribution. We can use the properties of the Normal distribution (Chapter 7) to make inferences about these variables after transforming the data by taking logs.
- If a data set has a Lognormal distribution, we can use the geometric mean (Chapter 5) as a summary measure of location.

Discrete probability distributions

The random variable that defines the probability distribution is discrete. The sum of the probabilities of all possible mutually exclusive events is one.

The Binomial distribution

- Suppose, in a given situation, there are only two outcomes, 'success' and 'failure'. For example, we may be interested in whether a woman conceives (a success) or does not conceive (a failure) after *in vitro* fertilization (IVF). If we look at $n = 100$ unrelated women undergoing IVF (each with the same probability of conceiving), the Binomial random variable is the observed number of conceptions (successes). Often this concept is explained in terms of n independent repetitions of a trial (e.g. 100 tosses of a coin) in which the outcome is either success (e.g. head) or failure.

- The two parameters that describe the Binomial distribution are n, the number of individuals in the sample (or repetitions of a trial), and π, the true probability of success for each individual (or in each trial).
- Its **mean** (the value for the random variable that we *expect* if we look at n individuals, or repeat the trial n times) is $n\pi$. Its **variance** is $n\pi(1 - \pi)$.
- When n is small, the distribution is skewed to the right if $\pi < 0.5$ and to the left if $\pi > 0.5$. The distribution becomes more symmetrical as the sample size increases (Fig. 8.4) and approximates the Normal distribution if both $n\pi$ and $n(1 - \pi)$ are greater than 5.
- We can use the properties of the Binomial distribution when making inferences about **proportions**. In particular, we often use the Normal approximation to the Binomial distribution when analysing proportions.

The Poisson distribution

- The Poisson random variable is the **count** of the number of events that occur independently and randomly in time or space at some average rate, μ. For example, the number of hospital admissions per day typically follows the Poisson distribution. We can use our knowledge of the Poisson distribution to calculate the probability of a certain number of admissions on any particular day.
- The parameter that describes the Poisson distribution is the **mean**, i.e. the average rate, μ.
- The **mean** equals the **variance** in the Poisson distribution.
- It is a right-skewed distribution if the mean is small, but becomes more symmetrical as the mean increases, when it approximates a Normal distribution.

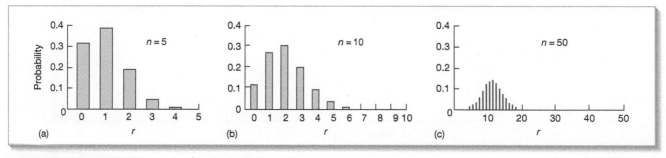

Figure 8.4 Binomial distribution showing the number of successes, r, when the probability of success is $\pi = 0.20$ for sample sizes (a) $n = 5$, (b) $n = 10$ and (c) $n = 50$. (NB in Chapter 23, the observed seroprevalence of HHV-8 was $p = 0.185 \approx 0.2$, and the sample size was 271: the proportion was assumed to follow a Normal distribution.)

9 Transformations

Why transform?

The observations in our investigation may not comply with the requirements of the intended statistical analysis (Chapter 35).

- A variable may not be Normally distributed, a **distributional** requirement for many different analyses.
- The spread of the observations in each of a number of groups may be different (constant variance is an assumption about a **parameter** in the comparison of means using the unpaired t-test and analysis of variance – Chapters 21 and 22).
- Two variables may not be linearly related (**linearity** is an assumption in many regression analyses – Chapters 27–33 and 42).

It is often helpful to **transform** our data to satisfy the assumptions underlying the proposed statistical techniques.

How do we transform?

We convert our raw data into transformed data by taking the same mathematical transformation of each observation. Suppose we have n observations ($y_1, y_2, …, y_n$) on a variable, y, and we decide that the log transformation is suitable. We take the log of each observation to produce ($\log y_1, \log y_2, …, \log y_n$). If we call the transformed variable z, then $z_i = \log y_i$ for each i ($i = 1, 2, …, n$), and our transformed data may be written ($z_1, z_2, …, z_n$).

We check that the transformation has achieved its purpose of producing a data set that satisfies the assumptions of the planned statistical analysis (e.g. by plotting a histogram of the transformed data – Chapter 35), and proceed to analyse the transformed data ($z_1, z_2, …, z_n$). We may back-transform any summary measures (such as the mean) to the original scale of measurement; we then rely on the conclusions we draw from hypothesis tests (Chapter 17) on the transformed data.

Typical transformations

The logarithmic transformation, $z = \log y$

When log transforming data, we can choose to take logs to base 10 ($\log_{10} y$, the 'common' log) or to base e ($\log_e y$ or $\ln y$, the 'natural' or Naperian log where $e = 2.718$), or to any other base, but must be consistent for a particular variable in a data set. Note that we cannot take the log of a negative number or of zero. The back-transformation of a log is called the antilog; the antilog of a Naperian log is the exponential, e.

- If y is skewed to the right, $z = \log y$ is often approximately **Normally distributed** (Fig. 9.1a). Then y has a Lognormal distribution (Chapter 8).
- If there is an exponential relationship between y and another variable, x, so that the resulting curve bends upward when y (on the vertical axis) is plotted against x (on the horizontal axis), then the relationship between $z = \log y$ and x is approximately **linear** (Fig. 9.1b).
- Suppose we have different groups of observations, each comprising measurements of a continuous variable, y. We may find that the groups that have the higher values of y also have larger variances. In particular, if the coefficient of variation (the standard deviation divided by the mean) of y is constant for all the groups, the log transformation, $z = \log y$, produces groups that have **similar variances** (Fig. 9.1c).

In medicine, the log transformation is frequently used because many variables have right-skewed distributions and

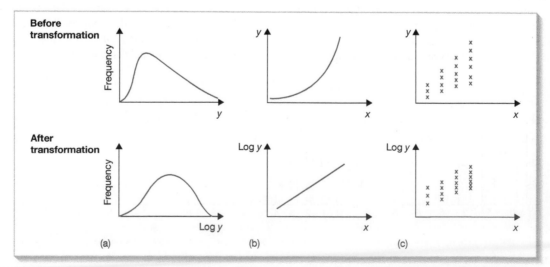

Figure 9.1 The effects of the logarithmic transformation: (a) Normalizing, (b) linearizing, (c) variance stabilizing.

Medical Statistics at a Glance, Fourth Edition. Aviva Petrie and Caroline Sabin. © 2020 Aviva Petrie and Caroline Sabin. Published 2020 by John Wiley & Sons Ltd.
Companion Website: www.medstatsaag.com

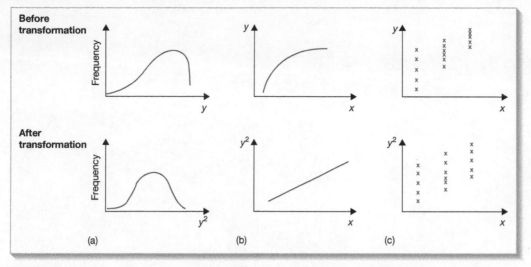

Figure 9.2 The effect of the square transformation: (a) Normalizing, (b) linearizing, (c) variance stabilizing.

because the results have a logical interpretation. For example, if the raw data are log transformed, then the difference in two means on the log scale is equal to the ratio of the two means on the original scale. Taking the antilog of the 95% confidence limits (Chapter 11) for the mean of log transformed data gives a 95% confidence interval for the geometric mean (Chapter 5). If we take a $\log_{10}$ transformation of an explanatory variable in regression analysis (Chapter 29), a unit increase in the variable on the log scale represents a 10-fold increase in the variable on the original scale. Note that a log transformation of the outcome variable in a regression analysis allows for back-transformation of the regression coefficients, but the effect is multiplicative rather than additive on the original scale (Chapters 30 and 31).

The square root transformation, $z = \sqrt{y}$

This transformation has properties that are similar to those of the log transformation, although the results after they have been back-transformed are more complicated to interpret. In addition to its **Normalizing** and **linearizing** abilities, it is effective at **stabilizing variance** if the variance increases with increasing values of y, i.e. if the variance divided by the mean is constant. We often apply the square root transformation if y is the count of a rare event occurring in time or space, i.e. it is a Poisson variable (Chapter 8). Remember, we cannot take the square root of a negative number.

The reciprocal transformation, $z = 1/y$

We often apply the reciprocal transformation to survival times unless we are using special techniques for survival analysis (Chapter 41). The reciprocal transformation has properties that are similar to those of the log transformation. In addition to its **Normalizing** and **linearizing** abilities, it is more effective at **stabilizing variance** than the log transformation if the variance increases very markedly with increasing values of y, i.e. if the variance divided by the (mean)^4 is constant. Note that we cannot take the reciprocal of zero.

The square transformation, $z = y^2$

The square transformation achieves the reverse of the log transformation.

- If y is skewed to the left, the distribution of $z = y^2$ is often approximately **Normal** (Fig. 9.2a).
- If the relationship between two variables, x and y, is such that a line curving downward is produced when we plot y against x, then the relationship between $z = y^2$ and x is approximately **linear** (Fig. 9.2b).
- If the variance of a continuous variable, y, tends to decrease as the value of y increases, then the square transformation, $z = y^2$, **stabilizes the variance** (Fig. 9.2c).

The logit (logistic) transformation, $z = \ln \dfrac{p}{1-p}$

This is the transformation we apply most often to each proportion, p, in a set of proportions. We cannot take the logit transformation if either $p = 0$ or $p = 1$ because the corresponding logit values are $-\infty$ and $+\infty$. One solution is to take p as $1/(2n)$ instead of 0, and as $\{1 - 1/(2n)\}$ instead of 1, where n is the sample size.

The logit transformation **linearizes** a sigmoid curve (Fig. 9.3). See Chapter 30 for the use of the logit transformation in regression analysis.

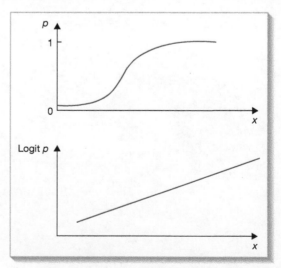

Figure 9.3 The effect of the logit transformation on a sigmoid curve

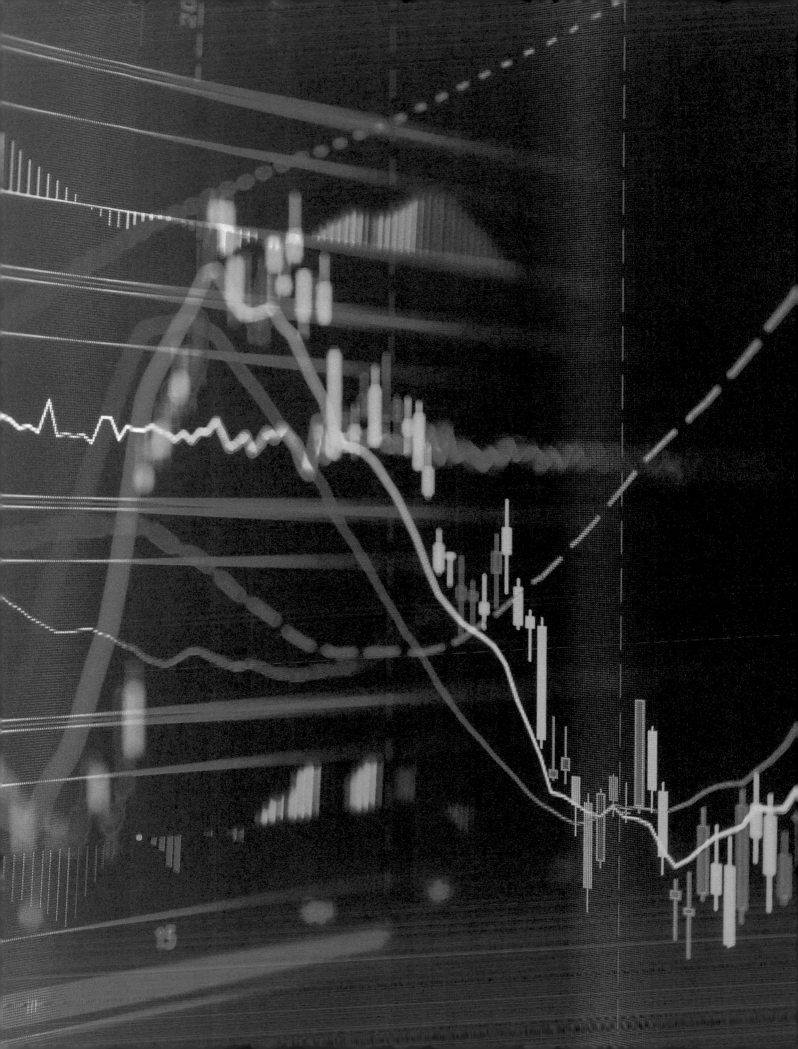

Sampling and estimation

Part 2

Chapters

10 Sampling and sampling distributions

By the end of this chapter, you should be able to:
- Explain what is meant by statistical inference and sampling error
- Explain how to obtain a representative sample
- Distinguish between point and interval estimates of a parameter
- List the properties of the sampling distribution of the mean
- List the properties of the sampling distribution of the proportion
- Explain what is meant by a standard error
- State the relationship between the standard error of the mean (SEM) and the standard deviation (SD)
- Distinguish between the uses of the SEM and the SD

Relevant Workbook questions: MCQs 18 and 19 available online

Why do we sample?

In statistics, a **population** represents the entire group of individuals in whom we are interested. Generally it is costly and labour-intensive to study the entire population and, in some cases, may be impossible because the population may be hypothetical (e.g. patients who may receive a treatment in the future). Therefore we collect data on a **sample** of individuals who we believe are **representative** of this population (i.e. they have similar characteristics to the individuals in the population), and use them to draw conclusions (i.e. make **inferences**) about the population.

When we take a sample of the population, we have to recognize that the information in the sample may not fully reflect what is true in the population. We have introduced **sampling error** by studying only some of the population. In this chapter we show how to use theoretical probability distributions (Chapters 7 and 8) to quantify this error.

Obtaining a representative sample

Ideally, we aim for a **random sample**. A list of all individuals from the population is drawn up (the **sampling frame**), and individuals are selected randomly from this list, i.e. every possible sample of a given size in the population has an equal probability of being chosen. Sometimes, we may have difficulty in constructing this list or the costs involved may be prohibitive, and then we take a **convenience sample**. For example, when studying patients with a particular clinical condition, we may choose a single hospital, and investigate some or all of the patients with the condition in that hospital. Very occasionally, non-random schemes, such as **quota sampling** or **systematic sampling**, may be used. Although the statistical tests described in this book assume that individuals are selected for the sample randomly, the methods are generally reasonable as long as the sample is **representative** of the population.

Point estimates

We are often interested in the value of a **parameter** in the population (Chapter 7), such as a mean or a proportion. Parameters are usually denoted by letters of the Greek alphabet. For example, we usually refer to the population mean as μ and the population standard deviation as σ. We estimate the value of the parameter using the data collected from the sample. This estimate is referred to as the **sample statistic** and is a **point estimate** of the parameter (i.e. it takes a single value) as opposed to an **interval estimate** (Chapter 11) which takes a range of values.

Sampling variation

If we were to take repeated samples of the same size from a population, it is unlikely that the estimates of the population parameter would be exactly the same in every sample. However, our estimates should all be close to the true value of the parameter in the population, and the estimates themselves should be similar to each other. By quantifying the variability of these estimates, we obtain information on the precision of our estimate and can thereby assess the sampling error. *In reality, we usually only take one sample from the population.* However, we still make use of our knowledge of the theoretical distribution of sample estimates to draw inferences about the population parameter.

Sampling distribution of the mean

Suppose we are interested in estimating the population mean; we could take many repeated samples of size n from the population, and estimate the mean in each sample. A histogram of the estimates of these means would show their distribution (Fig. 10.1); this is the **sampling distribution of the mean**. We can show the following:
- If the sample size is reasonably large, the estimates of the mean follow a **Normal** distribution, whatever the distribution of the original data in the population (this comes from a theorem known as the *Central Limit Theorem*).
- If the sample size is small, the estimates of the mean follow a Normal distribution provided the data in the population follow a Normal distribution.
- The mean of the estimates is an **unbiased** estimate of the true mean in the population, i.e. the mean of the estimates equals the true population mean.
- The variability of the distribution is measured by the standard deviation of the estimates; this is known as the **standard error of the mean** (often denoted by SEM). If we know the population standard deviation (σ), then the standard error of the mean is given by

$$SEM = \sigma / \sqrt{n}$$

Medical Statistics at a Glance, Fourth Edition. Aviva Petrie and Caroline Sabin. © 2020 Aviva Petrie and Caroline Sabin. Published 2020 by John Wiley & Sons Ltd.
Companion Website: www.medstatsaag.com

When we only have one sample, as is customary, our best estimate of the population mean is the sample mean, and because we rarely know the standard deviation in the population, we estimate the standard error of the mean by

$$\text{SEM} = s/\sqrt{n}$$

where s is the standard deviation of the observations in the sample (Chapter 6). The SEM provides a measure of the precision of our estimate.

Interpreting standard errors

- A **large** standard error indicates that the estimate is *imprecise*.
- A **small** standard error indicates that the estimate is *precise*.

The standard error is reduced, i.e. we obtain a more precise estimate, if:

- the size of the sample is increased (Fig. 10.1);
- the data are less variable.

SD or SEM?

Although these two parameters seem to be similar, they are used for different purposes. The standard deviation (SD) describes the variation in the data values and should be quoted if you wish to illustrate variability in the data. In contrast, the standard error describes the precision of the sample mean, and should be quoted if you are interested in the mean of a set of data values.

Sampling distribution of the proportion

We may be interested in the proportion of individuals in a population who possess some characteristic. Having taken a sample of size n from the population, our best estimate, p, of the population proportion, π, is given by

$$p = r/n$$

where r is the number of individuals in the sample with the characteristic. If we were to take repeated samples of size n from our population and plot the estimates of the proportion as a histogram, the resulting **sampling distribution of the proportion** would approximate a Normal distribution with mean value π. The standard deviation of this distribution of estimated proportions is the **standard error of the proportion**. When we take only a single sample, it is estimated by

$$\text{SE}(p) = \sqrt{\frac{p(1-p)}{n}}$$

This provides a measure of the precision of our estimate of π; a small standard error indicates a precise estimate.

Example

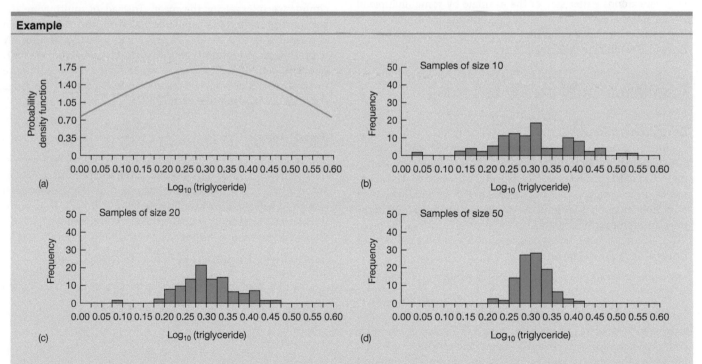

Figure 10.1 (a) Theoretical Normal distribution of $\log_{10}$ (triglyceride levels) in $\log_{10}$ (mmol/L) with mean = $0.31\log_{10}$ (mmol/L) and standard deviation = $0.24\log_{10}$ (mmol/L), and the observed distributions of the means of 100 random samples of size (b) 10, (c) 20 and (d) 50 taken from this theoretical distribution.

11 Confidence intervals

Once we have taken a sample from our population, we obtain a point estimate (Chapter 10) of the parameter of interest, and calculate its standard error to indicate the precision of the estimate. However, to most people the standard error is not, by itself, particularly useful. It is more helpful to incorporate this measure of precision into an **interval estimate** for the population parameter. We do this by making use of our knowledge of the theoretical probability distribution of the sample statistic to calculate a **confidence interval** for the parameter. Generally the confidence interval extends either side of the estimate by some multiple of the standard error; the two values (the **confidence limits**) which define the interval are generally separated by a comma, a dash or the word 'to' and are contained in brackets.

Confidence interval for the mean
Using the Normal distribution
In Chapter 10 we stated that, if we take repeated samples of a given size taken from a population, the sample means follow a Normal distribution if the sample size is large. Therefore we can make use of the properties of the Normal distribution when considering the sample mean. In particular, 95% of the distribution of sample means lies within 1.96 standard deviations (SD) of the population mean. We call this SD the standard error of the mean (SEM), and when we have a single sample, the 95% **confidence interval (CI) for the mean** is

(Sample mean − (1.96 × SEM) to Sample mean + (1.96 × SEM))

If we were to repeat the experiment many times, the range of values determined in this way would contain the true population mean on 95% of occasions. This range is known as the 95% confidence interval for the mean. We usually interpret this confidence interval as the range of values within which we are 95% confident that the true population mean lies. Although not strictly correct (the population mean is a fixed value and therefore cannot have a probability attached to it), we will interpret the confidence interval in this way as it is conceptually easier to understand.

Using the t-distribution
Strictly, we should only use the Normal distribution in the calculation if we know the value of the variance, σ^2, in the population. Furthermore, if the sample size is small, the sample mean only follows a Normal distribution if the underlying population data are Normally distributed. Where the data are not Normally distributed, and/or we do not know the population variance but estimate it by s^2, the sample mean follows a t-distribution (Chapter 8). We calculate the 95% confidence interval for the mean as

(Sample mean − ($t_{0.05}$ × SEM) to Sample mean + ($t_{0.05}$ × SEM))

i.e. it is Sample mean $\pm t_{0.05} \times \dfrac{s}{\sqrt{n}}$

where $t_{0.05}$ is the **percentage point** (percentile) of the t-distribution with $(n-1)$ degrees of freedom which gives a two-tailed probability (Chapter 17) of 0.05 (Appendix A2). This generally provides a slightly wider confidence interval than that using the Normal distribution to allow for the extra uncertainty that we have introduced by estimating the population standard deviation and/or because of the small sample size. When the sample size is large, the difference between the two distributions is negligible. *Therefore, we always use the t-distribution when calculating a confidence interval for the mean even if the sample size is large.*

By convention we usually quote 95% confidence intervals. We could calculate other confidence intervals, e.g. a 99% confidence interval for the mean. Instead of multiplying the standard error by the tabulated value of the t-distribution corresponding to a two-tailed probability of 0.05, we multiply it by that corresponding to a two-tailed probability of 0.01. The 99% confidence interval is wider than a 95% confidence interval, to reflect our increased confidence that the range includes the true population mean.

Confidence interval for the proportion
The sampling distribution of a proportion follows a Binomial distribution (Chapter 8). However, if the sample size, n, is reasonably large, then the sampling distribution of the proportion is approximately Normal with mean π. We estimate π by the proportion in the sample, $p = r/n$ (where r is the number of individuals in the sample with the characteristic of interest), and its standard error is estimated by $\sqrt{\dfrac{p(1-p)}{n}}$ (Chapter 10).

The 95% confidence interval for the proportion is estimated by

$$\left(p - \left[1.96 \times \sqrt{\frac{p(1-p)}{n}} \right] \text{ to } p + \left[1.96 \times \sqrt{\frac{p(1-p)}{n}} \right] \right)$$

If the sample size is small (usually when np or $n(1-p)$ is less than 5) then we have to use the Binomial distribution to calculate exact confidence intervals[1]. Note that if p is expressed as a percentage, we replace $(1-p)$ by $(100-p)$.

Interpretation of confidence intervals
When interpreting a confidence interval we are interested in a number of issues.
- **How wide is it?** A wide interval indicates that the estimate is imprecise; a narrow one indicates a precise estimate. The width

of the confidence interval depends on the size of the standard error, which in turn depends on the sample size and, when considering a numerical variable, the variability of the data. Therefore, small studies on variable data give wider confidence intervals than larger studies on less variable data.

- **What clinical implications can be derived from it?** The upper and lower limits provide a way of assessing whether the results are clinically important (see Example).
- **Does it include any values of particular interest?** We can check whether a hypothesized value for the population parameter falls within the confidence interval. If so, then our results are consistent with this hypothesized value. If not, then it is unlikely (for a 95% confidence interval, the chance is at most 5%) that the parameter has this value.

Degrees of freedom

You will come across the term 'degrees of freedom' in statistics. In general they can be calculated as the sample size minus the number of constraints in a particular calculation; these constraints may be the parameters that have to be estimated. As a simple illustration, consider a set of three numbers that add up to a particular total (T). Two of the numbers are 'free' to take any value but the remaining number is fixed by the constraint imposed by T. Therefore the numbers have two degrees of freedom. Similarly, the degrees of freedom of the sample variance, $s^2 = \dfrac{\sum (x - \bar{x})^2}{n-1}$ (Chapter 6), are the sample size minus one, because we have to calculate the sample mean ($\bar{x}$), an estimate of the population mean, in order to evaluate s^2.

Bootstrapping and jackknifing

Bootstrapping is a computer-intensive simulation process which we can use to derive a confidence interval for a parameter if we do not want to make assumptions about the sampling distribution of its estimate (e.g. the Normal distribution for the sample mean). From the original sample, we create a large number of random samples (usually at least 1000), each of the same size as the original sample, by sampling with replacement, i.e. by allowing an individual who has been selected to be 'replaced' so that, potentially, this individual can be included more than once in a given sample. Every sample provides an estimate of the parameter, and we use the variability of the distribution of these estimates to obtain a confidence interval for the parameter, for example, by considering relevant percentiles (e.g. the 2.5th and 97.5th percentiles to provide a 95% confidence interval).

Jackknifing is a similar technique to bootstrapping. However, rather than creating random samples of the original sample, we remove one observation from the original sample of size n and then compute the estimated parameter on the remaining $(n-1)$ observations. This process is repeated, removing each observation in turn, giving us n estimates of the parameter. As with bootstrapping, we use the variability of the estimates to obtain the confidence interval.

Bootstrapping and jackknifing may both be used when generating and validating prognostic scores (Chapter 46).

Reference

1 Lentner, C (ed.) (1982) *Geigy Scientific Tables*. 8th edition, Volume 2. Basle: Ciba-Geigy.Confidence interval for the mean

---

Example

Confidence interval for the mean
We are interested in determining the mean age at first birth in women who have bleeding disorders. In a sample of 49 such women who had given birth by the end of 1997 (Chapter 2):

Mean age at birth of child, $\bar{x} = 27.01$ years

Standard deviation, $s = 5.1282$ years

Standard error, $\text{SEM} = \dfrac{5.1282}{\sqrt{49}} = 0.7326$ years

The variable is approximately Normally distributed but, because the population variance is unknown, we use the t-distribution to calculate the confidence interval. The 95% confidence interval for the mean is:

$$27.01 \pm (2.011 \times 0.7326) = (25.54, 28.48) \text{ years}$$

where 2.011 is the percentage point of the t-distribution with $(49 - 1) = 48$ degrees of freedom giving a two-tailed probability of 0.05 (Appendix A2).

We are 95% certain that the true mean age at first birth in women with bleeding disorders in the population lies between 25.54 and 28.48 years. This range is fairly narrow, reflecting a precise estimate. In the general population, the mean age at first birth in 1997 was 26.8 years. As 26.8 falls into our confidence interval, there is no evidence that women with bleeding disorders tend to give birth at an older age than other women.

Note that the 99% confidence interval (25.05, 28.97 years) is slightly wider than the 95% confidence interval, reflecting our increased confidence that the population mean lies in the interval.

Confidence interval for the proportion
Of the 64 women included in the study, 27 (42.2%) reported that they experienced bleeding gums at least once a week. This is a relatively high percentage, and may provide a way of identifying undiagnosed women with bleeding disorders in the general population. We calculate a 95% confidence interval for the proportion with bleeding gums in the population.

Sample proportion $= 27/64 = 0.422$

Standard error of proportion $= \sqrt{\dfrac{0.422(1 - 0.422)}{64}} = 0.0617$

95% confidence interval $= 0.422 \pm (1.96 \times 0.0617) = (0.301, 0.543)$

We are 95% certain that the true percentage of women with bleeding disorders in the population who experience bleeding gums this frequently lies between 30.1% and 54.3%. This is a fairly wide confidence interval, suggesting poor precision; a larger sample size would enable us to obtain a more precise estimate. However, the upper and lower limits of this confidence interval both indicate that a substantial percentage of these women are likely to experience bleeding gums. We would need to obtain an estimate of the frequency of this complaint in the general population before drawing any conclusions about its value for identifying undiagnosed women with bleeding disorders.

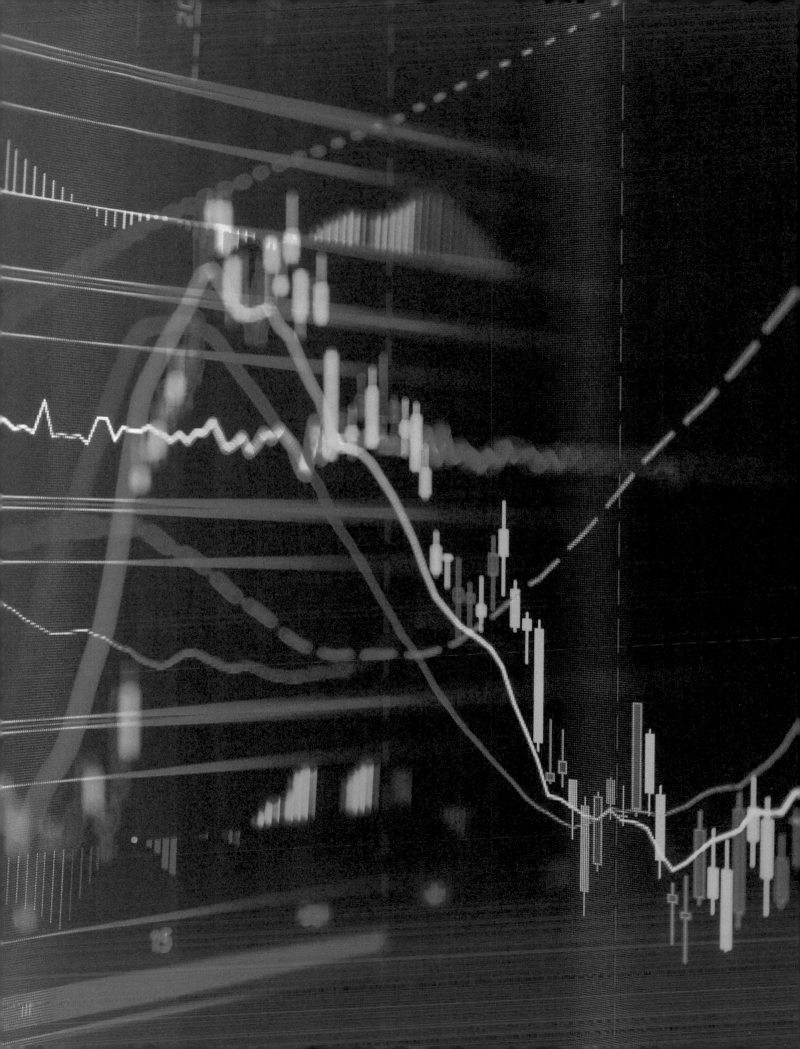

Study design

Part 3

Chapters

12 Study design I

Learning objectives

By the end of this chapter, you should be able to:
- Distinguish between experimental and observational studies, and between cross-sectional and longitudinal studies
- Explain what is meant by the unit of observation
- Explain the terms: control group, epidemiological study, cluster randomized trial, ecological study, multicentre study, survey, census
- List the criteria for assessing causality in observational studies
- Describe the time course of cross-sectional, repeated cross-sectional, cohort, case–control and experimental studies
- List the typical uses of these various types of study
- Distinguish between prevalence and incidence

Relevant Workbook questions: MCQs 22, 23, 27, 31, 32, 33 and 39 available online

Study design is vitally important as poorly designed studies may give misleading results. Large amounts of data from a poor study will not compensate for problems in its design. In this chapter and in Chapter 13 we discuss some of the main aspects of study design. In Chapters 14–16 we discuss specific types of study: clinical trials, cohort studies and case–control studies.

The aims of any study should be clearly stated at the outset. We may wish to estimate a parameter in the population such as the risk of some event (Chapter 15), to consider associations between a particular aetiological factor and an outcome of interest, or to evaluate the effect of an intervention such as a new treatment. There may be a number of possible designs for any such study. The ultimate choice of design will depend not only on the aims but also on the resources available and ethical considerations (Table 12.1).

Experimental or observational studies

- **Experimental** studies involve the investigator intervening in some way to affect the outcome. The clinical trial (Chapter 14) is an example of an experimental study in which the investigator introduces some form of treatment. Other examples include animal studies or laboratory studies that are carried out under experimental conditions. Experimental studies provide the most convincing evidence for any hypothesis as it is generally possible to control for factors that may affect the outcome (see also Chapter 40). However, these studies are not always feasible or, if they involve humans or animals, may be unethical.
- **Observational** studies, e.g. cohort (Chapter 15) or case–control (Chapter 16) studies, are those in which the investigator does nothing to affect the outcome but simply observes what happens. These studies may provide poorer information than experimental studies because it is often impossible to control for all factors that affect the outcome. However, in some

Table 12.1 Study designs.

Type of study	Timing	Form	Action in past time	Action in present time (starting point)	Action in future time	Typical uses
Cross-sectional	Cross-sectional	Observational		Collect all information		• Prevalence estimates • Reference ranges and diagnostic tests • Current health status of a group
Repeated cross-sectional	Cross-sectional	Observational		Collect all information	Collect all information → Collect all information	• Changes over time
Cohort (Chapter 15)	Longitudinal (usually prospective)	Observational		Define cohort and assess risk factors → follow	Observe outcomes	• Prognosis and natural history (what will happen to someone with disease) • Aetiology
Case–control (Chapter 16)	Longitudinal (retrospective)	Observational	Assess risk factors ← trace	Define cases and controls (i.e. outcome)		• Aetiology (particularly for rare diseases)
Experiment	Longitudinal (prospective)	Experimental		Apply intervention → follow	Observe outcomes	• Clinical trial to assess therapy (Chapter 14) • Trial to assess preventative measure, e.g. large-scale vaccine trial • Laboratory experiment

Medical Statistics at a Glance, Fourth Edition. Aviva Petrie and Caroline Sabin. © 2020 Aviva Petrie and Caroline Sabin. Published 2020 by John Wiley & Sons Ltd.
Companion Website: www.medstatsaag.com

situations, they may be the only types of study that are helpful or possible. **Epidemiological studies**, which assess the relationship between factors of interest and disease in the population, are observational.

Defining the unit of observation

The **unit of observation** is the 'individual' or smallest group of 'individuals' that can be regarded as independent for the purposes of analysis, i.e. its response of interest is unaffected by those of the other units of observation. In medical studies, whether experimental or observational, investigators are usually interested in the outcomes of an individual person. For example, in a clinical trial (Chapter 14), the unit of observation is usually the individual patient as his/her response to treatment is believed not to be affected by the responses to treatment experienced by other patients in the trial. However, for some studies, it may be appropriate to consider different units of observation. For example:

• In dental studies, the unit of observation may be the patient's mouth rather than an individual tooth, as the teeth within a patient's mouth are not independent of each other.

• In some experimental studies, particularly laboratory studies, it may be necessary to pool material from different individuals (e.g. mice). It is then impossible to assess each individual separately and the pooled material (e.g. that in the well of a tissue culture plate) becomes the unit of observation.

• A **cluster randomized trial** (Chapter 14) is an example of an experimental study where the unit of observation is a group of individuals, such as all the children in a class.

• An **ecological study** is a particular type of epidemiological study in which the unit of observation is a community or group of individuals rather than the individual. For example, we may compare national mortality rates from breast cancer across a number of different countries to see whether mortality rates appear to be higher in some countries than others, or whether mortality rates are correlated with other national characteristics. While any associations identified in this way may provide interesting hypotheses for further research, care should always be taken when interpreting the results from such studies owing to the potential for bias (see the ecological fallacy in Chapter 34).

Multicentre studies

A multicentre study, which may be experimental or observational, enrols a number of individuals from each of two or more centres (e.g. hospital clinic, general practice). While these centres may be of a different type and/or size, the same study protocol will be used in all centres. If management practices vary across centres, it is likely that the outcomes experienced by two individuals within the same centre will be more similar than those experienced by two individuals in different centres. The analysis of a multicentre study, which is usually performed in a single coordinating centre, should always take account of any centre 'effects', either through an analysis suitable for clustered data (Chapter 42), or by adjustment for the centre in a multivariable regression analysis (Chapter 33).

Assessing causality

In medical research we are generally interested in whether exposure to a factor *causes* an effect (e.g. whether smoking causes lung cancer). Although the most convincing evidence for the causal role of a factor in disease usually comes from randomized controlled trials (Chapter 14), information from observational studies may be used provided a number of criteria are met. The most well-known criteria for assessing causation were proposed by Hill[1].

1 The cause must precede the effect.

2 The association should be plausible, i.e. the results should be biologically sensible.

3 There should be consistent results from a number of studies.

4 The association between the cause and the effect should be strong.

5 There should be a dose–response relationship with the effect, i.e. higher levels of the effect should lead to more severe disease or more rapid disease onset.

6 Removing the factor of interest should reduce the risk of disease.

Cross-sectional or longitudinal studies

• A **cross-sectional** study is carried out at a single point in time. A **survey** is a type of cross-sectional study where, usually, the aim is to describe individuals' beliefs in or attitudes towards a particular issue in a large sample of the population. A **census** is a particular type of survey in which the entire target population is investigated. In a medical setting, a cross-sectional study is particularly suitable for estimating the **point prevalence** of a condition in the population.

$$\text{Point prevalence} = \frac{\text{Number with the disease at a single time point}}{\text{Total number studied at the same time point}}$$

As we do not know when the events occurred prior to the study, we can only say that there is an association between the factor of interest and disease, and not that the factor is likely to have *caused* disease (i.e. we have not demonstrated that Hill's criterion 1 has been satisfied). Furthermore, we cannot estimate the **incidence** of the disease, i.e. the rate of new events in a particular period (Chapter 31). In addition, because cross-sectional studies are only carried out at one point in time, we cannot consider trends over time. However, these studies are generally quick and cheap to perform.

• A **repeated cross-sectional** study may be carried out at different time points to assess trends over time. However, as this study is likely to include different groups of individuals at each time point, it can be difficult to assess whether apparent changes over time simply reflect differences in the groups of individuals studied.

• A **longitudinal study** follows a sample of individuals over time. This type of study is usually **prospective** in that individuals are followed forward from some point in time (Chapters 14 and 15). Sometimes a **retrospective** study, in which individuals are selected and factors that have occurred in their past are identified (Chapter 16), are also perceived as longitudinal. Longitudinal studies generally take longer to carry out than cross-sectional studies, thus requiring more resources, and, if they rely on patient memory or medical records, may be subject to bias (Chapter 34).

Experimental studies are prospective as they consider the impact of an intervention on an outcome that will happen in the future. However, observational studies may be either prospective or retrospective.

Controls

The use of a comparison group, or **control group**, is important when designing a study and interpreting any research findings. For example, when assessing the causal role of a particular factor for a disease, the risk (Chapter 15) or odds (Chapter 16) should be compared in those who are exposed and in those who are unexposed to the factor of interest. See also 'Treatment comparisons' in Chapter 14.

Bias

When there is a systematic difference between the results from a study and the true state of affairs, bias is said to have occurred. Bias and methods to reduce its impact are described in detail in Chapter 34.

Reference

1   Hill, A.B. (1965) The environment and disease: association or causation? *Proceedings of the Royal Society of Medicine*, 58, 295.

13 Study design II

Learning objectives

By the end of this chapter, you should be able to:
- Describe how to increase the precision of an estimate
- Explain the principles of blocking (stratification)
- Distinguish between parallel and cross-over designs
- Describe the features of a factorial experiment
- Explain what is meant by an interaction between factors
- Explain the terms: study endpoint, surrogate marker, composite endpoint

Relevant Workbook questions: MCQs 24, 25, 26, 29 and 60 available online

Variation

Variation in data may be caused by biological factors (e.g. sex, age) or measurement 'errors' (e.g. observer variation), or it may be **unexplainable random variation** (see also Chapter 39). We measure the impact of variation in the data on the estimation of a population parameter by using the standard error (Chapter 10). When the measurement of a variable is subject to considerable variation, estimates relating to that variable will be imprecise, with large standard errors. Clearly, it is desirable to reduce the impact of variation as far as possible, and thereby increase the precision of our estimates. There are various ways in which we can do this, as described in this chapter.

Replication

Our estimates are more precise if we take replicates (e.g. two or three measurements of a given variable for every individual on each occasion). However, as replicate measurements are not independent, we must take care when analysing these data. A simple approach is to use the mean of each set of replicates in the analysis in place of the original measurements. Alternatively, we can use methods that specifically deal with replicated measurements (Chapters 41 and 42).

Sample size

The choice of an appropriate size for a study is a crucial aspect of study design. With an increased sample size, the standard error of an estimate will be reduced, leading to increased precision and study power (Chapter 18). Sample size calculations (Chapter 36) should be carried out before starting the study.

In any type of study, it is important that the sample size included in the final study analysis is as close as possible to the planned sample size to ensure that the study is sufficiently powered (Chapter 18). This means that **response rates** should be as high as possible in cross-sectional studies and surveys. In clinical trials and cohort studies, attempts should be made to minimize any loss to follow-up; this will also help attenuate any biases (Chapter 34) that may be introduced if non-responders or cohort drop-outs differ in any respect to responders or those remaining in the trial or cohort.

Particular study designs

Modifications of simple study designs can lead to more precise estimates. Essentially, we are comparing the effect of one or more '**treatments**' on **experimental units**. The experimental unit (i.e. the unit of observation in an experiment – Chapter 12) is the 'individual' or the smallest group of 'individuals' whose response of interest is not affected by that of any other units, such as an individual patient, volume of blood or skin patch. If experimental units are assigned randomly (i.e. by chance) to treatments (Chapter 14) and there are no other refinements to the design, we have a **complete randomized design**. Although this design is straightforward to analyse, it is inefficient if there is substantial variation between the experimental units. In this situation, we can incorporate **blocking** and/or use a **cross-over design** to reduce the impact of this variation.

Blocking (stratification)

It is often possible to group experimental units that share similar characteristics into a homogeneous **block** or **stratum** (e.g. the blocks may represent different age groups). The variation between units in a block is less than that between units in different blocks. The individuals within each block are randomly assigned to treatments; we compare treatments within each block rather than making an overall comparison between the individuals in different blocks. We can therefore assess the effects of treatment more precisely than if there was no blocking.

Parallel and cross-over designs (Fig. 13.1)

Generally, we make comparisons between individuals in different groups. For example, most clinical trials (Chapter 14) are **parallel** trials, in which each patient receives one of the two (or occasionally more) treatments that are being compared, i.e. they result in *between-individual* comparisons.

Because there is usually less variation in a measurement within an individual than between different individuals (Chapter 6), in some situations it may be preferable to consider using each individual as his/her own control. These *within-individual* comparisons provide more precise comparisons than those from between-individual designs, and fewer individuals are required for the study to achieve the same level of precision. In a clinical trial setting, the **cross-over** design[1] is an example of a within-individual comparison; if there are two treatments, each individual gets both treatments, one after the other in a random order to eliminate any effect of calendar time. The treatment periods are separated by a **washout period**, which allows any residual effects (**carry-over**) of the previous treatment to dissipate. We analyse the difference in the responses on the two treatments for each individual. This design can only be used when the treatment temporarily alleviates symptoms rather than provides a cure, and the response time is not prolonged.

Medical Statistics at a Glance, Fourth Edition. Aviva Petrie and Caroline Sabin. © 2020 Aviva Petrie and Caroline Sabin. Published 2020 by John Wiley & Sons Ltd.
Companion Website: www.medstatsaag.com

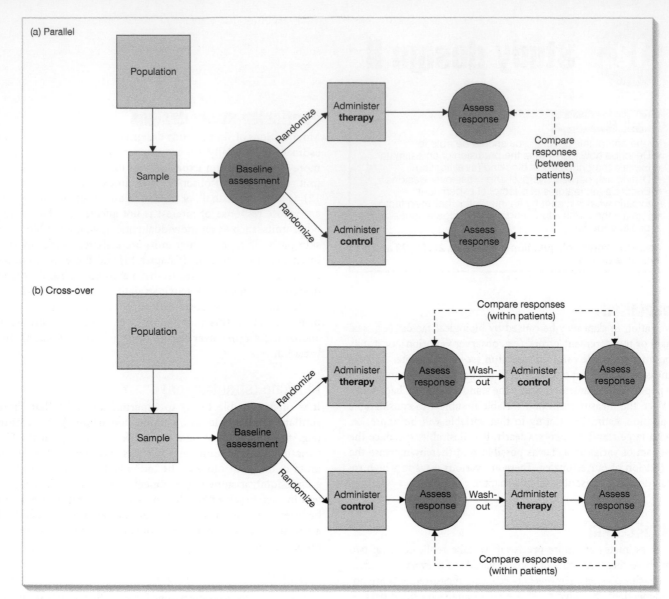

(a) Parallel

(b) Cross-over

Figure 13.1 (a) Parallel, and (b) cross-over designs.

Factorial experiments

When we are interested in more than one factor, separate studies that assess the effect of varying one factor at a time may be inefficient and costly. **Factorial designs** allow the simultaneous analysis of any number of **factors** of interest. The simplest design, a 2×2 factorial experiment, considers two factors (e.g. two different treatments), each at two **levels** (e.g. either active or inactive treatment). As an example, consider the US Lantus for C-reactive Protein Reduction in Early Treatment of Type 2 Diabetes (LANCET) trial[2], designed to assess the importance of insulin glargine and metformin for achieving glycaemic control in patients who have type 2 diabetes with suboptimal glycaemic control and elevated levels of high sensitivity C-reactive protein (hsCRP). A 2×2 factorial design was used, with the two factors being the different compounds. For metformin, the two levels indicated whether the patient received the active compound or its placebo (Chapter 14); as the insulin glargine was provided in an open-label manner, the two levels for this compound were whether the patient received the active compound or no compound. Table 13.1 shows the possible treatment combinations,

Table 13.1 Active treatment combinations.

Insulin glargine	Active metformin	
	No	**Yes**
No	Metformin placebo	Metformin
Yes	Insulin glargine + metformin placebo	Insulin glargine + metformin

We assess the effect of the level of metformin by comparing patients in the left-hand column with those in the right-hand column. Similarly, we assess the effect of the level of insulin glargine by comparing patients in the top row with those in the bottom row. In addition, we can test whether the two factors are **interactive**, i.e. when the effect of metformin is different for the two levels of insulin glargine. If the effects differ, we then say that there is an **interaction** between the two factors (Chapter 33). In this example, an interaction would suggest that the combination of insulin glargine and metformin together is more (or less) effective than would be expected by simply adding the separate effects of each drug. This design, therefore, provides additional information to two separate studies and is a more efficient use of resources, requiring a smaller sample size to obtain estimates with a given degree of precision.

Choosing an appropriate study endpoint

A study **endpoint**, which must be specified before the data are collected, is a clearly defined outcome for an individual. It should relate to the relevant hypothesis under study and have clinical/biological relevance. Study endpoints may be *clinical* (e.g. death, onset of fever) or may be based on **surrogate markers** (e.g. the presence of the tumour marker CA125 for ovarian cancer, measurement of HIV viral load for AIDS). Surrogate marker endpoints are often biomarkers that are used as a substitute for a clinical endpoint when it is difficult, expensive or time-consuming to measure the clinical endpoint. Occasionally, a **composite endpoint** may be defined – this usually requires the participant to experience one or more of a number of possible endpoints. For example, a cardiovascular endpoint may be defined if any of the following events occur: a myocardial infarction, death due to cardiovascular disease or stroke. However, analyses involving composite endpoints may be difficult to interpret, particularly if the components of the endpoint are associated with different prognoses, and care should be taken when choosing and analysing this type of endpoint.

Further issues surrounding the choice of an appropriate study endpoint for a clinical trial are described in Chapter 14.

References

1 Senn, S. (2003) *Cross-over Trials in Clinical Research*. 2nd edition. Chichester: Wiley.
2 Pradhan, A.D., Everett, B.M., Cook, N.R., Rifai, N. and Ridker, P.M. (2009) Effects of initiating insulin and metformin on glycemic control and inflammatory biomarkers among patients with type 2 diabetes. The LANCET Randomized Trial. *JAMA*, 302, 1186–1196.

14 Clinical trials

Learning objectives

By the end of this chapter, you should be able to:
- Define 'clinical trial' and distinguish between Phase I/II and Phase III clinical trials
- Explain the importance of a control treatment and distinguish between positive and negative controls
- Explain what is meant by a placebo
- Distinguish between primary and secondary endpoints
- Explain why it is important to randomly allocate individuals to treatment groups and describe different forms of randomization
- Explain why it is important to incorporate blinding (masking)
- Distinguish between double- and single-blind trials
- Discuss the ethical issues arising from a randomized controlled trial (RCT)
- Explain the principles of a sequential trial
- Distinguish between on-treatment analysis and analysis by intention-to-treat (ITT)
- Describe the contents of a protocol
- Apply the CONSORT Statement guidelines

Relevant Workbook questions: MCQs 24, 25, 27 and 28; and SQ 5 available online

A **clinical trial**[1] is any form of planned experimental study designed, in general, to evaluate the effect of a new treatment on a clinical outcome in humans. Clinical trials may either be pre-clinical studies, small clinical studies to investigate effect and safety (**Phase I/II trials**) or full evaluations of the new treatment (**Phase III trials**). In this chapter we discuss the main aspects of Phase III trials, all of which should be reported in any publication. Guidance for reporting randomized controlled trials may be found in the CONSORT guidelines – we provide its checklist and recommended flow chart in Appendix D (Table D2 and Fig. D1). (See Fig 14.1 for an example of a flow chart.) Further relevant information and any updates may be obtained from the CONSORT website (www.equator-network.org/reporting-guidelines/consort/ and www.consort-statement.org). CONSORT is one component of the EQUATOR initiative (Appendix D), promoting the responsible reporting of health research studies (www.equator-network.org).

Treatment comparisons

Clinical trials are prospective studies in that we are interested in measuring the impact of a treatment given now on a future possible outcome. In general, clinical trials evaluate new interventions (e.g. type or dose of drug; surgical procedure). Throughout this chapter we assume, for simplicity, that only one *new* treatment is being evaluated in a trial.

An important feature of a clinical trial is that it should be comparative (Chapter 12). Without a **control** treatment, it is impossible to be sure that any response is due solely to the effect of the treatment, and the importance of the new treatment can be overstated. The control may be the standard treatment (a **positive control**) or, if one does not exist, it may be a **negative control**, which can be a **placebo** (a treatment that looks and tastes like the new therapy but that does not contain any active compound) or the absence of treatment if ethical considerations permit.

Primary and secondary endpoints

When choosing the endpoint at the planning stage of a study (Chapter 13), we must decide which outcome most accurately reflects the benefit of the new therapy. This is known as the **primary endpoint** of the study and usually relates to treatment *efficacy*. **Secondary endpoints**, which often relate to *toxicity*, are of interest and should also be considered at the outset. Generally, all these endpoints are analysed at the end of the study. However, we may wish to carry out some pre-planned **interim analyses** (for example, to ensure that no major toxicities have occurred requiring the trial to be stopped). Care should be taken when comparing treatments at these times owing to the problems of multiple hypothesis testing (Chapter 18). An independent **Data Safety and Monitoring Committee** (DSMC) often takes responsibility for the interpretation of interim analyses, the results of which should generally be treated confidentially and not circulated to other trial investigators unless the trial is stopped.

Subgroup analyses

There is often a temptation to assess the effect of a new treatment in various subgroups of patients in the trial (e.g. in men and women separately; in older and younger individuals). Owing to the problems with multiple hypothesis testing and reduced study power (Chapter 18), these should be avoided unless they are pre-planned, the study sample size has been calculated accordingly, and appropriate statistical methods have been used for analysis.

Treatment allocation

Once a patient has been formally entered into a clinical trial, she or he is allocated to a treatment group. In general, patients are allocated in a random manner (i.e. based on chance), using a process known as **random allocation** or **randomization**. This is often performed using a computer-generated list of random numbers or by using a table of random numbers (Appendix A12). For example, to allocate patients to two treatments, we might follow a sequence of random numbers and allocate the patient to treatment A if the number is even (treating zero as even) and to treatment B if it is odd. This process promotes similarity between the treatment groups in terms of baseline characteristics at entry to the trial (i.e. it avoids **allocation bias** and, consequently, **confounding** (Chapter 34)), maximizing the efficiency of the trial. If a baseline characteristic is not evenly distributed in the treatment groups (evaluated by examining the appropriate summary measures, e.g. the means and standard deviations), the discrepancy must be due to chance if

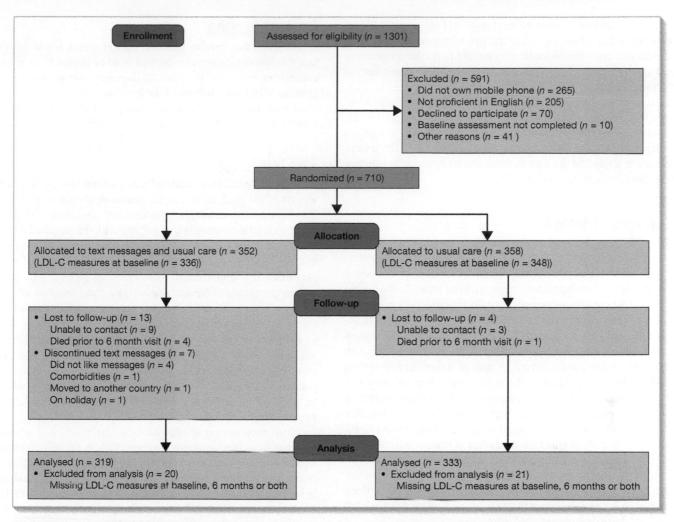

Figure 14.1 Trial profile example (based on Fig. D1). Adapted from Chow, C.K., Redfern, J., Hillis, G.S., et al. (2015) Effect of lifestyle-focused text messaging on risk factor modification in patients with coronary heart disease. A randomized clinical trial. *JAMA*, **314(12)**, 1255–1263 (see the example in Chapter 40). Reproduced with permission of American Medical Association.

randomization has been used. Therefore, it is inappropriate to perform a formal statistical hypothesis test (such as the *t*-test, Chapter 21) to compare the parameters of any baseline characteristic in the treatment groups because the hypothesis test assesses whether the difference between the groups is due to chance.

Trials in which patients are randomized to receive either the new treatment or a control treatment are known as **randomized controlled trials** (often referred to as **RCTs**), and are regarded as optimal. **Systematic allocation**, whereby patients are allocated to treatment groups systematically rather than randomly, possibly by day of visit or date of birth, should be avoided where possible; the clinician may be able to determine the proposed treatment for a particular patient before he or she is entered into the trial, and this may influence his/her decision as to whether to include a patient in the trial.

Refinements of simple randomization include the following:
• **Stratified randomization**, which controls for the effects of important factors (e.g. age, sex) by helping to ensure that each factor is equally distributed across treatment groups. The patients are stratified by one or more of these factors and a separate randomization list is used in each stratum.
• **Blocked or restricted randomization**, which ensures roughly equal-sized treatment groups at the end of patient

recruitment. This is achieved by choosing relatively small block sizes (e.g. 6 or 9) that are multiples of the number of treatments, and allocating equal numbers of patients to the different treatments in each block, using some modified form of randomization.
• **Cluster randomization**, whereby we randomly allocate a *group* or *cluster* of individuals, rather than each individual, to a treatment. This may be necessary when it is infeasible to randomize individuals separately within each cluster (e.g. fluoride in drinking water) or when the response to treatment of one individual may affect that of other individuals in the same cluster. For example, suppose we wish to evaluate the effects of a GP-led health education programme to improve the diet and lifestyle of people at high risk of heart disease. To achieve this, we could compare relevant outcomes (e.g. the average change in weight and blood pressure at the end of 1 year) in individuals who are randomized either to receive the programme (the new 'treatment') or not to receive the programme (the control 'treatment'). Unfortunately, it may be difficult in this situation to randomize individual patients to the two 'treatments' as it may be impractical for a doctor to switch randomly between the type of care that he/she provides in the same clinic. Furthermore, even if individual randomization were feasible, there is likely to be dissemination of the information about the programme to those individuals

who were randomized not to receive it, and responses will not be independent of each other in the two treatment groups. Thus all patients, even the controls, may benefit from the programme and any comparison of outcomes between those on and not on the programme is likely to be diluted. In these instances, it is usually the doctor who is randomized to the treatment group rather than the individual patients in his/her care. We should take care when planning the sample size, because the unit of investigation (Chapter 12) is the group and not the individual in the group, and when analysing the data in these cluster randomized studies (see also Chapters 36, 41 and 42)[2].

Sequential trials

Most clinical trials have sample sizes that are predetermined at the outset (Chapter 36), i.e. they are *fixed-size* designs. **A sequential design** may be used occasionally when the time interval between a treatment and an outcome is expected to be short. In the simple situation where we are comparing two treatments (e.g. a novel and a control treatment), individuals are randomized to treatment in 'pairs', one to each of the treatments. Once the treatment outcomes of both members of the pair are known, *all the data currently available* are analysed. A formal statistical rule is then used to determine whether the trial should stop (if there is a clear difference between the treatments or it becomes obvious that a difference between them will not be detected) or whether another pair of individuals should be recruited and randomized. The main benefit of this type of design is that, when there is a large treatment effect, the trial will require fewer patients than a standard fixed-size parallel design (Chapter 13). However, mainly because of the requirement for the time interval between the treatment and outcome to be short, and other practical difficulties, these designs are used infrequently.

Blinding or masking

There may be **assessment bias** when patients and/or clinicians are aware of the treatment allocation, particularly if the response is subjective. An awareness of the treatment allocation may influence the recording of signs of improvement or adverse events. Therefore, where possible, all participants (clinicians, patients, assessors) in a trial should be **blinded** or **masked** to the treatment allocation and to the randomization list. A trial in which the patient, the treatment team and the assessor are unaware of the treatment allocation is a **double-blind trial**. Trials in which it is impossible to blind the patient may be **single-blind** providing the clinician and/or assessor is blind to the treatment allocation.

Patient issues

As clinical trials involve humans, patient issues are of importance. In particular, any clinical trial must be passed by an **ethics committee** who judge that the trial does not contravene the Declaration of Helsinki. **Informed patient consent** must be obtained from each patient (or from the legal guardian or parent if the patient is a minor) before she or he is entered into a trial.

The protocol

Before any clinical trial is carried out, a written description of all aspects of the trial, known as the **protocol**, should be prepared. This includes information on the aims and objectives of the trial, along with a definition of which patients are to be recruited (**inclusion** and **exclusion criteria**), treatment schedules, data collection and analysis, contingency plans should problems arise, and study personnel. It is important to recruit enough patients into a trial so that the chance of correctly detecting a true treatment effect is sufficiently high. Therefore, before carrying out any clinical trial, the optimal **trial size** should be calculated (Chapter 36).

Protocol deviations occur when patients who enter the trial but do not conform to the protocol criteria, e.g. patients who were incorrectly recruited into or who withdrew from the study, and patients who switched treatments. To avoid bias, the study should be analysed on an **intention-to-treat** (ITT) basis, in which all patients on whom we have information are analysed in the groups to which they were originally allocated, irrespective of whether they followed the treatment regimen. Where possible, attempts should be made to collect information on patients who withdraw from the trial. **On-treatment** (also called **per-protocol**) analyses, in which patients are only included in the analysis if they complete a *full* course of treatment as prescribed in the protocol, are not recommended as they often lead to biased treatment comparisons.

SPIRIT, another component of the EQUATOR network (Appendix D and Chapter 37), is an international initiative that aims to improve the quality of clinical trial protocols by providing evidence-based recommendations for a minimum set of scientific, ethical and administrative elements that should be addressed in a clinical trial protocol. Details may be found at www.spirit-statement.org and http://www.equator-network.org/reporting-guidelines/spirit-2013-statement-defining-standard-protocol-items-for-clinical-trials/.

References

1 Pocock, S.J. (1983) *Clinical Trials: A Practical Approach*. Chichester: Wiley.
2 Kerry, S.M. and Bland, J.M. (1998) Sample size in cluster randomisation. *British Medical Journal*, **316**, 549.

15 Cohort studies

A cohort study takes a group of individuals and usually follows them forward in time, the aim being to study whether exposure to a particular aetiological factor will affect the incidence of a disease outcome in the future (Fig. 15.1). If so, the factor is generally known as a **risk factor** for the disease outcome. For example, a number of cohort studies have investigated the relationship between dietary factors and cancer. Although most cohort studies are prospective, **historical** cohorts are occasionally used: these are identified retrospectively and relevant information relating to outcomes and exposures of interest up to the present day ascertained using medical records and memory. However, while these studies are often quicker and cheaper to perform than prospective cohort studies, the quality of historical studies may be poor as the information collected may be unreliable.

Cohort studies can either be fixed or dynamic. If individuals leave a **fixed** cohort, they are not replaced. In **dynamic** cohorts, individuals may drop out of the cohort, and new individuals may join as they become eligible.

In this chapter we discuss the main aspects of cohort studies. The STROBE statement, another component of the EQUATOR network (Appendix D and Chapter 14), is a set of recommendations to improve the reporting of observational studies, with particular reference to cohort, case–control (Chapter 16) and cross-sectional (Chapter 12) studies. We provide the STROBE checklist in Table D2 (Appendix D). Further relevant information and any updates may be obtained from the STROBE website (www.equator-network.org/reporting-guidelines/strobe/ and www.strobe-statement.org).

Selection of cohorts

The cohort should be representative of the population to which the results will be generalized. It is often advantageous if the individuals can be recruited from a similar source, such as a particular occupational group (e.g. civil servants, medical practitioners), as information on mortality and morbidity can be easily obtained from records held at the place of work, and individuals can be re-contacted when necessary. However, such a cohort may not be truly representative of the general population, and may be healthier. Cohorts can also be recruited from GP lists, ensuring that a group of individuals

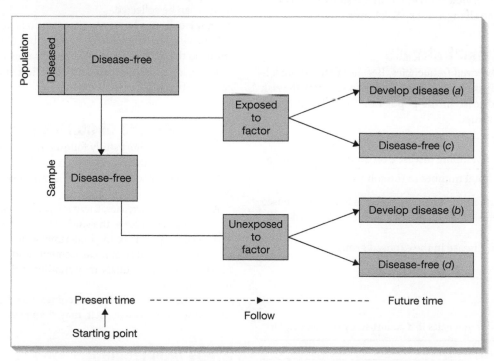

Figure 15.1 Diagrammatic representation of a cohort study (frequencies in parentheses, see Table 15.1).

with different health states is included in the study. However, these patients tend to be of similar social backgrounds because they live in the same area.

When trying to assess the aetiological effect of a risk factor, individuals recruited to cohorts should be disease-free at the start of the study. This is to ensure that any exposure to the risk factor occurs before the outcome, thus enabling a causal role for the factor to be postulated. Because individuals are disease-free at the start of the study, we often see a **healthy entrant** effect. Mortality rates in the first period of the study are then often lower than would be expected in the general population. This will be apparent when mortality rates start to increase suddenly a few years into the study.

Follow-up of individuals

When following individuals over time, there is always the problem that they may be **lost to follow-up**. Individuals may move without leaving a forwarding address, or they may decide that they wish to leave the study. The benefits of a cohort study are reduced if a large number of individuals is lost to follow-up. We should thus find ways to minimize these drop-outs, e.g. by maintaining regular contact with the individuals.

Information on outcomes and exposures

It is important to obtain full and accurate information on disease outcomes, e.g. mortality and illness from different causes. This may entail searching through disease registries, mortality statistics and GP and hospital records.

Exposure to the risks of interest may change over the study period. For example, when assessing the relationship between alcohol consumption and heart disease, an individual's typical alcohol consumption is likely to change over time. Therefore it is important to re-interview individuals in the study on repeated occasions to examine changes in exposure over time.

Analysis of cohort studies

Table 15.1 shows observed frequencies. Because patients are followed longitudinally over time, it is possible to estimate the **risk** of developing the disease in the population, by calculating the risk in the sample studied.

Estimated risk of disease

$$= \frac{\text{Number developing disease over study period}}{\text{Total number in the cohort}} = \frac{a+b}{n}$$

The risk of disease in the individuals exposed and unexposed to the factor of interest in the population can be estimated in the same way.

Estimated risk of disease in the exposed group:

$$\text{risk}_{\text{exp}} = a/(a+c)$$

Estimated risk of disease in the unexposed group:

$$\text{risk}_{\text{unexp}} = b/(b+d)$$

Then, **estimated relative risk** $= \dfrac{\text{risk}_{\text{exp}}}{\text{risk}_{\text{unexp}}}$

$$= \frac{a/(a+c)}{b/(b+d)}$$

The **relative risk** (RR) indicates the increased (or decreased) risk of disease associated with exposure to the factor of interest. A relative risk of one indicates that the risk is the same in the exposed and unexposed groups. A relative risk greater than one indicates that there is an increased risk in the exposed group compared with the unexposed group; a relative risk less than one indicates a reduction in the risk of disease in the exposed group. For example, a relative risk of two would indicate that individuals in the exposed group had twice the risk of disease of those in the unexposed group.

A relative risk should always be interpreted alongside the underlying risk of the disease. Even a large relative risk may have limited clinical implications when the underlying risk of disease is very small.

A confidence interval for the relative risk should be calculated, and we can use it, or determine a test statistic, to test the null hypothesis that the true RR = 1. These calculations are easily performed on a computer and therefore we omit details.

Advantages of cohort studies

• The time sequence of events can be assessed.
• They can provide information on a wide range of disease outcomes.
• The incidence/risk of disease can be measured directly.
• Very detailed information on exposure to a wide range of factors can be collected.
• They can be used to study exposure to factors that are rare.
• Exposure can be measured at a number of time points in each study, so that changes in exposure over time can be studied.
• There is reduced **recall** and **selection bias** compared with case–control studies (Chapter 16).

Disadvantages of cohort studies

• In general, a cohort study follows individuals for long periods of time, and it is therefore costly to perform.
• Where the outcome of interest is rare, a very large sample size is required.
• As follow-up increases, there is often increased loss of patients as they migrate or leave the study, leading to biased results.
• As a consequence of the long time-scale, it is often difficult to maintain consistency of measurements and outcomes over time. Furthermore, individuals may modify their behaviour after an initial interview.
• It is possible that disease outcomes and their probabilities, or the aetiology of disease itself, may change over time.

Study management

Although cohort studies are usually less regulated than clinical trials (Chapter 14), it is still helpful to prepare a study protocol at the outset of any cohort study. It is important to pay particular attention to the following aspects of study management when preparing this document.

Table 15.1 Observed frequencies in a cohort study (see Fig. 15.1).

| | Exposed to factor | | |
Disease of interest	Yes	No	Total
Yes	a	b	$a+b$
No	c	d	$c+d$
Total	$a+c$	$b+d$	$n=a+b+c+d$

- **The outcome of interest** – specify the outcome (e.g. obesity) and provide an unambiguous definition of it (e.g. body mass index > 30 kg/m^2). How will it be ascertained (e.g. through direct contact with patients, through access to hospital records or through linkage with national registries)?
- **The exposures of interest** – specify which exposure variables will be considered and give unambiguous definitions of them. How will the exposures be ascertained?
- **Monitoring of participants** – how will participants be monitored (e.g. by direct face-to-face visits, through postal questionnaires, through access to hospital records)? How frequently will participants be followed up? What information will be collected at each time point? Will any biological samples (e.g. blood, urine, biopsy samples) be collected?
- **The size of cohort and length of follow-up** – how frequently is the outcome likely to occur in those with and without the exposures of interest? How 'big' should the study be to ensure that the study is sufficiently large to demonstrate associations of interest? Note that in a cohort setting, the power of a study (Chapters 18 and 36) is largely determined by the number of events that occur; this can be increased either by increasing the size of the cohort or by lengthening the period of follow-up.
- **The definition and ascertainment of any potential confounders** (Chapter 34) **and/or effect modifiers** – specify which other important variables should be investigated and provide an unambiguous definition for each.
- **The plans for statistical analysis** – when is it anticipated that the statistical analysis of the cohort will be undertaken (e.g. after 5 years)?
- **The steps taken to reduce bias** (Chapter 34) – what steps will be taken to minimize drop-out from the cohort? What steps will be taken to ensure that the definition and ascertainment of outcomes, exposures and other key variables do not change over time?

- **The plans for quality control** – describe any statistical analyses that will be conducted at interim time points (Chapter 18) to ensure that:
  - loss to follow-up is not substantial;
  - the way in which exposures, outcomes and other key data are measured or ascertained has not changed over time; and
  - outcomes are occurring at the rate expected at the outset such that the study is 'on target' for the planned analyses.
- **The need for ethics committee approval and/or patient consent** – will these be required? If patient consent is required, how will this be collected?

Clinical cohorts

Sometimes we select a cohort of patients with the same clinical condition attending one or more hospitals and follow them (either as inpatients or outpatients) to see how many patients experience a resolution (in the case of a positive outcome of the condition) or some indication of disease progression such as death or relapse. The information we collect on each patient is usually that which is collected as part of routine clinical care. The aims of **clinical cohorts** (sometimes called **disease registers** or **observational databases**) may include describing the outcomes of individuals with the condition and assessing the effects of different approaches to treatment (e.g. different drugs or different treatment modalities). In contrast to randomized controlled trials (Chapter 14), which often include a highly selective sample of individuals who are willing to participate in the trial, clinical cohorts often include all patients with the condition at the hospitals in the study. Thus, outcomes from these cohorts are thought to more accurately reflect the outcomes that would be seen in clinical practice. However, as allocation to treatment in these studies is not randomized (Chapter 14), clinical cohorts are particularly prone to confounding bias (Chapter 34).

Example

The Avon Longitudinal Study of Parents and Children (ALSPAC) is a large cohort study that aims to investigate a wide range of influences on the health and development of children. The aim of this particular analysis was to determine whether there was an association between peer victimization at the age of 13 years and depression at 18 years. Whilst information on peer victimization was captured on the children at several ages, the present analysis comprised 6719 children who provided information on peer victimization at age 13 years. Information on depression was determined through a self-administered computerized clinical interview at 18 years of age. Of the 6719 children who provided information on peer victimization, 3898 completed the clinical interview at age 18 years, of whom 1446 (37.1%) reported occasional victimization and 683 (17.5%) reported frequent victimization. By the age of 18 years, 302 (7.7%) of these 3898 children had self-reported depression. The results, displayed in Table 15.2, show the number (and percentage) of those in the different peer victimization groups who did and did not have depression at age 18.

The estimated relative risk for depression in those reporting frequent victimization at age 13 years compared with those reporting no victimization at that age

$$= \frac{(101/683)}{(98/1769)} = 2.67$$

Table 15.2 Observed frequencies (percentages) in the peer victimization study.

Peer victimization at age 13 years	Depression at age 18 years		
	Yes	No	Total
No victimization	98 (5.5%)	1671 (94.5%)	1769
Occasional victimization	103 (7.1%)	1343 (92.9%)	1446
Frequent victimization	101 (14.8%)	582 (85.2%)	683
Total	302 (7.7%)	3596 (92.3%)	3898

It can be shown that the 95% confidence interval for the true relative risk is (2.05, 3.47).

We can interpret the relative risk to mean that an 18-year-old who reported frequent victimization at age 13 years is 2.67 times more likely to suffer from depression at age 18 years than an 18-year-old who reported no victimization at age 13 years. Alternatively, the risk of depression for an 18-year-old who reported frequent victimization at age 13 years is 167% greater than that of an 18-year-old who reported no victimization at age 13 years.

Data extracted from Bowes, L., Joinson, C., Wolke, D. and Lewis, G. (2015) Peer victimization during adolescence and its impact on depression in early adulthood: prospective cohort study in the United Kingdom. *British Medical Journal*, 350, h2469.

16 Case–control studies

A case–control study compares the characteristics of a group of patients with a particular disease outcome (the **cases**) to a group of individuals without the disease outcome (the **controls**), to see whether exposure to any factor occurred more or less frequently in the cases than the controls (Fig. 16.1). Such retrospective studies do not provide information on the prevalence or incidence of disease but may give clues as to which factors elevate or reduce the risk of disease. We discuss the main aspects of case–control studies in this chapter. The STROBE guidelines (see Chapter 15, www.equator-network.org/reporting-guidelines/strobe/ and www.strobe-statement.org) provide a checklist (Appendix D, Table D2) for the reporting of case–control studies.

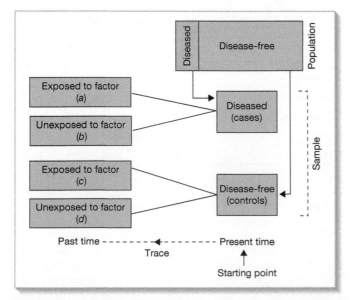

Figure 16.1 Diagrammatic representation of a case–control study (frequencies in parentheses, see Table 16.1).

Selection of cases

The eligibility criteria for cases should be precise and unambiguous (e.g. diabetes mellitus [World Health Organization criteria]: single fasting glucose concentration ≥ 7 mmol/L or venous plasma glucose measured 2 hours after ingestion of 75 g oral glucose load ≥ 11 mmol/L). In particular, it is important to define whether **incident** cases (patients who are recruited at the time of diagnosis) or **prevalent** cases (patients who were already diagnosed before entering the study) should be recruited. Prevalent cases may have had time to reflect on their history of exposure to known risk factors, especially if the disease is a well-publicized one such as cancer, and may have altered their behaviour after diagnosis. It is important to identify as many cases as possible so that the results carry more weight and the conclusions can be generalized to future populations. To this end, it may be necessary to access hospital lists and disease registries, and to include cases who died during the time period when cases and controls were recruited, because their exclusion may lead to a biased sample of cases.

Selection of controls

As with cases, the eligibility criteria for controls should also be precise and unambiguous. Controls should be screened at entry to the study to ensure that they do not have the disease of interest. Where possible, controls should be selected from the same source as cases. Controls are often selected from hospitals. However, as risk factors related to one disease outcome may also be related to other disease outcomes, the selection of hospital-based controls may over-select individuals who have been exposed to the risk factor of interest, and may, therefore, not always be appropriate. It is often acceptable to select controls from the general population, although they may not be as motivated to take part in such a study, and response rates may therefore be poorer in controls than cases. The use of neighbourhood controls may ensure that cases and controls are from similar social backgrounds. Of note, it is important to avoid the temptation to relax the criteria for eligibility of controls part-way through a study simply to speed up the process of recruitment.

Although most case–control studies include only a single control for each case (often referred to as a 1:1 case–control study), it is possible to include multiple controls for each case (a 1:n case–control study). Increased numbers of controls per case will provide the study with greater power (Chapter 18), although any such gains in power are likely to be fairly small beyond four controls per case[1]. Where a greater number of individuals are eligible to be selected as controls than is required, it is important to document how the controls should be selected (e.g. by random selection from all eligible individuals).

Identification of risk factors

As in any epidemiological study, the potential risk factors should be defined before conducting the study. The definition of these factors of interest should be clear and unambiguous (e.g. in a case–control study for the development of diabetes mellitus, where 'exercise' is the factor of interest, there should be a clear explanation of how exercise is to be measured and categorized). A pilot study may help to ensure that the definition will be feasible given the need to rely on retrospectively collected data and/or memory. Other factors that may have an impact on the outcome (i.e. case–control status), either as confounders (Chapter 34) and/or effect modifiers, should also be listed and defined.

Matching

Many case–control studies are **matched** in order to select cases and controls who are as similar as possible. We may have **frequency matching** on a *group* basis (i.e. the average value of each of the relevant potential risk factors of the whole group of cases should be similar to that of the whole group of controls) or we may have **pairwise matching** on an *individual* basis (i.e. each case is matched individually to a control who has similar potential risk factors). In general, when performing individual matching, it is useful to sex-match individuals (i.e. if the case is male, the control should also be male), and, sometimes, patients will be age-matched. However, it is important not to match on the basis of the risk factor of interest, or on any factor that falls on the causal pathway of the disease (Chapter 34), as this will remove the ability of the study to assess any relationship between the risk factor and the disease. Furthermore, it is important not to match on too many factors, as this may restrict the availability of suitable controls. Unfortunately, matching does mean that the effect on disease of the variables that have been used for matching cannot be studied.

Analysis of unmatched or group-matched case–control studies

Table 16.1 shows observed frequencies. Because patients are selected on the basis of their disease status, it is not possible to estimate the absolute risk of disease. We can calculate the **odds ratio (OR)**, which is given by

$$\text{Odds ratio} = \frac{\text{Odds of being a case in exposed group}}{\text{Odds of being a case in unexposed group}}$$

where, for example, the odds of being a case in the exposed group is equal to

$$\frac{\text{Probability of being a case in the exposed group}}{\text{Probability of not being a case in the exposed group}}$$

The odds of being a case in the exposed and unexposed samples are

$$\text{odds}_{\text{exp}} = \frac{\left(\dfrac{a}{a+c}\right)}{\left(\dfrac{c}{a+c}\right)} = \frac{a}{c} \quad \text{odds}_{\text{unexp}} = \frac{\left(\dfrac{b}{b+d}\right)}{\left(\dfrac{d}{b+d}\right)} = \frac{b}{d}$$

and therefore the **estimated odds ratio** $= \dfrac{a/c}{b/d} = \dfrac{a \times d}{b \times c}$

When a disease is rare, the odds ratio is an estimate of the relative risk. It is interpreted in a similar way to the relative risk, i.e. it gives an indication of the increased (or decreased) odds associated with exposure to the factor of interest. An odds ratio of one indicates that the odds of disease is the same in the exposed and unexposed groups; an odds ratio greater than one indicates that the odds of disease is greater in the exposed group than in the unexposed group, etc. Confidence intervals and hypothesis tests can also be generated for the odds ratio.

Analysis of individually matched case–control studies

Where possible, the analysis of individually matched case–control studies should allow for the fact that cases and controls are linked to each other as a result of the matching. Further details of methods of analysis for matched studies can be found in Chapter 30 ('Conditional logistic regression') and in Breslow and Day[2].

Advantages of case–control studies
- They are generally relatively quick, cheap and easy to perform.
- They are particularly suitable for rare diseases.
- A wide range of risk factors can be investigated in each study.
- There is no loss to follow-up.

Disadvantages of case–control studies
- **Recall bias**, when cases have a differential ability to remember certain details about their histories, is a potential problem. For example, a lung cancer patient may well remember the occasional period when she or he smoked, whereas a control may not remember a similar period. When preparing the protocol for a case–control study, it is important to describe any attempts that will be made to reduce the possibility of recall bias by ensuring that exposure data are collected in an identical manner from cases and controls.
- If the onset of disease preceded exposure to the risk factor, causation cannot be inferred.
- Case–control studies are not suitable when exposures to the risk factor are rare.

References
1 Grimes, D.A. and Schulz, K.F. (2005) Compared to what? Finding controls for case–control studies. *Lancet*, **365**, 1429–1433.
2 Breslow, N.E. and Day, N.E. (1980) *Statistical Methods in Cancer Research. Volume I – The Analysis of Case-Control Studies.* Lyon: International Agency for Cancer Research.

Table 16.1 Observed frequencies (see Fig. 16.1).

Disease status	Exposed to factor		
	Yes	No	Total
Case	a	b	$a+b$
Control	c	d	$c+d$
Total	$a+c$	$b+d$	$n = a+b+c+d$

Example

A total of 171 patients who had started a long-term oxygen therapy for pulmonary fibrosis (PF) in Sweden between February 1997 and April 2000 were investigated in this unmatched case–control study. They were compared with 719 control participants randomly selected from the general population of the same age range as the patients with PF. Interest was centred on whether cumulative smoking exposure (measured up to 10 years before the diagnosis of PF in the cases) was associated with the risk of PF. The results in Table 16.2 show the number of ever smokers and never smokers in the case and control groups.

The observed odds ratio = (119 × 344)/(52 × 375) = 2.10.

It can be shown that the 95% confidence interval for the odds ratio is (1.47, 3.00).

Thus the odds of having PF in the Swedish population who had ever smoked was 2.10 times greater than that of never smokers, i.e. having ever smoked increased the odds of PF by 110%.

Table 16.2 Observed frequencies in the pulmonary fibrosis study.

	Current/ ex-smoker	Never smoked	Total
Pulmonary fibrosis (cases)	119	52	171
No pulmonary fibrosis (controls)	375	344	719
Total	494	396	890

Data extracted from Ekstrom, M., Gustafson, T., Boman, K., *et al.* (2014) Effects of smoking, gender and occupational exposure on the risk of severe pulmonary fibrosis: a population-based case-control study. *BMJ Open*, **4**, e004018.

Hypothesis testing

Part 4

Chapters

17 Hypothesis testing

We often gather sample data in order to assess how much evidence there is against a specific hypothesis about the population. When performing descriptive analyses (Chapters 4–6) we may see trends that appear to support or refute this hypothesis. However, we do not know if these trends reflect real associations or are simply a result of random fluctuations caused by the variability present in any data set. We use a process known as **hypothesis testing** (or **significance testing**) to quantify our belief against a particular hypothesis.

This chapter describes the format of hypothesis testing in general; details of specific hypothesis tests are given in subsequent chapters. For easy reference, each hypothesis test is contained in a similarly formatted box.

Hypothesis testing – a general overview

We define five stages when carrying out a hypothesis test:
1 Define the *null* and *alternative hypotheses* under study.
2 Collect relevant data from a sample of individuals.
3 Calculate the value of the *test statistic* specific to the null hypothesis.
4 Compare the value of the test statistic to values from a known probability distribution.
5 Interpret the *P*-value and results.

Defining the null and alternative hypotheses

We usually test the **null hypothesis** (H_0) which assumes *no effect* (e.g. the difference in means equals zero) in the *population*. For example, if we are interested in comparing smoking rates in men and women in the population, the null hypothesis would be:

H_0: smoking rates are the same in men and women in the population

We then define the **alternative hypothesis** (H_1) which holds if the null hypothesis is not true. The alternative hypothesis relates more directly to the theory we wish to investigate. So, in the example, we might have:

H_1: smoking rates are different in men and women in the population

We have not specified any direction for the difference in smoking rates, i.e. we have not stated whether men have higher or lower rates than women in the population. This leads to what is known as a **two-tailed test** because we allow for either eventuality, and is recommended as we are rarely certain, *in advance*, of the direction of any difference, if one exists. In some, very rare, circumstances, we may carry out a **one-tailed test** in which a direction of effect is specified in H_1. This might apply if we are considering a disease from which all untreated individuals die (a new drug cannot make things worse) or if we are conducting a trial of equivalence or non-inferiority (see last section in this chapter).

Obtaining the test statistic

After collecting the data, we substitute values from our sample into a formula, specific to the test we are using, to determine a value for the **test statistic**. This reflects the amount of evidence in the data *against* the null hypothesis – usually, the larger the value, ignoring its sign, the stronger the evidence.

Obtaining the *P*-value

All test statistics follow known theoretical probability distributions (Chapters 7 and 8). We relate the value of the test statistic obtained from the sample to the known distribution to obtain the **P-value**, the area in both (or occasionally one) tails of the probability distribution. Most computer packages provide the two-tailed *P*-value automatically. **The *P*-value is the probability of obtaining our results, or something more extreme, if the null hypothesis is true.** The null hypothesis relates to the population of interest, rather than the sample. Therefore, the null hypothesis is either true or false and we *cannot* interpret the *P*-value as the probability that the null hypothesis is true.

Using the *P*-value

We must make a decision about how much evidence we require to enable us to decide to reject the null hypothesis in favour of the alternative. The smaller the *P*-value, the greater the evidence against the null hypothesis.
- Conventionally, we consider that if the *P*-value is less than 0.05, there is sufficient evidence to reject the null hypothesis, as there is only a small chance of the results occurring if the null hypothesis were true. We then *reject* the null hypothesis and say that the results are **significant** at the 5% level (Fig. 17.1).
- In contrast, if the *P*-value is equal to or greater than 0.05, we usually conclude that there is insufficient evidence to reject the null hypothesis. We *do not reject* the null hypothesis, and we say that the results are **not significant** at the 5% level (Fig. 17.1). This does not mean that the null hypothesis is true; simply that we do not have enough evidence to reject it.

Medical Statistics at a Glance, Fourth Edition. Aviva Petrie and Caroline Sabin. © 2020 Aviva Petrie and Caroline Sabin. Published 2020 by John Wiley & Sons Ltd.
Companion Website: www.medstatsaag.com

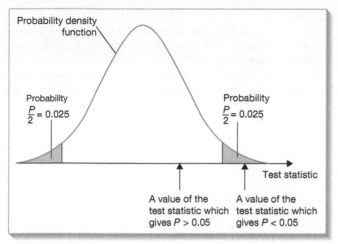

Figure 17.1 Probability distribution of the test statistic showing a two-tailed probability, $P = 0.05$.

The choice of 5% is arbitrary. On 5% of occasions we will incorrectly reject the null hypothesis when it is true. In situations in which the clinical implications of incorrectly rejecting the null hypothesis are severe, we may require stronger evidence before rejecting the null hypothesis (e.g. we may decide to reject the null hypothesis if the P-value is less than 0.01 or 0.001). The selected cut-off for the P-value (e.g. 0.05 or 0.01) is called the **significance level** of the test; it must be chosen before the data are collected.

Quoting a result only as significant at a certain cut-off level (e.g. stating only that $P < 0.05$) can be misleading. For example, if $P = 0.04$ we would reject H_0; however, if $P = 0.06$ we would not reject it. Are these really different? Therefore, we recommend quoting the exact P-value, often obtained from the computer output.

Non-parametric tests

Hypothesis tests which are based on knowledge of the probability distributions that the data follow are known as **parametric tests**. Often data do not conform to the assumptions that underlie these methods (Chapter 35). In these instances we can use **non-parametric tests** (sometimes referred to as **distribution-free** tests or **rank methods**). These tests generally replace the data with their ranks (i.e. the numbers 1, 2, 3, etc., describing their position in the ordered data set) and make no assumptions about the probability distribution that the data follow.

Non-parametric tests are particularly useful when the sample size is small (so that it is impossible to assess the distribution of the data), and/or when the data are measured on a categorical scale. However, non-parametric tests are generally wasteful of information; consequently they have less power (Chapter 18) to detect a real effect than the equivalent parametric test if all the assumptions underlying the parametric test are satisfied. Furthermore, they are primarily significance tests that often do not provide estimates of the effects of interest; they lead to decisions rather than an appreciation or understanding of the data.

Which test?

Deciding which statistical test to use depends on the design of the study, the type of variable and the distribution that the data being studied follow. The flow chart on the inside back cover will aid your decision.

Hypothesis tests versus confidence intervals

Confidence intervals (Chapter 11) and hypothesis tests are closely linked. The primary aim of a hypothesis test is to make a decision and provide an exact P-value. A confidence interval quantifies the effect of interest (e.g. the difference in means) and enables us to assess the clinical implications of the results. However, because it provides a range of plausible values for the true effect, it can also be used to make a decision although an exact P-value is not provided. For example, if the hypothesized value for the effect (e.g. zero) lies outside the 95% confidence interval then we believe the hypothesized value is implausible and would reject H_0. In this instance, we know that the P-value is less than 0.05 but do not know its exact value.

Equivalence and non-inferiority trials

In most randomized controlled trials (Chapter 14) of two or more different treatment strategies, we are usually interested in demonstrating the **superiority** of at least one treatment over the other(s). However, in some situations we may believe that a new treatment (e.g. drug) may be no more effective clinically than an existing treatment but will have other important benefits, perhaps in terms of reduced side effects, pill burden or costs. Then, we may wish to show simply that the efficacy of the new treatment is similar to (in an **equivalence** trial) or not *substantially* worse than (in a **non-inferiority** trial) that of the existing treatment. A **bioequivalence trial** is a particular type of randomized trial in which we are interested in showing that the rate and extent of absorption of a new formulation of a drug is the same as that of an old formulation, when the two drugs are given at the same dose.

When carrying out an equivalence or non-inferiority trial, the hypothesis testing procedure used in the usual superiority trial, testing the null hypothesis that the two treatments are the same, is irrelevant. This is because (i) a non-significant result does not imply non-inferiority or equivalence, and (ii) even if a statistically significant effect is detected, it may be clinically unimportant. Instead, we essentially reverse the null and alternative hypotheses in an equivalence trial, so that the null hypothesis expresses a difference and the alternative hypothesis expresses equivalence.

Rather than calculating test statistics, we generally approach the problem of assessing equivalence and non-inferiority[1] by determining whether the confidence interval for the effect of interest (e.g. the difference in means between two treatment groups) lies wholly or partly within a predefined **equivalence range** (i.e. the range of values, determined by clinical experts, that corresponds to an effect of no clinical importance). If the whole of the confidence interval for the effect of interest lies within the equivalence range, then we conclude that the two treatments are equivalent; in this situation, even if the upper and lower limits of the confidence interval suggest there is benefit of one treatment over the other, it is unlikely to have any clinical importance. In a non-inferiority trial, we want to show that the new treatment is not substantially worse than the standard one. (If the new treatment turns out to be better than the standard, this would be an added bonus!) In this situation, if the lower limit of the appropriate confidence interval does not fall below the lower limit of the equivalence range, we conclude that the new treatment is not inferior.

Unless otherwise specified, the hypothesis tests in subsequent chapters are tests of superiority. Note that the methods for determining sample size described in Chapter 36 do not apply to equivalence or non-inferiority trials. The sample size required for an equivalence or non-inferiority trial[2] is generally greater than that of the comparable superiority trial if all factors that affect sample size (e.g. significance level, power) are the same.

References

1 John, B., Jarvis, P., Lewis, J.A. and Ebbutt, A.F. (1996) Trials to assess equivalence: the importance of rigorous methods. *British Medical Journal*, **313**, 36–39.

2 Julious, S.A. (2004) Tutorial in biostatistics: sample sizes for clinical trials with Normal data. *Statistics in Medicine*, **23**, 1921–1986.

18 Errors in hypothesis testing

Making a decision

Most hypothesis tests in medical statistics compare groups of people who are exposed to a variety of experiences. We may, for example, be interested in comparing the effectiveness of two forms of treatment for reducing 5-year mortality from breast cancer. For a given outcome (e.g. death), we call the *comparison of interest* (e.g. the difference in 5-year mortality rates) the **effect** of interest or, if relevant, the **treatment effect**. We express the null hypothesis in terms of no effect (e.g. the 5-year mortality from breast cancer is the same in two treatment groups); the two-sided alternative hypothesis is that the effect is not zero. We perform a hypothesis test that enables us to decide whether we have enough evidence to reject the null hypothesis (Chapter 17). We can make one of two decisions; either we reject the null hypothesis, or we do not reject it.

Making the wrong decision

Although we hope we will draw the correct conclusion about the null hypothesis, we have to recognize that, because we only have a sample of information, we may make the wrong decision when we reject/do not reject the null hypothesis. The possible mistakes we can make are shown in Table 18.1.

- **Type I error** – *we reject the null hypothesis when it is true*, and conclude that there is an effect when, in reality, there is none. The maximum chance (probability) of making a Type I error is denoted by α (alpha). This is the significance level of the test (Chapter 17); we reject the null hypothesis if our P-value is less than the significance level, i.e. if $P < \alpha$.

Table 18.1 The consequences of hypothesis testing.

	Reject H_0	**Do not reject H_0**
H_0 **true**	Type I error	No error
H_0 **false**	No error	Type II error

We must decide on the value of α before we collect our data. We usually assign a conventional value of 0.05 to it, although we might choose a more restrictive value such as 0.01 (if we are particularly concerned about the consequences of incorrectly rejecting the null hypothesis) or a less restrictive value such as 0.10 (if we do not want to miss a real effect). Our chance of making a Type I error will never exceed our chosen significance level, say $\alpha = 0.05$, because we will only reject the null hypothesis if $P < 0.05$. If we find that $P \geq 0.05$, we will not reject the null hypothesis, and, consequently, not make a Type I error.

- **Type II error** – *we do not reject the null hypothesis when it is false*, and conclude that there is no evidence of an effect when one really exists. The chance (probability) of making a Type II error is denoted by β (beta); its complement, $(1 - \beta)$, is the **power** of the test. The power, therefore, is the *probability of rejecting the null hypothesis when it is false*; i.e. it is the chance (usually expressed as a percentage) of detecting, as statistically significant, a real treatment effect of a given size.

Ideally, we should like the power of our test to be 100%; we must recognize, however, that this is impossible because there is always a chance, albeit slim, that we could make a Type II error. Fortunately, however, we know which factors affect power, and thus we can control the power of a test by giving consideration to them.

Power and related factors

It is essential that we know the power of a proposed test at the planning stage of our investigation. Clearly, we should only embark on a study if we believe that it has a 'good' chance of detecting a clinically relevant effect, if one exists (by 'good' we mean that the power should be at least 80%). It is ethically irresponsible, and wasteful of time and resources, to undertake a clinical trial that has, say, only a 40% chance of detecting a real treatment effect.

A number of factors have a direct bearing on power for a given test.

- The **sample size** – power increases with increasing sample size. This means that a large sample has a greater ability than a small sample to detect a clinically important effect if it exists. When the sample size is very small, the test may have an inadequate power to detect a particular effect. We explain how to choose sample size, with power considerations, in Chapter 36. The methods can also be used to evaluate the power of the test for a specified sample size.
- The **variability of the observations**: – power increases as the variability of the observations decreases (Fig. 18.1).
- The **effect of interest** – the power of the test is greater for larger effects. A hypothesis test thus has a greater chance of detecting a large real effect than a small one.
- The **significance level** – the power is greater if the significance level is larger (this is equivalent to the probability of the Type I error (α) increasing as the probability of the Type II error (β)

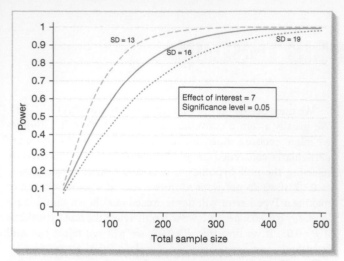

Figure 18.1 Power curves showing the relationship between power and the sample size in each of two groups for the comparison of two means using the unpaired *t*-test (Chapter 21). Each power curve relates to a two-sided test for which the significance level is 0.05, and the effect of interest (e.g. the difference between the treatment means) is 7 (e.g. 34 – 27). The assumed equal standard deviation of the measurements in the two groups is different for each power curve (see Example 1, Chapter 36).

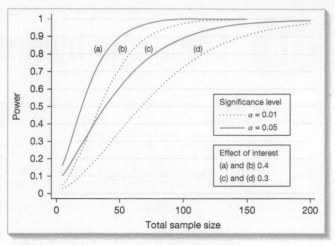

Figure 18.2 Power curves showing the relationship between power and the sample size in each of two groups for the comparison of two proportions using the Chi-squared test (Chapter 24). Curves are drawn when the effect of interest (e.g. the difference in the proportions with the characteristic of interest in the two treatment groups is either 0.4 (the upper two curves, e.g. 0.5 - 0.1) or 0.3 (the lower two curves, e.g. 0.5 - 0.2); the significance level of the two-sided test is either 0.05 or 0.01 (see Example 2, Chapter 36).

decreases). So, we are more likely to detect a real effect if we decide at the planning stage that we will regard our *P*-value as significant if it is less than 0.05 rather than less than 0.01. We can see this relationship between power and the significance level in Fig. 18.2.

Note that an inspection of the confidence interval (Chapter 11) for the effect of interest gives an indication of whether the power of the test was adequate. A wide confidence interval results from a small sample and/or data with substantial variability, and is a suggestion of low power.

Multiple hypothesis testing

The problem

Often, we want to carry out a number of significance tests on a data set. Unfortunately, the Type I error rate increases dramatically as the number of comparisons made increases, leading to spurious conclusions. In particular, if the significance level for a test is 0.05, the test has a 5% chance of erroneously rejecting the null hypothesis. However, if we perform 20 such tests, the probability that at least one of them will give a false positive result is 64%. In the situation where some of our multiple comparison findings are significant, a problem arises in that we cannot identify which, if any, are falsely positive.

Examples

Situations that involve **multiple comparisons** within a data set include:
- **Subgroup analyses** – these should be avoided as spurious results may arise because:
  - the power of the treatment comparison within a subgroup may be low (due to a small sample size) so that a real treatment effect is not detected as statistically significant;
  - often, the subgroups are not identified for biological or clinical reasons at the design stage of the study but are selected only after the data have been analysed; or
  - in a randomized clinical trial, bias may occur because the individuals have not been randomized to the different treatments within a subgroup (Chapters 14 and 34).
- **Multiple comparisons for a single outcome variable** – typical examples include making all pairwise comparisons between:
  - three or more treatment groups (such as A *vs* B, A *vs* C and B *vs* C for treatment groups A, B and C); or
  - three or more time points when each individual has the response variable measured at multiple time points.
- **Multiple outcome variables** – when different endpoints can be used to evaluate a treatment effect (Chapter 14).
- **Interim analyses** – when treatment comparisons are made at predetermined intermediate stages of a study (Chapter 14).
- **Data dredging** – to make comparisons and look for relationships in a 'fishing expedition', with no specification of the relationships of specific interest *a priori*.

Solutions

Ideally we should only perform a small number of tests, chosen to relate to the primary aims of the study and specified at the design stage of the study. We may also consider the following (as relevant).
- Use a method to adjust (i.e. increase) the *P*-value obtained from each test to take account of the number of tests performed and then relate this adjusted *P*-value to the conventional cut-off for significance of 0.05 (Chapter 22). For example, the simple **Bonferroni** approach (often regarded as rather conservative) multiplies each *P*-value by the number of tests carried out. Note that the value of performing this type of adjustment for multiple testing remains a subject of debate for cohort studies.
- Use a more stringent significance level for each test (e.g. 0.01 instead of the conventional 0.05).

- Only perform a subgroup analysis if the test for an *interaction* (Chapters 13 and 33) between the treatment and the factor defining the subgroups (e.g. sex) produces a significant result. Previously planned subgroup analysis may be a prerequisite to ensure that these tests are suitably powered (Chapter 18).
- Undertake multiple pairwise treatment comparisons only if the overall treatment effect is significant (e.g. in an analysis of variance) and then adjust the *P*-values by using a *post hoc* multiple comparison method, limiting the procedure to those comparisons that are of interest (Chapter 22).
- Use special methods for clustered data if each individual has repeated measurements, such as at multiple time points (Chapters 41 and 42).

- If there are multiple outcomes, combine them, appropriately, into a single composite endpoint (Chapter 13) or perform a **multivariate analysis**[1] in which we consider simultaneously the effects of one or more explanatory variables on more than one outcome variable.
- Choose a lower significance level (the significance level for each repeated test is called the *nominal* significance level) for interim analyses in a trial to ensure that the required overall significance level (typically 0.05) is maintained[2].

References

1 Tabachnick, B.G. and Fidell, L.S. (2013) *Using Multivariate Statistics*. 6th edition. Harlow: Pearson.
2 Pocock, S.J. (1983) *Clinical Trials: A Practical Approach*. Chichester: John Wiley & Sons.

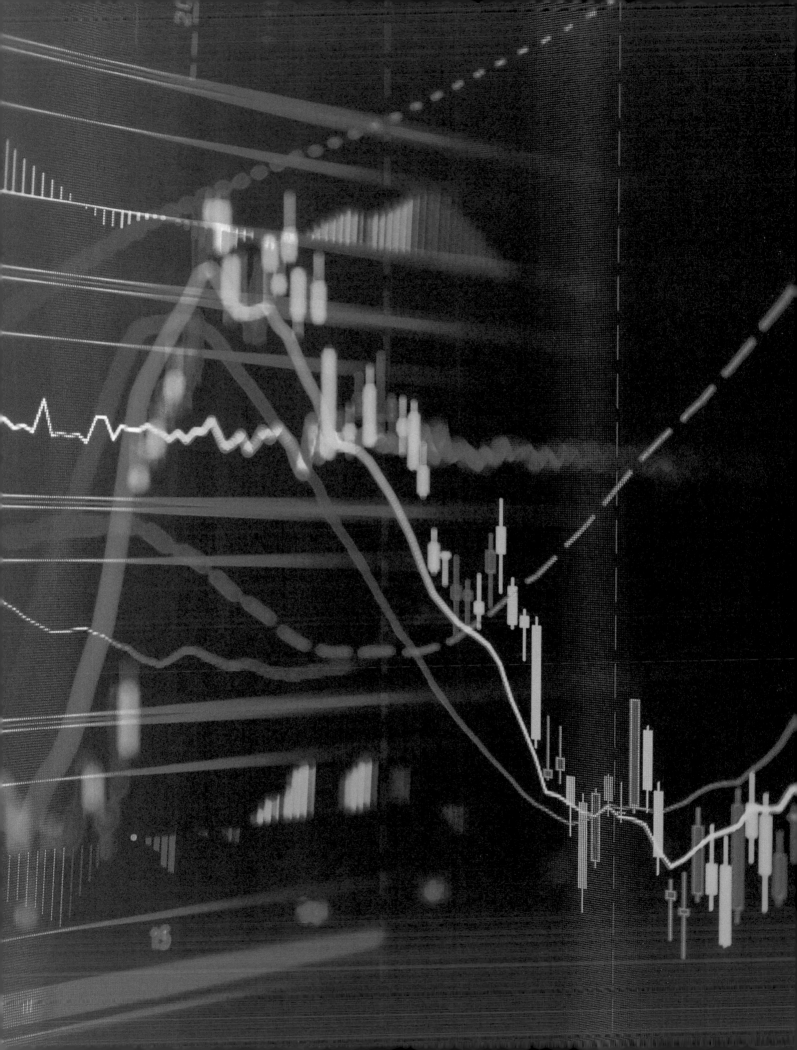

Basic techniques for analysing data

Part 5

Chapters

19 Numerical data: a single group

The problem

We have a sample from a single group of individuals and one numerical or ordinal variable of interest. We are interested in whether the average of this variable takes a particular value. For example, we may have a sample of patients with a specific medical condition. We have been monitoring triglyceride levels in the blood of healthy individuals and know that they have a geometric mean of 1.74 mmol/L. We wish to know whether the average level in the population from which our patients come is the same as this value.

The one-sample *t*-test

Assumptions

In the population of interest, the variable is Normally distributed with a given (usually unknown) variance. In addition, we have taken a reasonable sample size so that we can check the assumption of Normality (Chapter 35).

Rationale

We are interested in whether the mean, μ, of the variable in the population of interest differs from some hypothesized value, μ_1. We use a test statistic that is based on the difference between the sample mean, $\bar{x}$, and μ_1. Assuming that we do not know the population variance, then this test statistic, often referred to as *t*, follows the *t*-distribution. If we do know the population variance, or the sample size is very large, then an alternative test (often called a *z*-test), based on the Normal distribution, may be used. However, in these situations, results from both tests are virtually identical.

Additional notation

Our sample is of size n and the estimated standard deviation is s.

---

1 **Define the null and alternative hypotheses under study**

H_0: the mean in the population, μ, equals μ_1

H_1: the mean in the population does not equal μ_1.

2 **Collect relevant data from a sample of individuals**

---

3 **Calculate the value of the test statistic specific to H_0**

$$t = \frac{(\bar{x} - \mu_1)}{s/\sqrt{n}}$$

which follows the *t*-distribution with $(n-1)$ degrees of freedom.

4 **Compare the value of the test statistic to values from a known probability distribution**

Refer *t* to Appendix A2.

5 **Interpret the *P*-value and results**

Interpret the *P*-value and calculate a confidence interval for the true mean in the population (Chapter 11).

The 95% confidence interval is given by

$$\bar{x} \pm t_{0.05} \times \left(s/\sqrt{n}\right)$$

where $t_{0.05}$ is the percentage point of the *t*-distribution with $(n-1)$ degrees of freedom which gives a two-tailed probability of 0.05.

Interpretation and use of the confidence interval

The 95% confidence interval provides a range of values in which we are 95% certain that the true population mean lies. If the 95% confidence interval does not include the hypothesized value for the mean, μ_1, we reject the null hypothesis at the 5% level. If, however, the confidence interval includes μ_1, then we fail to reject the null hypothesis at that level.

If the assumptions are not satisfied

We may be concerned that the variable does not follow a Normal distribution in the population. Whereas the *t*-test is relatively **robust** (Chapter 35) to some degree of non-Normality, extreme skewness may be a concern. We can either transform the data, so that the variable is Normally distributed (Chapter 9), or use a non-parametric test such as the sign test or Wilcoxon signed ranks test (Chapter 20).

The sign test

Rationale

The sign test is a simple test based on the median of the distribution. We have some hypothesized value, λ, for the median in the population. If our sample comes from this population, then approximately half of the values in our sample should be greater than λ and half should be less than λ (after excluding any values which equal λ). The sign test considers the number of values in our sample that are greater (or less) than λ.

The sign test is a simple test; we can use a more powerful test, the Wilcoxon signed ranks test (Chapter 20), which takes into account the ranks of the data as well as their signs when carrying out such an analysis.

continued

Medical Statistics at a Glance, Fourth Edition. Aviva Petrie and Caroline Sabin. © 2020 Aviva Petrie and Caroline Sabin. Published 2020 by John Wiley & Sons Ltd.
Companion Website: www.medstatsaag.com

1 Define the null and alternative hypotheses under study

H_0: the median in the population equals λ

H_1: the median in the population does not equal λ.

2 Collect relevant data from a sample of individuals

3 Calculate the value of the test statistic specific to H_0

Ignore all values that are equal to λ, leaving n' values. Count the values that are greater than λ. Similarly, count the values that are less than λ. (In practice this will often involve calculating the difference between each value in the sample and λ, and noting its sign.) Consider r, the smaller of these two counts.

- If $n' \leq 10$, the test statistic is r

- If $n' > 10$, calculate $z = \dfrac{\left| r - \dfrac{n'}{2} \right| - \dfrac{1}{2}}{\dfrac{\sqrt{n'}}{2}}$

where $n'/2$ is the number of values above (or below) the median that we would expect if the null hypothesis were true. The vertical bars indicate that we take the absolute (i.e. the positive) value of the number inside the bars. The distribution of z is approximately Normal. The subtraction of ½ in the formula for z is a **continuity correction**, which we have to include to allow for the fact that we are relating a discrete value (r) to a continuous distribution (the Normal distribution).

4 Compare the value of the test statistic to values from a known probability distribution

- If $n' \leq 10$, refer r to Appendix A6
- If $n' > 10$, refer z to Appendix A1.

5 Interpret the P-value and results

Interpret the P-value and calculate a confidence interval for the median – some statistical packages provide this automatically; if not, we can rank the values in order of size and refer to Appendix A7 to identify the ranks of the values that are to be used to define the limits of the confidence interval. In general, confidence intervals for the median will be wider than those for the mean.

Example

There is some evidence that high blood triglyceride levels are associated with heart disease. As part of a large cohort study on heart disease, triglyceride levels were available in 232 men who developed heart disease over the 5 years after recruitment. We are interested in whether the average triglyceride level in the population of men from which this sample is chosen is the same as that in the general population. A **one-sample t-test** was performed to investigate this. Triglyceride levels are skewed to the right (Fig. 8.3a) but log triglyceride levels are approximately Normally distributed (Fig. 8.3b), so we performed our analysis on the log values. In the men in the general population, previous studies have shown that the mean of the log values equals $0.24\log_{10}$ (mmol/L), equivalent to a geometric mean of 1.74 mmol/L.

1 H_0: the mean $\log_{10}$ (triglyceride level) in the population of men who develop heart disease equals $0.24\log_{10}$ (mmol/L)

H_1: the mean $\log_{10}$ (triglyceride level) in the population of men who develop heart disease does not equal $0.24\log_{10}$ (mmol/L).

2 Sample size, $n = 232$

Mean of log values, $\bar{x} = 0.31\log_{10}$(mmol/L)

Standard deviation of log values, $s = 0.23\log_{10}$ (mmol/L).

3 Test statistic, $t = \dfrac{0.31 - 0.24}{0.23/\sqrt{232}} = 4.64$

4 We refer t to Appendix A2 with 231 degrees of freedom: $P < 0.001$.

5 There is strong evidence to reject the null hypothesis that the geometric mean triglyceride level in the population of men who develop heart disease equals 1.74 mmol/L. The geometric mean triglyceride level in the population of men who develop heart disease is estimated as antilog$_{10}$ $(0.31) = 10^{0.31}$, which equals 2.04 mmol/L. The 95% confidence interval for the geometric mean triglyceride level ranges from 1.90 to 2.19 mmol/L (i.e. antilog$_{10}$[$0.31 \pm 1.96 \times 0.23/\sqrt{232}$]). Therefore, in this population of patients, the geometric mean triglyceride level is significantly higher than that in the general population.

We can use the **sign test** to carry out a similar analysis on the untransformed triglyceride levels as this does not make any distributional assumptions. We assume that the median and geometric mean triglyceride level in the male population are similar.

1 H_0: the median triglyceride level in the population of men who develop heart disease equals 1.74 mmol/L

H_1: the median triglyceride level in the population of men who develop heart disease does not equal 1.74 mmol/L.

2 In this data set, the median value equals 1.94 mmol/L.

3 We investigate the differences between each value and 1.74. There are 231 non-zero differences, of which 135 are positive and 96 are negative. Therefore, $r = 96$. As the number of non-zero differences is greater than 10, we calculate

$$z = \frac{\left| 96 - \dfrac{231}{2} \right| - \dfrac{1}{2}}{\dfrac{\sqrt{231}}{2}} = 2.50$$

4 We refer z to Appendix A1: $P = 0.012$.

5 There is evidence to reject the null hypothesis that the median triglyceride level in the population of men who develop heart disease equals 1.74 mmol/L. Therefore, in this population of patients, the median triglyceride level is significantly higher than that in the general population. The formula in Appendix A7 indicates that the 95% confidence interval for the population median is given by the 101st and 132nd ranked values; these are 1.77 and 2.16 mmol/L.

Data kindly provided by Dr F.C. Lampe, Ms M. Walker and Dr P. Whincup, Department of Primary Care and Population Sciences, Royal Free and University College Medical School, London, UK.

20 Numerical data: two related groups

Learning objectives

By the end of this chapter, you should be able to:
- Describe different circumstances in which two groups of data are related
- Explain the rationale of the paired *t*-test
- Explain how to perform the paired *t*-test
- State the assumption underlying the paired *t*-test and explain how to proceed if it is not satisfied
- Explain the rationale of the Wilcoxon signed ranks test
- Explain how to perform the Wilcoxon signed ranks test

Relevant Workbook questions: MCQs 35, 39, 40, 41 and 42; and SQs 7 and 8 available online

The problem

We have two samples that are related to each other and one numerical or ordinal variable of interest.
- The variable may be measured on each individual in two circumstances. For example, in a cross-over trial (Chapter 13), each patient has two measurements on the variable, one while taking active treatment and one while taking placebo.
- The individuals in each sample may be different, but are linked to each other in some way. For example, patients in one group may be individually matched to patients in the other group in a case–control study (Chapter 16).

Such data are known as paired data. It is important to take account of the dependence between the two samples when analysing the data, otherwise the advantages of pairing (Chapter 13) are lost. We do this by considering the difference between the values for each pair, thereby reducing our two samples to a single sample of differences.

The paired *t*-test

Assumption

In the population of interest, the individual differences are Normally distributed with a given (usually unknown) variance. We have a reasonable sample size so that we can check the assumption of Normality.

Rationale

If the two sets of measurements were the same, then we would expect the mean of the differences between each pair of measurements to be zero in the population of interest. Therefore, our test statistic simplifies to a one-sample *t*-test (Chapter 19) on the differences, where the hypothesized value for the mean difference in the population is zero.

Additional notation

Because of the paired nature of the data, our two samples must be of the same size, n. We have n differences, $d_1, d_2, d_3, ..., d_n$: their sample mean is $\bar{d}$ and estimated standard deviation s_d.

1 Define the null and alternative hypotheses under study

H_0: the mean difference in the population equals zero

H_1: the mean difference in the population does not equal zero.

2 Collect relevant data from two related samples

3 Calculate the value of the test statistic specific to H_0

$$t = \frac{(\bar{d} - 0)}{\text{SE}(\bar{d})} = \frac{\bar{d}}{s_d / \sqrt{n}}$$

which follows the *t*-distribution with $(n-1)$ degrees of freedom.

4 Compare the value of the test statistic to values from a known probability distribution

Refer t to Appendix A2.

5 Interpret the *P*-value and results

Interpret the *P*-value and calculate a confidence interval for the true mean difference in the population. The 95% confidence interval is given by

$$\bar{d} \pm t_{0.05} \times (s_d/\sqrt{n})$$

where $t_{0.05}$ is the percentage point of the *t*-distribution with $(n-1)$ degrees of freedom, which gives a two-tailed probability of 0.05.

If the assumption is not satisfied

If the differences do not follow a Normal distribution, the assumption underlying the *t*-test is not satisfied. We can either transform the data (Chapter 9) or use a non-parametric test such as the sign test (Chapter 19) or Wilcoxon signed ranks test to assess whether the differences are centred around zero.

The Wilcoxon signed ranks test

Rationale

In Chapter 19 we explained how to use the **sign test** on a single sample of numerical measurements to test the null hypothesis that the population median equals a particular value. We can also use the sign test when we have **paired** observations, the pair representing matched individuals (e.g. in a case–control study, Chapter 16) or measurements made on the same individual in different circumstances (as in a cross-over trial of two treatments, A and B, Chapter 13). For each pair, we evaluate the **difference** in the measurements. The sign test can be used to assess whether the median difference in the population equals zero by considering the differences in the sample and observing how many are greater (or less) than zero. However, the sign test does not incorporate information on the sizes of these differences.

The **Wilcoxon signed ranks test** takes account not only of the signs of the differences but also their magnitude, and therefore is

Medical Statistics at a Glance, Fourth Edition. Aviva Petrie and Caroline Sabin. © 2020 Aviva Petrie and Caroline Sabin. Published 2020 by John Wiley & Sons Ltd.
Companion Website: www.medstatsaag.com

a more powerful test (Chapter 18). The individual difference is calculated for each pair of results. Ignoring zero differences, these are then classed as being either positive or negative. In addition, the differences are placed in order of size, ignoring their signs, and are **ranked** accordingly. The smallest difference thus gets the value 1, the second smallest gets the value 2, etc., up to the largest difference, which is assigned the value n', if there are n' non-zero differences. If two or more of the differences are the same, they each receive the mean of the ranks these values would have received if they had not been tied. Under the null hypothesis of no difference, the sums of the ranks relating to the positive and negative differences should be the same (see following box).

Wilcoxon signed ranks test

1 Define the null and alternative hypotheses under study

H_0: the median difference in the population equals zero

H_1: the median difference in the population does not equal zero.

2 Collect relevant data from two related samples

3 Calculate the value of the test statistic specific to H_0

Calculate the difference for each pair of results. Ignoring their signs, rank all n' non-zero differences, assigning the value 1 to the smallest difference and the value n' to the largest. Sum the ranks of the positive (T_+) and negative differences (T_-).

- If $n' \leq 25$, the test statistic, T, takes the value T_+ or T_-, whichever is smaller
- If $n' > 25$, calculate the test statistic z, where

$$z = \frac{\left| T - \frac{n'(n'+1)}{4} \right| - \frac{1}{2}}{\sqrt{\frac{n'(n'+1)(2n'+1)}{24}}}$$

z follows a Normal distribution (its value has to be adjusted if there are many tied values[1]).

4 Compare the value of the test statistic to values from a known probability distribution

- If $n' \leq 25$, refer T to Appendix A8
- If $n' > 25$, refer z to Appendix A1.

5 Interpret the P-value and results

Interpret the P-value and calculate a confidence interval for the median difference (Chapter 19) using all n differences in the sample.

Reference

1 Siegel, S. and Castellan, N.J. (1988) *Nonparametric Statistics for the Behavioural Sciences*. 2nd edition. New York: McGraw-Hill.

Example 1

It has been shown that a Palaeolithic diet (P) consisting of the typical food (lean meat, fish, fruits, vegetables, eggs and nuts) that our ancestors ate during the Palaeolithic era improves cardiovascular disease risk factors and glucose control compared with the currently recommended diabetes diet (D: a healthy eating plan rich in fruit, vegetables, wholegrain cereal products, fish and nuts, and low in dairy produce, fat, carbohydrates and calories) in patients with type 2 diabetes. To elucidate the mechanisms behind these effects, researchers evaluated fasting plasma concentrations of leptin (which plays a key role in the regulation of energy balance, is believed to be critical for glycaemic control, and tends to have higher values in individuals with type 2 diabetes) in a randomized cross-over pilot study of 14 patients with type 2 diabetes. Seven patients, chosen randomly, followed the Palaeolithic diet for 3 months and then switched to the usual diabetic diet for a further 3 months, and the remaining seven patients followed the diets in the reverse order. Baseline variables were similar in the two groups and no patient was treated with insulin. As the difference (D – P, at the end of each 3-month period) in fasting plasma leptin was approximately Normally distributed in this group of patients, a **paired t-test** was performed to compare the results. Full computer output is shown in Appendix C.

1 H_0: the mean difference in fasting plasma leptin in type 2 diabetic patients whilst on the diabetic diet and whilst on the Palaeolithic diet equals zero in the population

H_1: the mean difference in fasting plasma leptin in type 2 diabetic patients whilst on the diabetic and whilst on the Palaeolithic diet does not equal zero in the population.

2 Sample size, $n = 14$. The mean difference in fasting plasma leptin (D – P), $\bar{d} = 0.71$ ng/mL. Standard deviation of differences, $s_d = 0.83$ ng/mL.

3 Test statistic, $t = \dfrac{0.71}{0.83/\sqrt{14}} = 3.2$

4 We refer t to Appendix A2 with $(14 - 1) = 13$ degrees of freedom: $0.001 < P < 0.01$ (computer output gives $P = 0.007$).

5 There is evidence to reject the null hypothesis. The 95% confidence interval for the true mean difference in fasting plasma leptin is 0.23 to 1.19 ng/mL (i.e. $0.71 \pm 2.16 \times 0.83/\sqrt{14}$).

The fasting plasma leptin levels in patients on the Palaeolithic diet were significantly lower, on average, than the levels when these patients followed the standard diabetic diet. However, the sample size of this pilot study was small: long-term adequately powered (Chapter 18) trials investigating the effect of the Palaeolithic diet on fasting plasma levels of leptin are recommended.

Adapted from Fontes-Villalba, M., Lindeberg, S., Granfeldt, Y., *et al.* (2016) Palaeolithic diet decreases fasting plasma leptin concentrations more than a diabetes diet in patients with type 2 diabetes: a randomised cross-over trial. *Cardiovascular Diabetology* **15**, 80.

Example 2

Ten children with congenital hemiparesis aged between 8 and 17 years of age were given five treatments of 6 Hz primed, low-frequency, repetitive transcranial magnetic stimulation (rTMS) and five treatments of constraint-induced movement therapy (CIMT) on alternate weekdays for 2 weeks to assess the effect of rTMS combined with CIMT on promoting recovery of the paretic hand. The primary outcome of the study was the Assisting Hand Assessment (AHA) score which is derived from a test for children with unilateral limb dysfunction that assesses total body function and activity. Each of the 22 AHA test items was assessed by an ordinal score (from 1 to 4): the sum of these scores therefore ranges from 22 to 88 points, with higher scores indicating better ability. The data in Table 20.1 show the AHA scores of these children, pre- and post-treatment, and Fig. 20.1 shows the linked pairs of results. As there were only 10 children in this group and because the differences were clearly not Normally distributed, a **Wilcoxon signed ranks test** was performed to investigate whether there was a difference in the AHA scores pre- and post-treatment.

Table 20.1 AHA scores pre- and post-treatment with rTMS and CIMT.

Child	1	2	3	4	5	6	7	8	9	10
AHA pre-treatment	84	49	38	65	47	54	58	55	69	71
AHA post-treatment	87	56	42	74	53	58	66	62	69	79
Difference (post-minus pre-treatment)	3	7	4	9	6	4	8	7	0	8

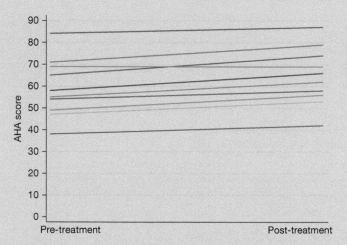

Figure 20.1 Change in AHA scores in 10 patients before and after treatment with rTMS and CIMT.

1 H_0: the median of the AHA score differences (post- minus pre-treatment) equals zero in the population of children with congenital hemiparesis receiving rTMS with CIMT

H_1: the median of the AHA score differences (post- minus pre-treatment) does not equal zero in the population of children with congenital hemiparesis receiving rTMS with CIMT.

2 The AHA scores pre- and post-treatment in each child receiving rTMS with CIMT are shown in Table 20.1.

3 There is one zero difference; of the remaining $n' = 9$ differences, all are positive. The sum of the ranks of the positive differences, $T_+ = 1+2+3+4+5+6+7+8+9 = 45$.

4 As $n' < 25$, we refer T_+ to Appendix A8: $P < 0.01$ (computer output gives $P = 0.004$).

5 There is strong evidence to reject the null hypothesis of no change in AHA scores after treatment. The median AHA score difference (post- minus pre-treatment values, including the zero difference) is 6.5 (the arithmetic mean of 6 and 7). As the median is positive, this indicates that, on average, the AHA score is greater after treatment. Appendix A7 shows that the approximate 95% confidence interval for the median AHA score difference in the population is given by the 2nd and the 9th ranked differences (including the zero difference); these are 3 and 8.

N.b. the analysis, as described, is open to criticism as there was no control group (Chapter 14) of children who did not receive rTMS. However, this group of 10 treated children comprised only one component of a randomized controlled trial in which children with congenital hemiparesis were randomized to receive either 6 Hz primed, low-frequency, repetitive rTMS (10 children) or a sham rTMS treatment (9 children), each alternated daily with CIMT. We provide the analysis of the changes in AHA score pre- and post-treatment in the two groups in Chapter 21 (Example 2).

Gillick, B.T., Krach, L.E., Rich, T.L., *et al* (2014) Primed low-frequency repetitive transcranial magnetic stimulation and constraint-induced movement therapy in pediatric hemiparesis: a randomized trial. *Developmental Medicine and Child Neurology* **56(1)**, 44–52. Data kindly provided by Professor Gillick.

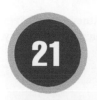

21 Numerical data: two unrelated groups

The problem

We have samples from two independent (unrelated) groups of individuals and one numerical or ordinal variable of interest. We are interested in whether the mean or distribution of the variable is the same in the two groups. For example, we may wish to compare the weights in two groups of children, each child being randomly allocated to receive either a dietary supplement or placebo.

The unpaired (two-sample) *t*-test

Assumptions

In the population, the variable is Normally distributed in each group and the variances of the two groups are the same. In addition, we have reasonable sample sizes so that we can check the assumptions of Normality and equal variances.

Rationale

We consider the difference in the means of the two groups. Under the null hypothesis that the population means in the two groups are the same, this difference will equal zero. Therefore, we use a test statistic that is based on the difference in the two sample means, and on the value of the difference in population means under the null hypothesis (i.e. zero). This test statistic, often referred to as *t*, follows the *t*-distribution.

Notation

Our two samples are of size n_1 and n_2. Their means are $\bar{x}_1$ and $\bar{x}_2$; their standard deviations are s_1 and s_2.

1 Define the null and alternative hypotheses under study

H_0: the population means in the two groups are equal

H_1: the population means in the two groups are not equal.

2 Collect relevant data from two samples of individuals

3 Calculate the value of the test statistic specific to H_0

If *s* is an estimate of the pooled standard deviation of the two groups,

$$s = \sqrt{\frac{(n_1 - 1)s_1^2 + (n_2 - 1)s_2^2}{n_1 + n_2 - 2}}$$

then the test statistic is given by *t*, where

$$t = \frac{(\bar{x}_1 - \bar{x}_2) - 0}{\text{SE}(\bar{x}_1 - \bar{x}_2)} = \frac{(\bar{x}_1 - \bar{x}_2)}{s\sqrt{\dfrac{1}{n_1} + \dfrac{1}{n_2}}}$$

which follows the *t*-distribution with $(n_1 + n_2 - 2)$ degrees of freedom.

4 Compare the value of the test statistic to values from a known probability distribution

Refer *t* to Appendix A2. When the sample sizes in the two groups are large, the *t*-distribution approximates a Normal distribution, and then we reject the null hypothesis at the 5% level if the absolute value (i.e. ignoring the sign) of *t* is greater than 1.96.

5 Interpret the *P*-value and results

Interpret the *P*-value and calculate a confidence interval for the difference in the two means. The 95% confidence interval, assuming equal variances, is given by

$$(\bar{x}_1 - \bar{x}_2) \pm t_{0.05} \times \text{SE}(\bar{x}_1 - x_2)$$

where $t_{0.05}$ is the percentage point of the *t*-distribution with $(n_1 + n_2 - 2)$ degrees of freedom, which gives a two-tailed probability of 0.05.

Interpretation of the confidence interval

The upper and lower limits of the confidence interval can be used to assess whether the difference between the two mean values is clinically important. For example, if the upper and/or lower limit is close to zero, this indicates that the true difference may be very small and clinically meaningless, even if the test is statistically significant.

If the assumptions are not satisfied

When the sample sizes are reasonably large, the *t*-test is fairly robust (Chapter 35) to departures from Normality. However, it is less robust to unequal variances. There is a modification of the unpaired *t*-test that allows for unequal variances, and results from it are often provided in computer output. However, if there are concerns that the assumptions are not satisfied, then the data can either be transformed (Chapter 9) to achieve approximate Normality and/or equal variances, or a non-parametric test such as the Wilcoxon rank sum test can be used.

continued

Medical Statistics at a Glance, Fourth Edition. Aviva Petrie and Caroline Sabin. © 2020 Aviva Petrie and Caroline Sabin. Published 2020 by John Wiley & Sons Ltd.
Companion Website: www.medstatsaag.com

The Wilcoxon rank sum (two-sample) test

Rationale

The **Wilcoxon rank sum test** makes no distributional assumptions and is the non-parametric equivalent to the unpaired *t*-test. The test is based on the sum of the ranks of the values in each of the two groups; these should be comparable after allowing for differences in sample size if the groups have similar distributions.

An equivalent test, known as the **Mann–Whitney *U* test**, gives identical results although it is slightly more complicated to carry out by hand.

Reference

1 Siegel, S. and Castellan, N.J. (1988) *Nonparametric Statistics for the Behavioural Sciences*. 2nd edition. New York: McGraw-Hill.

---

1 Define the null and alternative hypotheses under study

H_0: the two groups have the same distribution in the population

H_1: the two groups have different distributions in the population.

2 Collect relevant data from two samples of individuals

3 Calculate the value of the test statistic specific to H_0

All observations are ranked as if they were from a single sample. Tied observations are given the mean of the ranks the values would have received if they had not been tied. The sum of the ranks, T, is then calculated in the group with the smaller sample size.

- If the sample size in each group is 15 or less, T is the test statistic
- If at least one of the groups has a sample size of more than 15, calculate the test statistic

$$z = \frac{(T - \mu_t)}{\sigma_T}$$

which follows a Normal distribution, where

$$\mu_T = \frac{n_S(n_S + n_L + 1)}{2} \qquad \sigma_T = \sqrt{n_L \mu_T / 6}$$

and n_S and n_L are the sample sizes of the smaller and larger groups, respectively. z must be adjusted if there are many tied values[1].

4 Compare the value of the test statistic to values from a known probability distribution

- If the sample size in each group is 15 or less, refer T to Appendix A9
- If at least one of the groups has a sample size of more than 15, refer z to Appendix A1.

5 Interpret the *P*-value and results

Interpret the *P*-value and obtain a confidence interval for the difference in the two medians. This is time-consuming to calculate by hand so details have not been included; some statistical packages will provide the confidence interval. If this confidence interval is not included in the package, a confidence interval for the median in each of the two groups can be quoted.

Example 1

In order to determine the effect of regular prophylactic inhaled corticosteroids on wheezing episodes associated with viral infection in school-age children, a randomized double-blind controlled trial was carried out comparing inhaled beclomethasone dipropionate with placebo. In this investigation, the primary endpoint was the mean forced expiratory volume in 1 second (FEV1) over a 6-month period. After checking the assumptions of Normality and constant variance (see Fig. 4.2), we performed an **unpaired *t*-test** to compare the means in the two groups. The full computer output is shown in Appendix C.

1 H_0: the mean FEV1 in the population of school-age children is the same in the two treatment groups

H_1: the mean FEV1 in the population of school-age children is not the same in the two treatment groups.

2 Treated group: sample size, $n_1 = 50$; mean, $\bar{x}_1 = 1.64$ litres, standard deviation, $s_1 = 0.29$ litres

Placebo group: sample size, $n_2 = 48$; mean, $\bar{x}_2 = 1.54$ litres; standard deviation, $s_2 = 0.25$ litres.

3 Pooled standard deviation,

$$s = \sqrt{\frac{(49 \times 0.29^2) + (47 \times 0.25^2)}{(50 + 48 - 2)}} = 0.2670 \text{ litres}$$

Test statistic, $t = \dfrac{1.64 - 1.54}{0.2670 \times \sqrt{\dfrac{1}{50} + \dfrac{1}{48}}} = 1.9145$

4 We refer t to Appendix A2 with $50 + 48 - 2 = 96$ degrees of freedom. Because Appendix A2 is restricted to certain degrees of freedom, we have to **interpolate** (estimate the required value that lies between two known values). We therefore interpolate between the values relating to 50 and 100 degrees of freedom. Hence, $P > 0.05$ (computer output gives $P = 0.06$).

5 We have insufficient evidence to reject the null hypothesis at the 5% level. However, as the *P*-value is only just greater than 0.05, there may be an indication that the two population means are different. The estimated difference between the two means is $1.64 - 1.54 = 0.10$ litres. The 95% confidence interval for the true difference in the two means ranges from -0.007 to 0.207 litres

$$\left[= 0.10 \pm \left(1.99 \times 0.2670 \times \sqrt{\frac{1}{50} + \frac{1}{48}} \right) \right]$$

Data kindly provided by Dr I. Doull, Cystic Fibrosis/Respiratory Unit, Department of Child Health, University Hospital of Wales, Cardiff, UK, and Dr F.C. Lampe, Department of Primary Care and Population Sciences, Royal Free and University College Medical School, London, UK.

Example 2

Nineteen children with congenital hemiparesis aged between 8 and 17 years of age were randomized to receive either five treatments of 6 Hz primed, low-frequency, repetitive transcranial magnetic stimulation (rTMS) or five sham rTMS treatments, each alternated with five treatments of constraint-induced movement therapy (CIMT) on alternate weekdays for 2 weeks to assess the effect of rTMS on promoting recovery of the paretic hand. The primary outcome of the study was the Assisting Hand Assessment (AHA) score, as described in Chapter 20, Example 2. In that chapter, we compared the pre- and post-treatment AHA scores in the 10 children receiving rTMS with CIMT but were unable to draw conclusions about the effectiveness of rTMS because we had not included the sham treatment data. In this chapter, we assess the effectiveness of rTMS by comparing the distributions of the AHA score pre- and post-treatment differences in children receiving CIMT with either rTMS or the sham rTMS. Because of the small sample sizes and obviously skewed differences in AHA scores pre- and post-treatment (Fig. 21.1), we performed a **Wilcoxon rank sum test** to compare the distributions of the AHA score differences.

1 H_0: the distributions of AHA score differences (post-minus pre-treatment) in the two groups (test and sham rTMS) in the population of children with congenital hemiparesis are the same

H_1: the distributions of AHA score differences (post- minus pre-treatment) in the two groups (test and sham rTMS) in the population of children with congenital hemiparesis are not the same.

2 rTMS group: sample size, $n_L = 10$, AHA scores were 3, 7, 4, 9, 6, 4, 8, 7, 0, 8

Sham rTMS group: sample size, $n_S = 9$, AHA scores were 0, 2, 2, 1, 0, 4, 2, 6, 0

The ranked data are shown in Table 21.1 where tied values received the mean of the ranks they would have received had they not been tied.

3 Sum of the ranks in the rTMS group $= 2.5 + 9 + 11 + 11 + 13.5 + 15.5 + 15.5 + 17.5 + 17.5 + 19 = 132$

Sum of the ranks in the sham rTMS group $= 2.5 + 2.5 + 2.5 + 5 + 7 + 7 + 7 + 11 + 13.5 = 58$

4 Because there are 10 or fewer children in each group, we obtain the P-value from Appendix A9: $P < 0.01$ (computer output gives $P = 0.007$).

5 There is evidence to reject the null hypothesis that the distributions of the change in AHA score pre- and post-treatment are the same in the two groups. The median difference in AHA score in the rTMS group and the sham rTMS group is 6.5 (95% confidence interval 3.3 to 8) and 2 (95% confidence interval 0 to 3.8), respectively. We thus believe that primed low-frequency rTMS combined with CIMT is efficacious in paediatric hemiparesis.

Table 21.1 AHA score differences (post- minus pre-treatment) and their ranks in two groups of children with congenital hemiparesis.

rTMS	0								3	4	4		6		7	7	8	8	9
Sham rTMS		0	0	0	1	2	2	2				4		6					
Rank	2.5	2.5	2.5	2.5	5	7	7	7	9	11	11	11	13.5	13.5	15.5	15.5	17.5	17.5	19

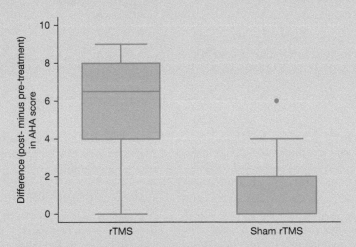

Figure 21.1 Box plot of AHA score differences (post- minus pre-treatment) in children with congenital hemiparesis receiving CIMT with either rTMS or sham rTMS.

Gillick, B.T., Krach, L.E., Rich, T.L., *et al.* (2014) Primed low-frequency repetitive transcranial magnetic stimulation and constraint-induced movement therapy in pediatric hemiparesis: a randomized trial. *Developmental Medicine and Child Neurology*, **56(1)**, 44–52. Data kindly provided by Professor Gillick.

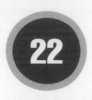

22 Numerical data: more than two groups

The problem

We have samples from a number of independent groups. We have a single numerical or ordinal variable and are interested in whether the average value of the variable varies in the different groups, e.g. whether the average platelet count varies in groups of women with different ethnic backgrounds. Although we could perform tests to compare the averages in each pair of groups, the high Type I error rate, resulting from the large number of comparisons, means that we may draw incorrect conclusions (Chapter 18). Therefore, we carry out a single **global** test to determine whether the averages differ in any groups.

One-way analysis of variance

Assumptions

The groups are defined by the *levels* of a single factor (e.g. different ethnic backgrounds). In the population of interest, the variable is Normally distributed in each group and the variance in every group is the same. We have a reasonable sample size so that we can check these assumptions.

Rationale

The one-way analysis of variance separates the total variability in the data into that which can be attributed to differences between the individuals from the different groups (the **between-group variation**) and to the random variation between the individuals within each group (the **within-group variation**, sometimes called **unexplained** or **residual** variation). These components of variation are measured using variances, hence the name **analysis of variance (ANOVA)**. Under the null hypothesis that the group means are the same, the between-group variance will be similar to the within-group variance. If, however, there are differences between the groups, then the between-group variance will be larger than the within-group variance. The test is based on the ratio of these two variances.

Notation

We have k independent samples, each derived from a different group. The sample sizes, means and standard deviations in each group are n_i, $\bar{x}_i$ and s_i, respectively ($i = 1, 2, \ldots, k$). The total sample size is $n = n_1 + n_2 + \ldots + n_k$.

---

1 Define the null and alternative hypotheses under study

H_0: all group means in the population are equal

H_1: at least one group mean in the population differs from the others.

2 Collect relevant data from samples of individuals

3 Calculate the value of the test statistic specific to H_0

The test statistic for ANOVA is a ratio, F, of the between-group variance to the within-group variance. This F-statistic follows the F-distribution (Chapter 8) with ($k - 1$, $n - k$) degrees of freedom in the numerator and denominator, respectively.

The calculations involved in ANOVA are complex and are not shown here. Most computer packages will output the values directly in an ANOVA table, which usually includes the F-ratio and P-value (see Example 1).

4 Compare the value of the test statistic to values from a known probability distribution

Refer the F-ratio to Appendix A5. Because the between-group variation is greater than or equal to the within-group variation, we look at the one-sided P-values.

5 Interpret the P-value and results

If we obtain a significant result at this initial stage, we may consider performing specific pairwise *post hoc* comparisons. We can use one of a number of special tests devised for this purpose (e.g. **Duncan's**, **Scheffé's**) or we can use the unpaired t-test (Chapter 21) adjusted for multiple hypothesis testing (Chapter 18). We can also calculate a confidence interval for each individual group mean (Chapter 11). Note that we use a pooled estimate of the variance of the values from *all* groups when calculating confidence intervals and performing t-tests. Most packages refer to this estimate of the variance as the **residual variance** or **residual mean square**; it is found in the ANOVA table.

Although the two tests appear to be different, the unpaired t-test and ANOVA give equivalent results when there are only two groups of individuals.

If the assumptions are not satisfied

Although ANOVA is relatively robust (Chapter 35) to moderate departures from Normality, it is not robust to unequal variances. Therefore, before carrying out the analysis, we check for Normality, and test whether the variances are similar in the groups either by 'eyeballing' them, or by using **Levene's** test or **Bartlett's** test (Chapter 35). If the assumptions are not satisfied, we can either transform the data (Chapter 9) or use the non-parametric equivalent of one-way ANOVA, the **Kruskal–Wallis** test.

Medical Statistics at a Glance, Fourth Edition. Aviva Petrie and Caroline Sabin. © 2020 Aviva Petrie and Caroline Sabin. Published 2020 by John Wiley & Sons Ltd.
Companion Website: www.medstatsaag.com

The Kruskal–Wallis test

Rationale

This non-parametric test is an extension of the Wilcoxon rank sum test (Chapter 21). Under the null hypothesis of no differences in the distributions between the groups, the sums of the ranks in each of the k groups should be comparable after allowing for any differences in sample size.

---

1 Define the null and alternative hypotheses under study

H_0: each group has the same distribution of values in the population

H_1: at least one group does not have the same distribution of values in the population.

2 Collect relevant data from samples of individuals

3 Calculate the value of the test statistic specific to H_0

Rank all n values and calculate the sum of the ranks in each of the groups: these sums are $R_1, \ldots R_k$. The test statistic (which should be modified if there are many tied values[1]) is given by

$$H = \frac{12}{n(n+1)} \sum \frac{R_i^2}{n_i} - 3(n+1)$$

---

continued

which follows a Chi-squared distribution with $(k-1)$ degrees of freedom.

4 Compare the value of the test statistic to values from a known probability distribution

Refer H to Appendix A3.

5 Interpret the P-value and results

Interpret the P-value and, if significant, perform two-sample non-parametric tests between pairs of groups, adjusting for multiple testing. Calculate a confidence interval for the median in each group.

We use one-way ANOVA or its non-parametric equivalent when the groups relate to a single factor and are independent. We can use other forms of ANOVA when the study design is more complex[2].

References

1 Siegel, S. and Castellan, N.J. (1988) *Nonparametric Statistics for the Behavioural Sciences.* 2nd edition. New York: McGraw-Hill.
2 Mickey, R.M., Dunn, O.J. and Clark, V.A. (2004) *Applied Statistics: Analysis of Variance and Regression.* 3rd edition. Chichester: Wiley.

Example 1

A total of 150 women of different ethnic backgrounds were included in a cross-sectional study of factors related to blood clotting. We compared mean platelet levels in the four groups using a **one-way ANOVA**. It was reasonable to assume Normality and constant variance, as shown in the computer output (Appendix C).

1 H_0: there are no differences in the mean platelet levels in the four groups in the population

H_1: at least one group mean platelet level differs from the others in the population.

2 The following table summarizes the data in each group.

Group	Sample size, n (%)	Mean ($\times 10^9$), $\bar{x}$	Standard deviation ($\times 10^9$), s	95% CI for mean (using pooled standard deviation – see point 3)
Caucasian	90 (60.0)	268.1	77.08	252.7 to 283.5
Afro-Caribbean	21 (14.0)	254.3	67.50	220.9 to 287.7
Mediterranean	19 (12.7)	281.1	71.09	245.7 to 316.5
Other	20 (13.3)	273.3	63.42	238.9 to 307.7

3 The following ANOVA table is extracted from the computer output:

Source	Sum of squares	df	Mean square	F-ratio	P-value
Between ethnic group	7711.967	3	2570.656	0.477	0.699
Within ethnic group	787289.533	146	5392.394		

Pooled standard deviation $= \sqrt{5392.394} \times 10^9 = 73.43 \times 10^9$.

4 The ANOVA table gives $P = 0.70$. (We could have referred F to Appendix A5 with (3, 146) degrees of freedom (df) to determine the P-value.)

5 There is insufficient evidence to reject the null hypothesis that the mean levels in the four groups in the population are the same.

Data kindly provided by Dr R.A. Kadir, University Department of Obstetrics and Gynaecology, and Professor C.A. Lee, Haemophilia Centre and Haemostasis Unit, Royal Free Hospital, London, UK.

Example 2

Quality-of-life scores, measured using the SF-36 questionnaire, were obtained in three groups of individuals: those with severe haemophilia, those with mild/moderate haemophilia, and normal controls. Each group comprised a sample of 20 individuals. Scores on the physical functioning scale (PFS), which can take values from 0 to 100, were compared in the three groups. As visual inspection of Fig. 22.1 showed that the data were not Normally distributed, we performed a **Kruskal–Wallis** test.

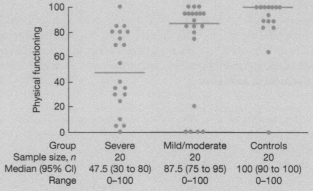

Group	Severe	Mild/moderate	Controls
Sample size, n	20	20	20
Median (95% CI)	47.5 (30 to 80)	87.5 (75 to 95)	100 (90 to 100)
Range	0–100	0–100	0–100

Figure 22.1 Dot plot showing physical functioning scores (from the SF-36 questionnaire) in individuals with severe and mild/moderate haemophilia and in normal controls. The horizontal bars are the medians.

1 H_0: each group has the same distribution of PFS scores in the population

H_1: at least one of the groups has a different distribution of PFS scores in the population.

2 The data are shown in Fig. 22.1.

3 Sum of ranks in severe haemophilia group = 372

Sum of ranks in mild/moderate haemophilia group = 599

Sum of ranks in normal control group = 859

$$H = \frac{12}{60(60+1)}\left(\frac{372^2}{20} + \frac{599^2}{20} + \frac{859^2}{20}\right) - 3(60+1) = 19.47$$

4 We refer H to Appendix A3: $P < 0.001$.

5 There is substantial evidence to reject the null hypothesis that the distribution of PFS scores is the same in the three groups. Pairwise comparisons were carried out using Wilcoxon rank sum tests, adjusting the P-values for the number of tests performed using the Bonferroni correction (Chapter 18). The individuals with severe and mild/moderate haemophilia both had significantly lower PFS scores than the controls ($P = 0.0003$ and $P = 0.03$, respectively) but the distributions of the scores in the haemophilia groups were not significantly different from each other ($P = 0.09$).

Data kindly provided by Dr A. Miners, Department of Primary Care and Population Sciences, Royal Free and University College Medical School, London, UK, and Dr C. Jenkinson, Health Services Research Unit, University of Oxford, Oxford, UK.

23 Categorical data: a single proportion

The problem

We have a single sample of n individuals; each individual either 'possesses' a characteristic of interest (e.g. is male, is pregnant, has died) or does not possess that characteristic (e.g. is female, is not pregnant, is still alive). A useful summary of the data is provided by the **proportion** of individuals with the characteristic. We are interested in determining whether the true proportion in the population of interest takes a particular value.

The test of a single proportion

Assumptions

Our sample of individuals is selected from the population of interest. Each individual either has or does not have the particular characteristic.

Notation

r individuals in our sample of size n have the characteristic. The estimated proportion with the characteristic is $p = r/n$. The proportion of individuals with the characteristic in the population is π. We are interested in determining whether π takes a particular value, π_1.

Rationale

The number of individuals with the characteristic follows the Binomial distribution (Chapter 8), but this can be approximated by the Normal distribution, providing np and $n(1-p)$ are each greater than 5.

Then p is approximately Normally distributed with:

$$\text{an estimated mean} = p \text{ and}$$

$$\text{an estimated standard deviation} = \sqrt{\frac{p(1-p)}{n}}$$

Therefore, our test statistic, which is based on p, also follows the Normal distribution.

1 Define the null and alternative hypotheses under study

H_0: the population proportion, π, is equal to a particular value, π_1

H_1: the population proportion, π, is not equal to π_1.

2 Collect relevant data from a sample of individuals

3 Calculate the value of the test statistic specific to H_0

$$z = \frac{|p - \pi_1| - \frac{1}{2n}}{\sqrt{\frac{\pi_1(1-\pi_1)}{n}}}$$

which follows a Normal distribution.

The $1/2n$ in the numerator is a **continuity correction**: it is included to make an allowance for the fact that we are approximating the discrete Binomial distribution by the continuous Normal distribution.

4 Compare the value of the test statistic to values from a known probability distribution

Refer z to Appendix A1.

5 Interpret the P-value and results

Interpret the P-value and calculate a confidence interval for the true population proportion, π. The 95% confidence interval for π is approximated by

$$p \pm 1.96\sqrt{\frac{p(1-p)}{n}}$$

We can use this confidence interval to assess the clinical or biological importance of the results. A wide confidence interval is an indication that our estimate has poor precision.

Medical Statistics at a Glance, Fourth Edition. Aviva Petrie and Caroline Sabin. © 2020 Aviva Petrie and Caroline Sabin. Published 2020 by John Wiley & Sons Ltd.
Companion Website: www.medstatsaag.com

The sign test applied to a proportion

Rationale

The sign test (Chapter 19) may be used if the response of interest can be expressed as a **preference** (e.g. in a cross-over trial, patients may have a preference for either treatment A or treatment B). If there is no preference overall, then we would expect the proportion preferring A, say, to equal ½. We use the sign test to assess whether this is so.

Although this formulation of the problem and its test statistic appear to be different from those of Chapter 19, both approaches to the sign test produce the same result.

---

1 Define the null and alternative hypotheses under study

H_0: the proportion, π, of preferences for A in the population is equal to ½

H_1: the proportion of preferences for A in the population is not equal to ½.

2 Collect relevant data from a sample of individuals

3 Calculate the value of the test statistic specific to H_0

Ignore any individuals who have no preference and reduce the sample size from n to n' accordingly. Then $p = r/n'$, where r is the number of preferences for A.

- If $n' \leq 10$, count r, the number of preferences for A
- If $n' > 10$, calculate the test statistic

$$z' = \frac{\left| p - \frac{1}{2} \right| - \frac{1}{2n'}}{\sqrt{\frac{0.5(1-0.5)}{n'}}}$$

z' follows the Normal distribution. Note that this formula is based on the test statistic, z, used in the previous box to test the null hypothesis that the population proportion equals π_1; here we replace n by n', and π_1 by ½.

4 Compare the value of the test statistic to values from a known probability distribution

- If $n' \leq 10$, refer r to Appendix A6
- If $n' > 10$, refer z' to Appendix A1.

5 Interpret the P-value and results

Interpret the P-value and calculate a confidence interval for the proportion of preferences for A (sample size = n) or for the proportion of preferences for A in those with a preference (sample size = n').

Example 1

Human herpesvirus 8 (HHV-8) has been linked to Kaposi's sarcoma, primary effusion lymphoma and certain types of multicentric Castleman's disease. It has been suggested that HHV-8 can be transmitted sexually. In order to assess the relationship between sexual behaviour and HHV-8 infection, the prevalence of antibodies to HHV-8 was determined in a group of 271 homosexual/bisexual men attending a London sexually transmitted disease clinic. In the blood donor population in the UK, the seroprevalence of HHV-8 has been documented to be 2.7%. Initially, the seroprevalence from this study was compared to 2.7% using a **single proportion** test.

---

1 H_0: the seroprevalence of HHV-8 in the population of homosexual/bisexual men equals 2.7%

H_1: the seroprevalence of HHV-8 in the population of homosexual/bisexual men does not equal 2.7%.

2 Sample size, $n = 271$; number who are seropositive to HHV-8, $r = 50$

Seroprevalence, $p = 50/271 = 0.185$ (i.e. 18.5%)

3 Test statistic is $z = \dfrac{|0.185 - 0.027| - \dfrac{1}{2 \times 271}}{\sqrt{\dfrac{0.027(1-0.027)}{271}}} = 15.86$

4 We refer z to Appendix A1: $P < 0.0001$.

5 There is substantial evidence that the seroprevalence of HHV-8 in homosexual/bisexual men attending sexually transmitted disease clinics in the UK is higher than that in the blood donor population. The 95% confidence interval for the seroprevalence of HHV-8 in the population of homosexual/bisexual men is 13.9% to 23.1%, calculated as

$$\left\{ 0.185 \pm 1.96 \times \sqrt{\frac{0.185 \times (1-0.185)}{271}} \right\} \times 100\%$$

Data kindly provided by Dr N.A. Smith, Dr D. Barlow and Dr B.S. Peters, Department of Genitourinary Medicine, Guy's and St Thomas' NHS Trust, London, and Dr J. Best, Department of Virology, Guy's, King's College and St Thomas' School of Medicine, King's College, London, UK.

Example 2

A randomized controlled, double-blind, cross-over trial was undertaken to assess treatment preference for pazopanib versus sunitinib in patients with metastatic renal cell carcinoma (RCC). A group of 169 patients with RCC, aged over 18 years and with no prior systemic therapy for their RCC, were randomly assigned to receive either pazopanib during period 1 followed by sunitinib in period 2 or the reverse. Each treatment period was 10 weeks and the two treatments were separated by a 2-week washout. Patient preference was assessed by questionnaire at the end of the two treatment periods. Of the 169 randomly assigned patients, 114 met the pre-specified intention-to-treat criteria for the analysis: exposure to both treatments, no disease progression before cross-over and completion of the preference questionnaire.

1 H_0: the proportion preferring pazopanib in the population equals 0.5

H_1: the proportion preferring pazopanib in the population does not equal 0.5

2 Of the 114 patients, 105 expressed a preference: 80 preferred pazopanib and 25 preferred sunitinib. Of those with a preference, the proportion preferring pazopanib, $p = 80/105 = 0.762$.

3 Test statistic is $z' = \dfrac{|0.762 - 0.5| - \dfrac{1}{2 \times 105}}{\sqrt{\dfrac{0.5(1 - 0.5)}{105}}} = 5.27$

4 We refer z' to Appendix A1: $P < 0.001$.

5 There is strong evidence to reject the null hypothesis that there is no preference for pazopanib in the population. The 95% confidence interval for the true proportion with a preference is estimated as 0.68 to 0.84, i.e. it is

$$0.762 \pm 1.96 \times \sqrt{\frac{0.762 \times (1 - 0.762)}{105}}$$

Therefore, at the very least, over two-thirds of the patients in the population with a preference prefer pazopanib to sunitinib.

Escudier, B., Porta, C., Bono, P., *et al.* (2014) Randomized, controlled, double-blind, cross-over trial assessing treatment preference for pazopanib versus sunitinib in patients with metastatic renal cell carcinoma: PISCES study. *Journal of Clinical Oncology*, **22(14)**, 1412–1421.

24 Categorical data: two proportions

The problems

- We have two independent groups of individuals (e.g. homosexual men with and without a history of gonorrhoea). We want to know whether the proportions of individuals with a characteristic (e.g. infected with human herpesvirus 8, HHV-8) are the same in the two groups.
- We have two related groups, e.g. individuals may be matched, or measured twice in different circumstances (say, before and after treatment). We want to know whether the proportions with a characteristic (e.g. raised test result) are the same in the two groups.

Independent groups: the Chi-squared test

Terminology

The data are obtained, initially, as **frequencies**, i.e. the numbers with and without the characteristic in each sample. A table in which the entries are frequencies is called a **contingency table**; when this table has two rows and two columns it is called a **2 × 2 table**. Table 24.1 shows the **observed** frequencies in the four cells corresponding to each row/column combination, the four **marginal totals** (the frequency in a specific row or column, e.g. $a + b$), and the **overall total**, n. We can calculate

(see 'Rationale' below) the frequency that we would expect in each of the four cells of the table if H_0 were true (the **expected frequencies**).

Table 24.1 Observed frequencies.

Characteristic	Group 1	Group 2	Total
Present	a	b	$a + b$
Absent	c	d	$c + d$
Total	$n_1 = a + c$	$n_2 = b + d$	$n = a + b + c + d$
Proportion with characteristic	$p_1 = \dfrac{a}{n_1}$	$p_2 = \dfrac{b}{n_2}$	$p = \dfrac{a + b}{n}$

Assumptions

We have samples of sizes n_1 and n_2 from two independent groups of individuals. We are interested in whether the proportions of individuals who possess the characteristic are the same in the two groups. Each individual is represented only once in the study. The rows (and columns) of the table are **mutually exclusive**, implying that each individual can belong in only one row and only one column. The usual, albeit conservative, approach requires that the expected frequency in each of the four cells is at least five.

Rationale

If the proportions with the characteristic in the two groups are equal, we can estimate the overall proportion of individuals with the characteristic by $p = (a + b)/n$; we **expect** $n_1 \times p$ of them to be in Group 1 and $n_2 \times p$ to be in Group 2. We evaluate expected numbers without the characteristic similarly. Therefore, *each expected frequency is the product of the two relevant marginal totals divided by the overall total*. A large discrepancy between the observed (O) and the corresponding expected (E) frequencies is an indication that the proportions in the two groups differ. The test statistic is based on this discrepancy.

---

1 Define the null and alternative hypotheses under study

H_0: the proportions of individuals with the characteristic are equal in the two groups in the population

H_1: these population proportions are not equal.

2 Collect relevant data from samples of individuals

---

continued

3 Calculate the value of the test statistic specific to H_0

$$\chi^2 = \sum \frac{\left(|O-E|-\frac{1}{2}\right)^2}{E}$$

where O and E are the observed and expected frequencies, respectively, in each of the four cells of the table. The vertical lines around $O-E$ indicate that we ignore its sign. The ½ in the numerator is the continuity correction (Chapter 19). The test statistic follows the Chi-squared distribution with 1 degree of freedom.

4 Compare the value of the test statistic to values from a known probability distribution

Refer χ^2 to Appendix A3.

5 Interpret the *P*-value and results

Interpret the *P*-value and calculate the confidence interval for the difference in the true population proportions. The 95% confidence interval is approximated by

$$(p_1 - p_2) \pm 1.96 \sqrt{\frac{p_1(1-p_1)}{n_1} + \frac{p_2(1-p_2)}{n_2}}$$

If the assumptions are not satisfied

If $E < 5$ in any one cell, we use **Fisher's exact test** to obtain a *P*-value that does not rely on the approximation to the Chi-squared distribution. This is best left to a computer program as the calculations are tedious to perform by hand.

Combining 2×2 tables

We should never combine contingency tables from separate studies (e.g. from different subgroups of the population, such as males/females, or from different populations, such as from the UK and USA) simply by adding the frequencies in the analogous cells of the two or more tables. If we were to do so and perform a Chi-squared test on the pooled data, this might lead to **Simpson's (reverse) paradox** when the direction of an association is reversed if data from subgroups are combined into a

Table 24.2 Observed frequencies of pairs in which the characteristic is present or absent.

	Circumstance 1		
Circumstance 2	Present	Absent	Total no. of pairs
Present	w	x	$w+x$
Absent	y	z	$y+z$
Total	$w+y$	$x+z$	$m = w+x+y+z$

single group. For example, from the analysis of two 2×2 tables, we may find that untreated males and untreated females each have a *lower* recovery rate than their treated counterparts, but when we analyse the combined 2×2 table for the whole group, there is a *higher* recovery rate for untreated patients compared with those on treatment. This paradox generally occurs because of an inappropriate weighting of the different subgroups when the data are pooled. There are a number of correct approaches to an analysis of such data, e.g. the Mantel–Haenszel procedure[1], logistic regression (Chapter 30) and meta-analysis (Chapter 43).

Related groups: McNemar's test

Assumptions

The two groups are related or dependent, e.g. each individual may be measured in two different circumstances. Every individual is classified according to whether the characteristic is present in both circumstances, one circumstance only, or in neither (Table 24.2).

Rationale

The observed proportions with the characteristic in the two circumstances are $(w+y)/m$ and $(w+x)/m$. They will differ if x and y differ. Therefore, to compare the proportions with the characteristic, we ignore those individuals who agree in the two circumstances, and concentrate on the discordant pairs, x and y.

1 Define the null and alternative hypotheses under study

H_0: the proportions with the characteristic are equal in the two groups in the population

H_1: these population proportions are not equal.

2 Collect relevant data from two samples

3 Calculate the value of the test statistic specific to H_0

$$\chi^2 = \frac{(|x-y|-1)^2}{x+y}$$

which follows the Chi-squared distribution with 1 degree of freedom. The 1 in the numerator is a continuity correction (Chapter 19).

4 Compare the value of the test statistic to values from a known probability distribution

Refer χ^2 to Appendix A3.

5 Interpret the *P*-value and results

Interpret the *P*-value and calculate the confidence interval for the difference in the true population proportions. The approximate 95% confidence interval is

$$\frac{x-y}{m} \pm \frac{1.96}{m} \sqrt{x+y-\frac{(x-y)^2}{m}}$$

Reference

1 Fleiss, J.L., Levin, B. and Paik, M.C. (2003) *Statistical Methods for Rates and Proportions*. 3rd edition. New York: John Wiley & Sons.

Example 1

In order to assess the relationship between sexual risk factors and HHV-8 infection (study described in Chapter 23), the prevalence of seropositivity to HHV-8 was compared in homosexual/bisexual men who had a previous history of gonorrhoea and in those who had not previously had gonorrhoea, using the **Chi-squared test**. A typical computer output is shown in Appendix C.

1 H_0: the seroprevalence of HHV-8 is the same in those with and without a history of gonorrhoea in the population

H_1: the seroprevalence is not the same in the two groups in the population.

2 The observed frequencies are shown in the following contingency table: 14/43 (32.6%) and 36/228 (15.8%) of those with and without a previous history of gonorrhoea are seropositive for HHV-8, respectively.

3 The expected frequencies are shown in the four cells of the contingency table.

The test statistic is

$$\chi^2 = \left\{ \frac{(|14-7.93|-\frac{1}{2})^2}{7.93} + \frac{(|36-42.07|-\frac{1}{2})^2}{42.07} + \frac{(|29-35.07|-\frac{1}{2})^2}{35.07} + \frac{(|192-185.93|-\frac{1}{2})^2}{185.93} \right\} = 5.70$$

4 We refer χ^2 to Appendix A3 with 1 degree of freedom: $0.01 < P < 0.05$ (computer output gives $P=0.017$).

5 There is evidence of a real difference in the seroprevalence in the two groups in the population. We estimate this difference as $32.6\% - 15.8\% = 16.8\%$. The 95% confidence interval for the true difference in the two percentages is 2.0% to 31.6%, i.e. $16.8 \pm 1.96 \times \sqrt{(32.6 \times 67.4)/43 + (15.8 \times 84.2)/228}$.

HHV-8	Previous history of gonorrhoea					Total observed
	Yes		No			
	Observed	Expected	Observed	Expected		
Seropositive	14	$(43 \times 50/271) = 7.93$	36	$(228 \times 50/271) = 42.07$		50
Seronegative	29	$(43 \times 221/271) = 35.07$	192	$(228 \times 221/271) = 185.93$		221
Total	43		228			271

Example 2

In order to evaluate emergency department (ED) patients' willingness to disclose substance use via either a computer kiosk or an in-person interview, Hankin *et al* conducted a cross-sectional study of 154 patients who attended an ED in Georgia, USA. Participants were asked about drug use using the Drug and Alcohol Screening Test (DAST-10) survey; reported drug use was classified as high risk in those scoring ≥ 3 on this survey. Participants undertook the survey firstly using a kiosk computer in the ED, and secondly as part of a face-to-face survey with a researcher in a private section of the ED or a private room. **McNemar's test** was used to compare the percentages of participants deemed at high risk using each of the two modalities.

1 H_0: the two modalities of assessment identify the same percentage of ED attendees exhibiting high-risk drug use in the population

H_1: these percentages are not equal.

2 The frequencies for the matched pairs are displayed in the table:

Face-to-face interview	Kiosk		Total
	High risk	Low risk	
High risk	5	3	8
Low risk	12	134	146
Total	17	137	154

3 Test statistic, $\chi^2 = \dfrac{(|12-3|-1)^2}{12+3} = 4.27$

4 We refer χ^2 to Appendix A3 with 1 degree of freedom: $0.001 < P < 0.01$ (computer output gives $P=0.009$).

5 There is evidence to reject the null hypothesis that the same percentage of ED attendees are detected as reporting high-risk drug use using the two modalities of assessment. The face-to-face interview has a tendency to fail to detect high-risk drug use. We estimate the difference in percentages of ED attendees detected as having high-risk drug use as $11.0\% - 5.2\% = 5.8\%$. An approximate confidence interval for the true difference in the percentages is given by 1.0% to 10.7%,

i.e. $\left\{ \dfrac{|12-3|}{154} \pm \dfrac{1.96}{154} \times \sqrt{(12+3) - \dfrac{(12-3)^2}{154}} \right\} \times 100\%$

Adapted from Hankin, A., Haley, L., Baugher, A., Colbert, K. and Houry, D. (2015) Kiosk versus in-person screening for alcohol and drug use in emergency department: patient preferences and disclosure. *Western Journal of Emergency Medicine*, **XVI**, 220–228.

25 Categorical data: more than two categories

Chi-squared test: large contingency tables

The problem

Individuals can be classified by two factors. For example, one factor may represent disease severity (mild, moderate, severe) and the other factor may represent blood group (A, B, O, AB). We are interested in whether the two factors are associated. Are individuals of a particular blood group likely to be more severely ill?

Assumptions

The data may be presented in an $r \times c$ contingency table with r rows and c columns (Table 25.1). The entries in the table are **frequencies**; each cell contains the number of individuals in a particular row and a particular column. Every individual is represented once, and can only belong in one row and in one column, i.e. the categories of each factor are mutually exclusive. At least 80% of the expected frequencies are greater than or equal to 5.

Rationale

The null hypothesis is that there is no association between the two factors. Note that if there are only two rows and two columns, then this test of no association is the same as that of two proportions (Chapter 24). We calculate the frequency that we expect in each cell of the contingency table if the null hypothesis is true. As explained in Chapter 24, the expected frequency in a particular cell is the product of the relevant row total and relevant column total, divided by the overall total. We calculate a test statistic that focuses on the discrepancy between the observed and expected frequencies in every cell of the table. If the overall discrepancy is large, then it is unlikely the null hypothesis is true.

1 Define the null and alternative hypotheses under study

H_0: there is no association between the categories of one factor and the categories of the other factor in the population

H_1: the two factors are associated in the population.

2 Collect relevant data from a sample of individuals

3 Calculate the value of the test statistic specific to H_0

$$\chi^2 = \sum \frac{(O - E)^2}{E}$$

where O and E are the observed and expected frequencies in each cell of the table. The test statistic follows the Chi-squared distribution with degrees of freedom equal to $(r-1) \times (c-1)$.

Because the approximation to the Chi-squared distribution is reasonable if the degrees of freedom are greater than 1, we do not need to include a continuity correction (as we did in Chapter 24).

4 Compare the value of the test statistic to values from a known probability distribution
Refer χ^2 to Appendix A3.

5 Interpret the P-value and results

If the assumptions are not satisfied

If more than 20% of the expected frequencies are less than 5, we try to combine, appropriately (i.e. so that it makes scientific sense), two or more rows and/or two or more columns of the contingency table. We then recalculate the expected frequencies of this reduced table, and carry on reducing the table, if necessary, to ensure that the $E \geq 5$ condition is satisfied. If we have reduced our table to a 2×2 table so that it can be reduced no further and we still have small expected frequencies, we use Fisher's exact test (Chapter 24) to evaluate the exact P-value. Some computer packages will compute the Fisher–Freeman–Halton exact P-values for larger contingency tables.

Chi-squared test for trend

The problem

Sometimes we investigate relationships in categorical data when one of the two factors has only two categories (e.g. the presence or absence of a characteristic) and the second factor can be categorized into k, say, mutually exclusive categories that are ordered in some sense. For example, one factor might be whether or not an individual responds to treatment, and the ordered categories of the other factor may represent four different age (in years) categories 65–69, 70–74, 75–79 and ≥ 80. We can then assess whether there is a trend in the proportions with the characteristic over the categories of the second factor. For example, we may wish to know whether the proportion responding to treatment tends to increase (say) with increasing age.

Note that we may obtain a significant result from this test even when a general test of association gives a non-significant result.

continued

Medical Statistics at a Glance, Fourth Edition. Aviva Petrie and Caroline Sabin. © 2020 Aviva Petrie and Caroline Sabin. Published 2020 by John Wiley & Sons Ltd.
Companion Website: www.medstatsaag.com

Table 25.1 Observed frequencies in an $r \times c$ table.

Row categories	Col 1	Col 2	Col 3	...	Col c	Total
Row 1	f_{11}	f_{12}	f_{13}	...	f_{1c}	R_1
Row 2	f_{21}	f_{22}	f_{23}	...	f_{2c}	R_2
Row 3	f_{31}	f_{32}	f_{33}	...	f_{3c}	R_3
...	...	...	...	...	...	...
Row r	f_{r1}	f_{r2}	f_{r3}	...	f_{rc}	R_r
Total	C_1	C_2	C_3	...	C_c	n

Table 25.2 Observed frequencies and assigned scores in a $2 \times k$ table.

Characteristic	Col 1	Col 2	Col 3	...	Col k	Total
Present	f_{11}	f_{12}	f_{13}	...	f_{1k}	R_1
Absent	f_{21}	f_{22}	f_{23}	...	f_{2k}	R_2
Total	C_1	C_2	C_3	...	C_k	n
Score	w_1	w_2	w_3	...	w_k	

1 Define the null and alternative hypotheses under study

H_0: there is no trend in the proportions with the characteristic in the population

H_1: there is a trend in the proportions in the population.

2 Collect relevant data from a sample of individuals

We estimate the proportion with the characteristic in each of the k categories. We assign a score to each of the column categories (Table 25.2). Typically, these are the successive values, 1, 2, 3, ..., k, but, depending on how we have classified the column factor, they could be numbers that in some way suggest the relative values of the ordered categories (e.g. the mid-point of the age range defining each category) or the trend we wish to investigate (e.g. linear or quadratic). The use of any equally spaced numbers (e.g. 1, 2, 3, ..., k) allows us to investigate a *linear trend*.

3 Calculate the value of the test statistic specific to H_0

$$\chi^2 = \frac{\left(\sum w_i f_{1i} - R_1 \sum \frac{w_i C_i}{n}\right)^2}{\frac{R_1}{n}\left(1 - \frac{R_1}{n}\right)\left(\sum C_i w_i^2 - n\left(\sum \frac{w_i C_i}{n}\right)^2\right)}$$

using the notation of Table 25.2, and where the sums extend over all the k categories. The test statistic follows the Chi-squared distribution with 1 degree of freedom.

4 Compare the value of the test statistic to values from a known probability distribution

Refer χ^2 to Appendix A3.

5 Interpret the *P*-value and results

Interpret the *P*-value and calculate a confidence interval for each of the k proportions (Chapter 11).

Note: an alternative approach to testing for a linear trend in proportions is to perform a logistic regression analysis (Chapters 30 and 33).

Example

A cross-sectional survey was carried out among schoolchildren aged 13–14 years living in southern Brazil, with the objective of investigating the relationship between body mass index (BMI; equal to the child's weight divided by his/her height^2, kg/m^2) and the prevalence of a number of asthma-related symptoms. A total of 4010 children (1933 males and 2077 females) were grouped into four BMI categories, defined by the percentiles of BMI (underweight (BMI < 5th percentile), normal weight (5th ≤ BMI < 85th), overweight (85th ≤ BMI < 95th) and obese (BMI ≥ 95th)) at the time of interview. We used the **Chi-squared test** to determine whether the prevalence of wheezing after exercise (an asthma-related symptom) differed in the four BMI groups.

1 H_0: there is no association between BMI and wheezing after exercise in the population of 13- and 14-year-old schoolchildren

H_1: there is an association between BMI and wheezing after exercise in the population of 13- and 14-year-old schoolchildren.

2 The observed frequencies (%) and expected frequencies are shown in the following contingency table.

3 Test statistic is

$$\chi^2 = \left[\frac{(23 - 32.0)^2}{32.0} + \dots + \frac{(197 - 208.6)^2}{208.6}\right] = 7.27$$

4 We refer χ^2 to Appendix A3 with 3 degrees of freedom: $0.05 < P < 0.10$ (computer output gives $P = 0.06$).

5 There is insufficient evidence to reject the null hypothesis of no association between BMI and wheezing after exercise in the population of 13- and 14-year-old teenagers. The estimated percentages (95% confidence intervals) with wheezing after exercise for the four successive BMI groups, starting with the underweight, are: 14% (9% to 19%), 19% (18% to 20%), 21% (17% to 25%) and 24% (19% to 29%).

continued

Wheezing after exercise	BMI group				
	Underweight	Normal	Overweight	Obese	Total
Yes					
Observed	23 (13.8%)	598 (18.9%)	86 (20.7%)	61 (23.6%)	768
Expected	32.0	606.9	79.7	49.4	
No					
Observed	144 (86.2%)	2571 (81.1%)	330 (79.3%)	197 (76.4%)	3242
Expected	135.0	2562.1	336.3	208.6	
Total	167	3169	416	258	4010

As the four BMI groups in this study are ordered, it is also possible to analyse these data using a **Chi-squared test for trend**, which takes into account the ordering of the groups.

We assign the scores of 1, 2, 3 and 4 to each of the four BMI groups, respectively, and test for a linear trend.

1 H_0: there is no linear association between BMI and wheezing after exercise in the 13- and 14-year-old population

  H_1: there is a linear association between BMI and wheezing after exercise in the 13- and 14-year-old population.

2 The data are displayed in the previous table. We assign scores of 1, 2, 3 and 4 to the four successive BMI groups.

3 Test statistic is χ^2.

4 We refer χ^2 to Appendix A3 with 1 degree of freedom: $0.01 < P < 0.05$ (computer output gives $P = 0.011$).

5 In contrast to the previous analysis that does not take ordering into account, when BMI is considered as an ordinal variable there is evidence to reject the null hypothesis of no linear association between BMI and wheezing after exercise in the percentage of 13- and 14-year-old schoolchildren. We can therefore infer that the percentages of 13- and 14-year-old schoolchildren with wheezing after exercise in southern Brazil increases significantly with increasing BMI. The estimated percentages (95% confidence interval) are 13.8% (8.6% to 19.0%), 18.9% (17.5% to 20.3%), 20.7% (16.8% to 24.6%) and 23.6% (18.4% to 28.8%) in the underweight, normal, overweight and obese schoolchildren, respectively.

$$\chi^2 = \frac{\left\{ [(1 \times 23) + \ldots + (4 \times 61)] - 768 \times \left[\left(\frac{1 \times 167}{4010} \right) + \ldots + \left(\frac{4 \times 258}{4010} \right) \right] \right\}^2}{\frac{768}{4010} \left(1 - \frac{768}{4010} \right) \times \left\{ [(167 \times 1^2) + \ldots + (258 \times 4^2)] - 4010 \times \left[\left(\frac{1 \times 167}{4010} \right) + \ldots + \left(\frac{4 \times 258}{4010} \right) \right]^2 \right\}} = 6.51$$

Adapted from Cassol, V., Rizzato, T., Teche, S.P., *et al.* (2005) [Prevalence and severity of asthma among adolescents and their relationship with the body mass index]. *Jornal de Pediatria (Rio J)*, **81**, 305–309.

26 Correlation

Correlation analysis is concerned with measuring the degree of association between two variables, x and y. Initially, we assume that both x and y are **numerical**, e.g. height and weight.

Suppose we have a pair of values, (x, y), measured on each of the n individuals in our sample. We can mark the point corresponding to each individual's pair of values on a two-dimensional **scatter diagram** (Chapter 4). Conventionally, we put the x variable on the horizontal axis, and the y variable on the vertical axis in this diagram. By plotting the points for all n individuals, we obtain a scatter of points that may suggest a relationship between the two variables.

Pearson correlation coefficient

We say that we have a **linear relationship** between x and y if a straight line drawn through the midst of the points provides the most appropriate approximation to the observed relationship. We measure how close the observations are to the straight line that best describes their linear relationship by calculating the **Pearson product moment correlation coefficient**, usually simply called the **correlation coefficient**. Its true value in the *population*, ρ (the Greek letter rho), is estimated in the *sample* by r, where

$$r = \frac{\sum(x - \bar{x})(x - \bar{y})}{\sqrt{\sum(x - \bar{x})^2 \sum(x - \bar{y})^2}}$$

which is usually obtained from computer output.

Properties

- r ranges from -1 to $+1$.
- Its **sign** indicates whether, in general, one variable increases as the other variable increases (positive r) or whether one variable decreases as the other increases (negative r) (Fig. 26.1).
- Its **magnitude** indicates how close the points are to the straight line. In particular if $r = +1$ or -1, then there is perfect correlation

with all the points lying on the line (this is most unusual, in practice); if $r = 0$, then there is no **linear** correlation (although there may be a non-linear relationship). The closer r is to the extremes, the greater the degree of linear association (Fig. 26.1).

- It is dimensionless, i.e. it has no units of measurement.
- Its value is valid only within the range of values of x and y in the sample. Its absolute value (ignoring sign) tends to increase as the range of values of x and/or y increases. Therefore, restricting the sample by imposing an upper or lower limit on the range of values of x or y or adding individuals to the sample who have values of x or y that are more extreme than those in the original sample will affect the magnitude of the correlation coefficient; furthermore, correlation coefficients should not be compared in populations which have a different range of values of x or of y.
- x and y can be interchanged without affecting the value of r.
- A correlation between x and y does not necessarily imply a 'cause and effect' relationship.
- r^2 represents the proportion of the variability of y that can be attributed to its linear relationship with x (Chapter 28).

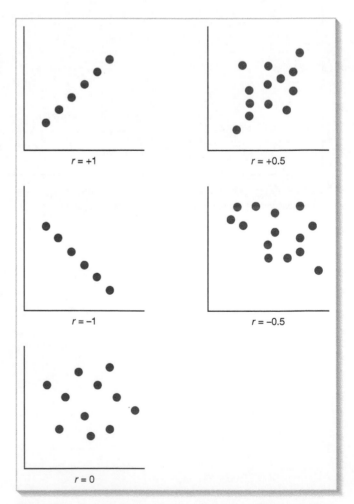

Figure 26.1 Five diagrams indicating values of r in different situations.

Medical Statistics at a Glance, Fourth Edition. Aviva Petrie and Caroline Sabin. © 2020 Aviva Petrie and Caroline Sabin. Published 2020 by John Wiley & Sons Ltd.
Companion Website: www.medstatsaag.com

When not to calculate r

It may be misleading to calculate r when:
- there is a non-linear relationship between the two variables (Fig. 26.2a), e.g. a quadratic relationship (Chapter 33);
- the data include more than one observation on each individual;
- one or more outliers are present (Fig. 26.2b);
- the data comprise subgroups of individuals for which the mean levels of the observations on at least one of the variables are different (Fig. 26.2c).

Hypothesis test for the Pearson correlation coefficient

We want to know whether there is any linear correlation between two numerical variables. Our sample consists of n independent pairs of values of x and y. We assume that at least one of the two variables is Normally distributed.

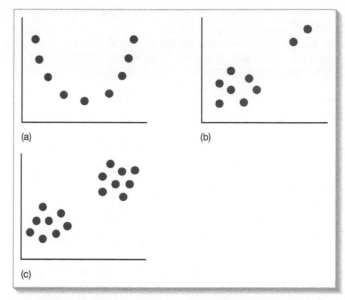

Figure 26.2 Diagrams showing when it is inappropriate to calculate the correlation coefficient. (a) Relationship not linear, $r = 0$. (b) In the presence of outlier(s). (c) Data comprise subgroups.

---

1 Define the null and alternative hypotheses under study

H_0: $\rho = 0$

H_1: $\rho \neq 0$.

2 Collect relevant data from a sample of individuals

3 Calculate the value of the test statistic specific to H_0

Calculate r.
- If $n \leq 150$, r is the test statistic
- If $n > 150$, calculate $T = r\sqrt{\dfrac{(n-2)}{(1-r^2)}}$

which follows a t-distribution with $n - 2$ degrees of freedom.

4 Compare the value of the test statistic to values from a known probability distribution
- If $n \leq 150$, refer r to Appendix A10
- If $n > 150$, refer T to Appendix A2.

5 Interpret the P-value and results

Calculate a confidence interval for ρ. *Provided both variables are approximately Normally distributed*, the approximate 95% confidence interval for ρ is

$$\left(\frac{e^{2z_1} - 1}{e^{2z_1} + 1}, \frac{e^{2z_2} - 1}{e^{2z_2} + 1} \right)$$

where $z_1 = z - \dfrac{1.96}{\sqrt{n-3}}$, $z_2 = z + \dfrac{1.96}{\sqrt{n-3}}$

and $z = 0.5\ln\left[\dfrac{(1+r)}{(1-r)}\right]$

Note that, if the sample size is large, H_0 may be rejected even if r is quite close to zero. Alternatively, even if r is large, H_0 may not be rejected if the sample size is small. For this reason, it is particularly helpful to calculate r^2, the proportion of the total variance of one variable explained by its linear relationship with the other. For example, if $r = 0.40$ then $P < 0.05$ for a sample size of 25, but the relationship is only explaining 16% ($= 0.40^2 \times 100$) of the variability of one variable.

Spearman's rank correlation coefficient

We calculate **Spearman's rank correlation coefficient**, a non-parametric equivalent to Pearson's correlation coefficient, if one or more of the following points is true:
- at least one of the variables, x or y, is measured on an ordinal scale;
- neither x nor y is Normally distributed;
- the sample size is small;
- we require a measure of the association between two variables when their relationship is non-linear.

Calculation

To estimate the population value of Spearman's rank correlation coefficient, ρ_s, by its sample value, r_s:

1 Arrange the values of x in increasing order, starting with the smallest value, and assign successive ranks (the numbers 1, 2, 3, …, n) to them. Tied values receive the mean of the ranks these values would have received had there been no ties.

2 Assign ranks to the values of y in a similar manner.

3 r_s is the Pearson correlation coefficient between the *ranks* of x and y.

Properties and hypothesis tests

These are the same as for Pearson's correlation coefficient, replacing r by r_s, except that:
- r_s provides a measure of association (not necessarily linear) between x and y;
- when testing the null hypothesis that $\rho_s = 0$, refer to Appendix A11 if the sample size is less than or equal to 10;
- we do not calculate r_s^2 (it does not represent the proportion of the total variation in one variable that can be attributed to its linear relationship with the other).

Example

As part of a study to investigate the factors associated with changes in blood pressure in children, information was collected on demographic and lifestyle factors, and clinical and anthropometric measures in 4245 children aged from 5 to 7 years. The relationship between height (cm) and systolic blood pressure (SBP, measured in mmHg) in a sample of 100 of these children is shown in the scatter diagram in Fig. 28.1; there is a tendency for taller children in the sample to have higher blood pressures. **Pearson's correlation coefficient** between these two variables was investigated. Appendix C contains a computer output from the analysis and Fig. 37.1 shows histograms of systolic blood pressure and height in this sample of children.

1 H_0: the population value of the Pearson correlation coefficient, ρ, is zero

H_1: the population value of the Pearson correlation coefficient, ρ, is not zero.

2 We can show (Fig. 37.1) that the sample values of both height and SBP are approximately Normally distributed.

3 We calculate r as 0.33. This is the test statistic since $n \le 150$.

4 We refer r to Appendix A10 with a sample size of 100: $P < 0.001$.

5 There is strong evidence to reject the null hypothesis; we conclude that there is a linear relationship between SBP and height in the population of such children. However, $r^2 = 0.33 \times 0.33 = 0.11$. Therefore, despite the highly significant result, the relationship between height and SBP explains only a small percentage, 11%, of the variation in SBP.

In order to determine the 95% confidence interval for the true correlation coefficient, we calculate

$$z = 0.5\ln\left(\frac{1.33}{0.67}\right) = 0.3428$$

$$z_1 = 0.3428 - \frac{1.96}{9.849} = 0.1438$$

$$z_2 = 0.3428 + \frac{1.96}{9.849} = 0.5418$$

Thus the confidence interval ranges from

$$\frac{(e^{2 \times 0.1438} - 1)}{(e^{2 \times 0.1438} + 1)} \text{ to } \frac{(e^{2 \times 0.5418} - 1)}{(e^{2 \times 0.5418} + 1)}, \text{ i.e. from } \frac{0.33}{2.33} \text{ to } \frac{1.96}{3.96}$$

We are thus 95% certain that ρ lies between 0.14 and 0.49.

As we might expect, given that each variable is Normally distributed, **Spearman's rank correlation coefficient** between these variables gave a comparable estimate of 0.32. To test H_0: $\rho_s = 0$, we refer this value to Appendix A10 and again find $P < 0.001$.

Data kindly provided by Ms O. Papacosta and Dr P. Whincup, Department of Primary Care and Population Sciences, Royal Free and University College Medical School, London, UK.

27 The theory of linear regression

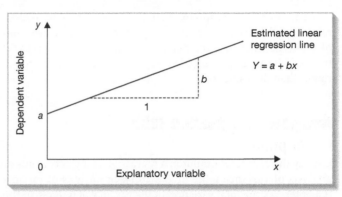

Figure 27.1 Estimated linear regression line showing the intercept, a, and the slope, b (the mean increase in Y for a unit increase in x).

What is linear regression?

To investigate the relationship between two numerical variables, x and y, we measure the values of x and y on each of the n individuals in our sample. We plot the points on a **scatter diagram** (Chapters 4 and 26), and say that we have a **linear** relationship if the data approximate a straight line. If we believe y is dependent on x, with a change in y being attributed to a change in x, rather than the other way round, we can determine the **linear regression line** (the **regression of y on x**) that best describes the straight line relationship between the two variables. In general, we describe the regression as **univariable** because we are concerned with only one x variable in the analysis; this contrasts with *multivariable* regression which involves two or more x's (see Chapters 29–31).

The regression line

The mathematical equation that estimates the **simple linear regression** line is

$$Y = a + bx$$

- x is called the **independent**, **predictor** or **explanatory** variable.
- For a given value of x, Y is the value of y (called the **dependent**, **outcome** or **response** variable) that lies on the estimated line. It is an estimate of the value we *expect* for y (i.e. its mean) if we know the value of x, and is called the **fitted** value of y.
- a is the **intercept** of the estimated line; it is the value of Y when $x = 0$ (Fig. 27.1).
- b is the **slope** or **gradient** of the estimated line; it represents the amount by which Y increases on average if we increase x by one unit (Fig. 27.1).

a and b are called the **regression coefficients** of the estimated line, although this term is often reserved only for b. We show how to evaluate these coefficients in Chapter 28. Simple linear regression can be extended to include more than one explanatory variable; in this case, it is known as **multivariable** or **multiple linear regression** (Chapter 29).

Method of least squares

We perform regression analysis using a sample of observations. a and b are the sample estimates of the true parameters, α and β, which define the linear regression line in the population. a and b are determined by the **method of least squares** (often called ordinary least squares, OLS) in such a way that the 'fit' of the line $Y = a + bx$ to the points in the scatter diagram is optimal. We assess this by considering the **residuals** (the vertical distance of each point from the line, i.e. **residual = observed y – fitted Y** (Fig. 27.2). The **line of best fit** is chosen so that the sum of the *squared* residuals is a *minimum*.

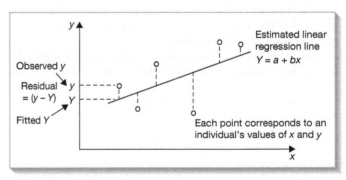

Figure 27.2 Estimated linear regression line showing the residual (vertical dashed line) for each point.

Assumptions

1 There is a linear relationship between x and y.
2 The observations in the sample are independent. The observations are independent if there is no more than one pair of observations on each individual.
3 For each value of x, there is a distribution of values of y in the population; this distribution is Normal. The mean of this distribution of y values lies on the true regression line (Fig. 27.3).

4 The variability of the distribution of the y values in the population is the same for all values of x, i.e. the variance, σ^2, is constant (Fig. 27.3).

5 The x variable can be measured without error. Note that we do not make any assumptions about the distribution of the x variable.

Many of the assumptions that underlie regression analysis relate to the distribution of the y population for a specified value of x, but they may be framed in terms of the residuals. It is easier to check the assumptions (Chapter 28) by studying the residuals rather than the values of y.

Analysis of variance table

Description

Usually the computer output in a regression analysis contains an **analysis of variance table** (Table 28.1). In analysis of variance (Chapter 22), the total variation of the variable of interest, in this case 'y', is partitioned into its two component parts. Because of the linear relationship of y on x, we expect y to vary as x varies; we call this the variation that is **due to** or **explained by the regression** (sometimes called simply the **model** or **regression** variation). The remaining variability is called the **residual error** or **unexplained** variation (sometimes called simply the **residual** or **error** variation). The residual variation should be as small as possible; if so, most of the variation in y will be explained by the regression, and the points will lie close to or on the line; i.e. the line is a **good fit**.

Purposes

The analysis of variance table enables us to do the following.
1 Assess how well the line fits the data points. From the information provided in the table, we can calculate the proportion of the total variation in y that is explained by the regression. This proportion, usually expressed as a percentage and denoted by R^2 (in simple linear regression it is r^2, the square of the correlation coefficient; Chapter 26), allows us to assess subjectively the **goodness of fit** of the regression equation.
2 Test the **null hypothesis** that the true slope of the line, β, is zero; a significant result indicates that there is evidence of a linear relationship between x and y.
3 Obtain an estimate of the **residual variance**. We need this for testing hypotheses about the slope or the intercept, and for

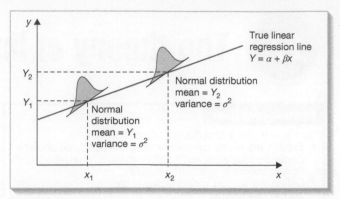

Figure 27.3 Illustration of assumptions made in linear regression.

calculating confidence intervals for these parameters and for predicted values of y.

We provide details of the more common procedures in Chapter 28, both in the main body of the text and in the Example.

Regression to the mean

The statistical use of the word 'regression' derives from a phenomenon known as **regression to the mean**, attributed to Sir Francis Galton in 1889. He demonstrated that although tall fathers tend to have tall sons, the average height of the sons is less than that of their tall fathers. The average height of the sons has 'regressed' or 'gone back' towards the mean height of all the fathers in the population. So, on average, tall fathers have shorter (but still tall) sons and short fathers have taller (but still short) sons.

We observe regression to the mean in **screening** (Chapter 38) and in **clinical trials** (Chapter 14), when a subgroup of patients may be selected for treatment because their levels of a certain variable, say cholesterol, are extremely high (or low). If the measurement is repeated some time later, the average value for the second reading for the subgroup is usually less than that of the first reading, tending towards (i.e. regressing to) the average of the age- and sex-matched population, irrespective of any treatment they may have received. Patients recruited into a clinical trial on the basis of a high cholesterol level on their first examination are thus likely to show a drop in cholesterol levels on average at their second examination, even if they remain untreated during this period.

28 Performing a linear regression analysis

The linear regression line

After selecting a sample of size n from our population and drawing a **scatter diagram** to confirm that the data approximate a straight line, we estimate the **regression of y on x** as

$$Y = a + bx$$

where Y is the estimated fitted or predicted value of y, a is the estimated intercept and b is the estimated slope that represents the mean change in Y for a unit change in x (Chapter 27).

Drawing the line

To draw the line $Y = a + bx$ on the scatter diagram, we choose three values of x (i.e. x_1, x_2 and x_3) along its range. We substitute x_1 in the equation to obtain the corresponding value of Y, namely $Y_1 = a + bx_1$; Y_1 is our estimated **fitted** value for x_1 which corresponds to the **observed** value, y_1. We repeat the procedure for x_2 and x_3 to obtain the corresponding values of Y_2 and Y_3. We plot these points on the scatter diagram and join them to produce a straight line.

Checking the assumptions

For each observed value of x, the **residual** is the observed y minus the corresponding fitted Y. Each residual may be either positive or negative. We can use the residuals to check the following assumptions underlying linear regression.

1 There is a linear relationship between x and y – *either* plot y against x (the data should approximate a straight line) *or* plot the residuals against x (we should observe a random scatter of points rather than any systematic pattern).

2 The observations are independent – the observations are independent if there is no more than one pair of observations on each individual.

3 The residuals are Normally distributed with a mean of zero – draw a histogram, stem-and-leaf plot, box-and-whisker plot (Chapter 4) or Normal plot (Chapter 35) of the residuals and 'eyeball' the result.

4 The residuals have the same variability (constant variance) for all the fitted values of y – plot the residuals against the fitted values, Y, of y; we should observe a random scatter of points. If the scatter of residuals progressively increases or decreases as Y increases, then this assumption is not satisfied.

5 The x variable can be measured without error.

Failure to satisfy the assumptions

If the linearity, Normality and/or constant variance assumptions are in doubt, we may be able to transform x or y (Chapter 9) and calculate a new regression line for which these assumptions are satisfied. It is not always possible to find a satisfactory transformation. The linearity and independence assumptions are the most important. If you are dubious about the Normality and/or constant variance assumptions, you may proceed, but the P-values in your hypothesis tests, and the estimates of the standard errors, may be affected. Note that the x variable is rarely measured without any error; provided the error is small, this is usually acceptable because the effect on the conclusions is minimal.

Outliers and influential points

- An **influential** observation will, if omitted, alter one or both of the parameter estimates (i.e. the slope and/or the intercept) in the model. Formal methods of detection are discussed briefly in Chapter 29. If these methods are not available, you may have to rely on intuition.
- An **outlier** (an observation that is inconsistent with most of the values in the data set (Chapter 3)) may or may not be an influential point, and can often be detected by looking at the scatter diagram or the residual plots (see also Chapter 29).

For both outliers and influential points, we fit the model with and without the suspect individual's data and note the effect on the estimate(s). Do not discard outliers or influential points routinely because their omission may affect the conclusions. Always investigate the reasons for their presence and report them.

Assessing goodness of fit

We can judge how well the line fits the data by calculating R^2 (usually expressed as a percentage), which is equal to the square of the correlation coefficient (Chapters 26 and 27). This represents the percentage of the variability of y that can be **explained** by its relationship with x. Its complement, $(100 - R^2)$, represents the percentage of the variation in y that is **unexplained** by the relationship. There is no formal test to assess R^2; we have to rely on subjective judgement to evaluate the fit of the regression line.

Medical Statistics at a Glance, Fourth Edition. Aviva Petrie and Caroline Sabin. © 2020 Aviva Petrie and Caroline Sabin. Published 2020 by John Wiley & Sons Ltd.
Companion Website: www.medstatsaag.com

Investigating the slope

If the slope of the line is zero, there is no linear relationship between x and y: changing x has no effect on y. There are two approaches, with identical results, to **testing the null hypothesis that the true slope, β, is zero**.

- *Examine the F-ratio* (equal to the ratio of the 'explained' to the 'unexplained' mean squares) in the analysis of variance table. It follows the F-distribution and has $(1, n-2)$ degrees of freedom in the numerator and denominator, respectively.

- *Calculate the test statistic* $= \dfrac{b}{SE(b)}$ which follows the t-distribution on $n-2$ degrees of freedom, where $SE(b)$ is the standard error of b.

In either case, a significant result, usually if $P < 0.05$, leads to rejection of the null hypothesis.

We calculate the **95% confidence interval** for β as $b \pm t_{0.05} \times SE(b)$, where $t_{0.05}$ is the percentage point of the t-distribution with $n-2$ degrees of freedom which gives a two-tailed probability of 0.05. This interval contains the true slope with 95% certainty. For large samples, say $n \geq 100$, we can approximate $t_{0.05}$ by 1.96.

Regression analysis is rarely performed by hand; computer output from most statistical packages will provide all of this information.

Using the line for prediction

We can use the regression line for predicting values of y for specific values of x within the observed range (never extrapolate beyond these limits). We predict the mean value of y for individuals who have a certain value of x by substituting that value of x into the equation of the line. So, if $x = x_0$, we predict y as $Y_0 = a + bx_0$. We use this estimated predicted value, and its standard error, to evaluate the confidence interval for the true mean value of y in the population. Repeating this procedure for various values of x allows us to construct confidence limits for the line. This is a band or region that contains the true line with, say, 95% certainty. Similarly, we can calculate a wider region within which we expect most (usually 95%) of the *observations* to lie.

Improving the interpretation of the model

In some situations the interpretation of the parameters in a regression model may be improved by **centring** or **scaling** (or **rescaling**) an explanatory variable, i.e. by subtraction of or division by a suitable constant.

- **Centring** – we generally choose to centre an explanatory variable when the intercept of the model does not provide a predicted value of the dependent variable for a meaningful individual (for example, when systolic blood pressure (SBP) in mmHg is regressed on height in cm as in the Example, the intercept represents the mean SBP when the height of a child is zero). We **centre** an explanatory variable by subtracting a fixed number from the value of the explanatory variable for each individual in the sample. This fixed number might be, for example, the lowest value of the explanatory variable observed in the sample; the intercept of the revised model then represents the predicted value of the outcome variable at this lowest value of the explanatory variable. Often, however, we centre by subtracting the sample mean of the explanatory variable from each value; the intercept of a regression model with the explanatory variable centred in this way is equal to the predicted or mean value of the outcome variable when the explanatory variable takes its mean value.

- **Scaling** – we may scale an explanatory variable if the interpretation of the coefficient for that variable does not reflect a clinically meaningful change in the measurement (e.g. if height were measured in mm rather than cm in the example, the regression coefficient would be a very small number representing the average change in SBP for a mm change in height). In this situation, a more meaningful regression coefficient is obtained by **scaling** the explanatory variable by dividing it by a suitable constant (e.g. height/10, so the rescaled variable is now measuring cm).

Note that centring only affects the intercept but does not affect the estimated regression coefficient for the explanatory variable; in contrast, scaling affects the estimated regression coefficient for the explanatory variable but not the intercept. Neither centring nor scaling affects the significance of the regression coefficient or the fit of the model.

Useful formulae for hand calculations

$$\bar{x} = \sum x/n \quad \text{and} \quad \bar{y} = \sum y/n$$

$$a = \bar{y} - b\bar{x}$$

$$b = \frac{\sum (x - \bar{x})(y - \bar{y})}{\sum (x - \bar{x})^2}$$

$$s_{res}^2 = \frac{\sum (y - Y)^2}{(n-2)}, \text{ the estimated residual variance}$$

$$SE(b) = \frac{s_{res}}{\sqrt{\sum (x - \bar{x})^2}}$$

Example

The relationship between height (measured in cm) and systolic blood pressure (SBP, measured in mmHg) in the 100 children described in Chapter 26 is shown in Fig. 28.1. We performed a **simple linear regression analysis** of SBP (the dependent variable) on height (the explanatory variable). Assumptions underlying this analysis are verified in Figs 28.2–28.4. A typical full computer output is shown in Appendix C. There is a significant linear relationship between height and SBP, as can be seen by the significant F-ratio in the analysis of variance table (Table 28.1). The R^2 of the model is 10.9% = 100 × (962.714)/ (8808.306), the sum of squares due to regression expressed as a percentage of the total sum of squares (it is also equal to the square of the correlation coefficient which is estimated as 0.33066 (Chapter 26 and Appendix C)). Thus the regression line is a poor fit since only approximately one-tenth of the variability in the SBP can be explained by the model; that is, by differences in the heights of the children.

The parameter estimate for 'Intercept' corresponds to a, and that for 'Height' corresponds to b (the slope of the regression line). So, the equation of the estimated regression line is

$$SBP = 46.28 + 0.48 \times height$$

In this example, the intercept is of no interest in its own right (it relates to the predicted blood pressure for a child who has a height of 0 cm – a nonsensical value and, in any case, clearly out of the range of values seen in the study). However, we can interpret the slope coefficient; in these children, SBP is predicted to increase by 0.48 mmHg, on average, for each cm increase in height.

$P = 0.0008$ (Table 28.2) for the hypothesis test for height (i.e. H_0: true slope equals zero) is identical to that obtained from the analysis of variance table (Table 28.1), as expected.

Since the sample size is large (it is 100), we can approximate $t_{0.05}$ by 1.96 and calculate the 95% confidence interval for the true slope as

$$b \pm 1.96 \times SE(b) = 0.48 \pm (1.96 \times 0.14)$$

Therefore, the 95% confidence interval for the slope ranges from 0.21 to 0.75 mmHg per cm increase in height. This confidence interval does not include zero, confirming the finding that the slope is significantly different from zero.

We can use the regression equation to predict the SBP we expect a child of a given height to have. For example, a child who is 115 cm tall has an estimated predicted SBP of 46.28 + (0.48 × 115) = 101.48 mmHg; a child who is 130 cm tall has an estimated predicted SBP of 46.28 + (0.48 × 130) = 108.68 mmHg.

Table 28.1 Analysis of variance table.

Source	Sum of squares	df	Mean square	F-ratio	P-value
Due to regression	962.714	1	962.714	12.030	0.0008
Residual error	7842.592	98	80.026		
Total	8805.306	99			

Note: the estimated residual variance is 80.026 mmHg, the residual mean square.

Table 28.2 Parameter estimates.

Variable	Parameter estimate	Standard error	Test statistic	P-value
Intercept	46.2817	16.7845	2.7574	0.0070
Height	0.4842	0.1396	3.4684	0.0008

continued

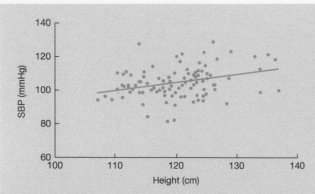

Figure 28.1 Scatter plot showing the relationship between systolic blood pressure (SBP) and height. The estimated regression line, SBP = 46.28 + 0.48 × height, is marked on the scatter plot.

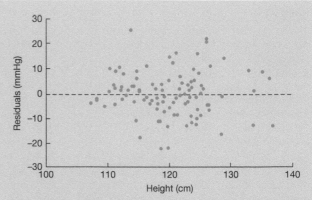

Figure 28.2 No relationship is apparent between the residuals and height, indicating that a linear relationship between height and systolic blood pressure is appropriate.

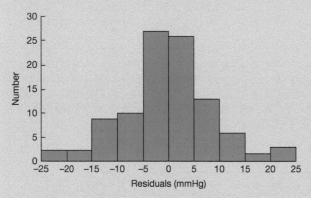

Figure 28.3 The distribution of the residuals is approximately Normal.

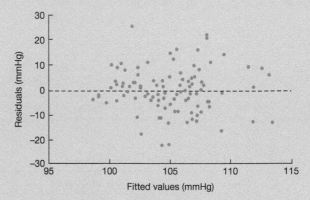

Figure 28.4 There is no tendency for the residuals to increase or decrease systematically with the fitted values. Hence the constant variance assumption is satisfied.

29 Multiple linear regression

What is it?

We may be interested in the effect of several explanatory variables, $x_1, x_2, ..., x_k$, on a response variable, y. If we believe that these x's may be interrelated, we should not look, in isolation, at the effect on y of changing the value of a single x, but should simultaneously take into account the values of the other x's. For example, as there is a strong relationship between a child's height and weight, we may want to know whether the relationship between height and systolic blood pressure (Chapter 28) is changed when we take the child's weight into account. **Multiple linear regression** allows us to investigate the joint effect of these explanatory variables on y; it is an example of a **multivariable** analysis where we relate a single outcome variable to two or more explanatory variables simultaneously. Note that, although the explanatory variables are sometimes called independent variables, this is a misnomer because they may be related.

We take a sample of n individuals, and measure the value of each of the variables on every individual. The multiple linear regression equation that estimates the relationships in the population is

$$Y = a + b_1 x_1 + b_2 x_2 + ... + b_k x_k$$

- x_i is the ith explanatory variable or **covariate** ($i = 1, 2, 3, ..., k$);
- Y is the estimated predicted, expected, mean or fitted value of y, which corresponds to a particular set of values of $x_1, x_2, ..., x_k$;
- a is a constant term, the estimated intercept; it is the value of Y when all the x's are zero;
- $b_1, b_2, ..., b_k$ are the estimated **partial regression coefficients**; b_1 represents the amount by which Y increases on average if we increase x_1 by one unit but keep all the other x's constant (i.e.

adjust or **control** for them). If there is a relationship between x_1 and the other x's, b_1 differs from the estimate of the regression coefficient obtained by regressing y on only x_1, because the latter approach does not adjust for the other variables. b_1 represents the effect of x_1 on y that is **independent** of the other x's.

Multiple linear regression analyses are invariably performed on the computer, and so we omit the formulae for these estimated parameters.

Why do it?

We perform a multiple regression analysis to be able to:
- identify explanatory variables that are associated with the dependent variable in order to promote understanding of the underlying process;
- determine the extent to which one or more of the explanatory variables is/are linearly related to the dependent variable, after adjusting for other variables that may be related to it; and
- possibly, predict the value of the dependent variable as accurately as possible from the explanatory variables.

Assumptions

The assumptions in multiple linear regression are the same (if we replace 'x' by 'each of the x's') as those in simple linear regression (Chapter 27), and they are checked in the same way. Failure to satisfy the linearity or independence assumptions is particularly important. We can transform (Chapter 9) the y variable and/or some or all of the x variables if the assumptions are in doubt, and then repeat the analysis (including checking the assumptions) on the transformed data.

Categorical explanatory variables

We can perform a multiple linear regression analysis using **categorical** explanatory variables. In particular, if we have a **binary** variable, x_1 (e.g. male = 0, female = 1), and we increase x_1 by one unit, we are 'changing' from males to females. b_1 thus represents the difference in the estimated mean values of y between females and males, after adjusting for the other x's.

If we have a **nominal** explanatory variable (Chapter 1) that has more than two categories of response, we have to create a number of **dummy** or **indicator** variables[1]. In general, for a nominal variable with k categories, we create $k - 1$ binary dummy variables. We choose one of the categories to represent our **reference category**, and each dummy variable allows us to compare one of the remaining $k - 1$ categories of the variable with the reference category. For example, we may be interested in comparing mean systolic blood pressure levels in individuals living in four countries in Europe (the Netherlands, UK, Spain and France). Suppose we choose our reference category to be the Netherlands. We generate one binary variable to identify those living in the UK; this variable takes the value 1 if the individual lives in the UK and 0 otherwise. We then generate binary variables to identify those living in Spain and France in a similar way. By default, those living in the Netherlands can then be identified since these individuals will have the value 0 for each of the three binary variables. In a multiple linear regression analysis, the regression coefficient for each of the other three countries represents the amount by which Y (systolic blood pressure) differs, on average, among those living in the relevant country *compared with* those living in the Netherlands. The intercept provides an estimate of the mean systolic blood pressure for those living in the Netherlands (when all of the other explanatory variables take the value zero). Some computer packages will create dummy variables automatically once it is specified that the variable is categorical.

If we have an **ordinal** explanatory variable and its three or more categories can be assigned values on a meaningful linear scale (e.g. social classes 1–5), then we can either use these values directly in the multiple linear regression equation (see also Chapter 33), or generate a series of dummy variables as for a nominal variable (but this does not make use of the ordering of the categories).

Analysis of covariance

An extension of analysis of variance (ANOVA, Chapter 22) is the **analysis of covariance (ANCOVA)**, in which we compare the response of interest between groups of individuals (e.g. two or more treatment groups) when other variables measured on each individual are taken into account. Such data can be analysed using multiple linear regression techniques by creating one or more dummy binary variables to differentiate between the groups. So, if we wish to compare the mean values of y in two treatment groups, while controlling for the effect of variables x_2, x_3, …, x_k (e.g. age, weight, etc.), we create a binary variable, x_1, to represent 'treatment' (e.g. $x_1 = 0$ for treatment A, $x_1 = 1$ for treatment B). In the multiple linear regression equation, b_1 is the estimated difference in the mean responses on y between treatments B and A, adjusting for the other x's.

Analysis of covariance is the preferred analysis for a randomized controlled trial comparing treatments when each individual in the study has a baseline and post-treatment follow-up measurement. In this instance, the response variable, y, is the follow-up measurement and two of the explanatory variables in the regression model are a binary variable representing treatment, x_1, and the individual's baseline level at the start of the study, x_2. This approach is generally better (i.e. has a greater power (Chapter 36)) than using either the change from baseline or the percentage change from baseline as the response variable.

Choice of explanatory variables

As a rule of thumb, we should not perform a multiple linear regression analysis if the number of variables is greater than the number of individuals divided by 10. Most computer packages have automatic procedures for selecting variables, e.g. stepwise selection (Chapter 33). These are particularly useful when many of the explanatory variables are related. A particular problem arises when **collinearity** is present, i.e. when pairs of explanatory variables are extremely highly correlated (Chapter 33).

Analysis

Most computer output contains the following items.

1 An assessment of goodness of fit

The **adjusted R^2** represents the proportion (often expressed as a percentage) of the variability of y that can be explained by its relationship with the x's. R^2 is adjusted so that models with different numbers of explanatory variables can be compared. If it has a low value (judged subjectively), the model is a poor fit. Goodness of fit is particularly important when we use the multiple linear regression equation for prediction.

2 The F-test in the ANOVA table

This tests the null hypothesis that all the partial regression coefficients in the population, $\beta_1, \beta_2, …, \beta_k$, are zero. A significant result indicates that there is a linear relationship between y and at least one of the x's.

3 The t-test of each partial regression coefficient, β_i ($i = 1, 2, …, k$)

Each t-test relates to one explanatory variable, and is relevant if we want to determine whether that explanatory variable affects the response variable, while controlling for the effects of the other covariates. To test H_0: $\beta_i = 0$, we calculate the test statistic $= \dfrac{b_i}{SE(b_i)}$, which follows the t-distribution with (n – *number of explanatory variables* – 1) degrees of freedom. Computer output includes the values of each b_i, $SE(b_i)$ and the related test statistic with its P-value. Sometimes the 95% confidence interval for β_i is included; if not, it can be calculated as $b_i \pm t_{0.05} \times SE(b_i)$.

Outliers and influential points

As discussed briefly in Chapter 28, an **outlier** (an observation that is inconsistent with most of the values in the data set (Chapter 3)) may or may not be **influential** (i.e. affect the parameter estimate(s) of the model if omitted). An outlier and/or influential observation may have one or both of the following:
- A large **residual** (a residual is the difference between the observed and predicted values of the outcome variable, y, for that individual's value(s) of the explanatory variable(s)).
- High **leverage** when the individual's value of x (or set of x's) is a long way from the mean value of x (or set of x's). High leverage values may be taken as those greater than $2(k+1)/n$ where k is the number of explanatory variables in the model and n is the number of individuals in the study.

We can determine suspect influential observations by, for example:
- investigating those individuals having large residuals, high leverage and/or values of **Cook's distance** (an overall measure of influence incorporating both residual and leverage values) greater than one or $4/n$ or very extreme relative to the others; or
- examining special diagnostic plots in which influential points may become apparent.

All influential points and outliers should be investigated thoroughly and checked for measurement and transcription errors.

Various methods are available for investigating model **sensitivity** – the extent to which estimates are affected by subsets of the data. Typically, we might fit the model with and without an influential point to assess the effect on the regression coefficients. However, we are rarely justified in removing influential observations or outliers from the data set providing the final model.

Reference

1   Armitage, P., Berry, G. and Matthews, J.N.S. (2001) *Statistical Methods in Medical Research*. 4th edition. Oxford: Blackwell Science.

Example

In Chapter 28 we studied the relationship between systolic blood pressure (SBP) and height in 100 children. It is known that height and weight are positively correlated. We therefore performed a **multiple linear regression analysis** to investigate the effects of height (cm), weight (kg) and sex (0 = boy, 1 = girl) on SBP (mmHg) in these children. Assumptions underlying this analysis are verified in Figs 29.1–29.4.

A typical output from a computer analysis of these data is contained in Appendix C. The analysis of variance table indicates that at least one of the explanatory variables is related to SBP ($F = 14.95$ with 3 and 96 degrees of freedom in the numerator and denominator, respectively, $P = 0.0001$). The adjusted R^2 value of 0.2972 indicates that 29.7% of the variability in SBP can be explained by the model – that is, by differences in the height, weight *and* sex of the children. Thus this provides a much better fit to the data than the simple linear regression in Chapter 28 in which $R^2 = 0.11$. Typical computer output contains the information in the following table about the explanatory variables in the model.

Variable	Parameter estimate	Standard error	95% CI for parameter	Test statistic	P-value
Intercept	79.4395	17.1182	(45.89 to 112.99)	4.6406	0.0001
Height	–0.0310	0.1717	(–0.37 to 0.31)	–0.1807	0.8570
Weight	1.1795	0.2614	(0.67 to 1.69)	4.5123	0.0001
Sex	4.2295	1.6105	(1.07 to 7.39)	2.6261	0.0101

The multiple linear regression equation is estimated by:

$$SBP = 79.44 - (0.03 \times height) + (1.18 \times weight) + (4.23 \times sex)$$

The relationship between weight and SBP is highly significant ($P < 0.0001$), with a 1 kg increase in weight being associated with a mean increase of 1.18 mmHg in SBP, after adjusting for height and sex. However, after adjusting for the weight and sex of the child, the relationship between height and SBP becomes non-significant ($P = 0.86$). This suggests that the significant relationship between height and SBP in the simple regression analysis reflects the fact that taller children tend to be heavier than shorter children. There is a significant relationship ($P = 0.01$) between sex and SBP; SBP in girls tends to be 4.23 mmHg higher, on average, than that in boys, even after taking account of possible differences in height and weight. Hence, both weight and sex are independent predictors of a child's SBP.

We can calculate the SBPs we would expect for children of given heights and weights. If the first child mentioned in Chapter 28 who is 115 cm tall is a girl and weighs 37 kg, she now has an estimated predicted SBP of $79.44 - (0.03 \times 115) + (1.18 \times 37) + (4.23 \times 1) = 123.88$ mmHg (higher than the 101.48 mmHg predicted in Chapter 28); if the second child who is 130 cm tall is a boy and weighs 30 kg, he now has an estimated predicted SBP of $79.44 - (0.03 \times 130) + (1.18 \times 30) + (4.23 \times 0) = 110.94$ mmHg (higher than the 108.68 mmHg predicted in Chapter 28).

continued

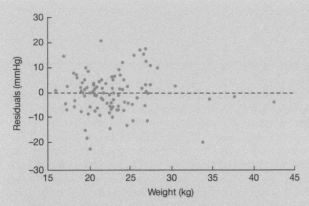

Figure 29.1 There is no systematic pattern to the residuals when plotted against weight. (Note that, similarly to Fig. 28.2, a plot of the residuals from this model against height also shows no systematic pattern.)

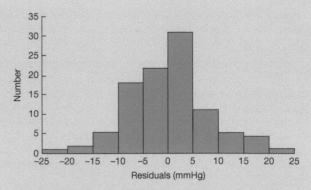

Figure 29.2 The distribution of the residuals is approximately Normal and the variance is slightly less than that from the simple regression model (Chapter 28), reflecting the improved fit of the multiple linear regression model over the simple model.

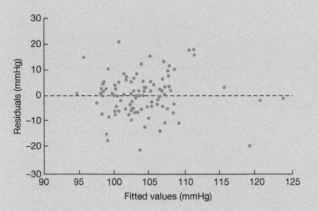

Figure 29.3 As with the univariable model, there is no tendency for the residuals to increase or decrease systematically with fitted values. Hence the constant variance assumption is satisfied.

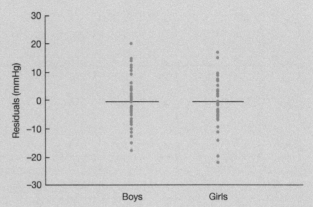

Figure 29.4 The distribution of the residuals is similar in boys and girls, suggesting that the model fits equally well in the two groups.

30 Binary outcomes and logistic regression

Learning objectives

By the end of this chapter, you should be able to:
- Explain why multiple linear regression analysis cannot be used for a binary outcome variable
- Define the logit of a proportion
- Define the multiple logistic regression equation
- Interpret the exponential of a logistic regression coefficient
- Calculate, from a logistic regression equation, the probability that a particular individual will have the outcome of interest
- Describe two ways of assessing whether a logistic regression coefficient is statistically significant
- Describe various ways of testing the overall model fit, assessing predictive efficiency and investigating the underlying assumptions of a logistic regression analysis
- Explain when the odds ratio is greater than and when it is less than the relative risk
- Explain the use of the following types of logistic regression: multinomial, ordinal, conditional

Relevant Workbook questions: MCQs 33, 46, 57 and 58; and SQs 4, 12 and 15 available online

Logistic regression is very similar to linear regression; we use it when we have a **binary outcome** of interest (e.g. the presence/absence of a symptom, or an individual who does/does not have a disease) and a number of explanatory variables. We perform a logistic regression analysis in order to do one or more of the following:

- Determine which explanatory variables influence the outcome.
- Evaluate the probability that an individual with a particular covariate pattern (i.e. a unique combination of values for the explanatory variables) will have the outcome of interest.
- Use this probability to assign the individual to an outcome group that reflects the individual's risk of the outcome (we usually use a cut-off of 0.5 for the probability for this purpose but we may choose a different cut-off if this better discriminates between the outcomes).
- Analyse an unmatched case–control study (Chapter 16) when the two outcomes are 'case' and 'control'.

Reasoning

We start by creating a binary variable to represent the two outcomes (e.g. 'has disease' = 1, 'does not have disease' = 0). However, we cannot use this as the dependent variable in a linear regression analysis since the Normality assumption is violated, and we cannot interpret predicted values that are not equal to zero or one. So, instead, we take the probability, p, that an individual is classified into the highest coded category (i.e. has disease) as the dependent variable, and, to overcome mathematical difficulties, use the logistic or logit transformation (Chapter 9) of it in the regression equation. The logit of this probability is the natural logarithm (i.e. to base e) of the odds of 'disease', i.e.

$$\text{logit}\,(p) = \ln\frac{p}{1-p}$$

The logistic regression equation

An iterative process, called maximum likelihood (Chapter 32), rather than ordinary least squares regression (so we cannot use linear regression software), produces, from the sample data, an estimated **logistic regression equation** of the form

$$\text{logit}\,(p) = a + b_1 x_1 + b_2 x_2 + \ldots + b_k x_k$$

where:
- x_i is the ith explanatory variable ($i = 1, 2, 3, \ldots, k$);
- p is the estimated value of the true probability that an individual with a particular set of values for $x_1, \ldots, x_k$ has the disease. p corresponds to the proportion with the disease; it has an underlying Binomial distribution (Chapter 8);
- a is the estimated constant term;
- $b_1, b_2, \ldots, b_k$ are the estimated **logistic regression coefficients**.

The exponential of a particular coefficient, for example, e^{b_1}, is an estimate of the **odds ratio** (Chapter 16). For a particular value of x_1, it is the estimated odds of disease for $(x_1 + 1)$ relative to the estimated odds of disease for x_1, while adjusting for all other x's in the equation (it is therefore often referred to as an **adjusted odds ratio**). If the odds ratio is equal to one (unity), then these two odds are the same, i.e. increasing the value of x_1 has no impact on the odds of disease. A value of the odds ratio above one indicates an increased odds of having the disease, and a value below one indicates a decreased odds of having the disease, as x_1 increases by one unit. When the disease is rare, the odds ratio can be interpreted as a **relative risk**.

We can manipulate the logistic regression equation to estimate the probability that an individual has the disease. For each individual, with a set of covariate values for $x_1, \ldots, x_k$, we calculate

$$z = a + b_1 x_1 + b_2 x_2 + \ldots + b_k x_k$$

Then, the probability that the individual has the disease is estimated as

$$p = \frac{e^z}{1 + e^z}$$

Generating a series of plots of these probabilities against the values of each of a number of covariates is often useful as an aid to interpreting the findings.

As the logistic regression model is fitted on a log scale, the effects of the x_i's are *multiplicative* on the odds of disease. This means that their combined effect is the product of their separate effects. Suppose, for example, x_1 and x_2 are two binary variables (each coded as 0 or 1) with estimated logistic coefficients b_1 and b_2, respectively, so that the corresponding estimated odds of disease for category 1 compared with category 0 for each variable is $\text{OR}_1 = e^{b_1}$ and $\text{OR}_2 = e^{b_2}$. To obtain the estimated odds of disease for an individual who has $x_1 = 1$ and $x_2 = 1$, compared with an individual who has $x_1 = 0$ and $x_2 = 0$, we multiply OR_1 by OR_2 (see Example). This concept is extended for numerical explanatory variables. The multiplicative effect on the odds scale

Medical Statistics at a Glance, Fourth Edition. Aviva Petrie and Caroline Sabin. © 2020 Aviva Petrie and Caroline Sabin. Published 2020 by John Wiley & Sons Ltd.
Companion Website: www.medstatsaag.com

is unlike the situation in linear regression where the effects of the x_i's on the dependent variable are additive.

Note that some statistical packages will, by default, model the probability that $p = 0$ (does not have disease) rather than $p = 1$. This will lead to the estimates from the logistic regression model being inverted (i.e. the estimate provided will be 1/OR). If this is the case, it is usually straightforward to modify these settings to ensure that the correct estimates are displayed.

The explanatory variables

Computer output for a logistic regression analysis generally includes, for each explanatory variable, the estimated logistic regression coefficient with standard error, the estimated odds ratio (i.e. the exponential of the coefficient) and a confidence interval for its true value. We can determine whether each variable is related to the outcome of interest (e.g. disease) by testing the null hypothesis that the relevant logistic regression coefficient is zero, which is equivalent to testing the hypothesis that the odds ratio of 'disease' associated with this variable is unity. This is usually achieved by performing one of the following tests.

• The **Wald test** – the test statistic, which follows the Standard Normal distribution, is equal to the estimated logistic regression coefficient divided by its standard error. Its square approximates the Chi-squared distribution with 1 degree of freedom.

• The **likelihood ratio test** (Chapter 32) – the test statistic is the **deviance** (also referred to as the **likelihood ratio statistic (LRS)** or **−2log likelihood**) for the full model *minus* the deviance for the full model excluding the relevant explanatory variable – this test statistic follows a Chi-squared distribution with 1 degree of freedom.

These tests give similar results if the sample size is large. Although the Wald test is less powerful (Chapter 18) and may produce biased results if there are insufficient data for each value of the explanatory variable, it is usually preferred because it is generally included in the computer output (which is not usually the case for the likelihood ratio test).

As in multiple linear regression, automatic selection procedures (Chapter 33) can be used to select the best combination of explanatory variables. As a rule of thumb, we should not perform a multiple logistic regression analysis if the number of responses in each of the two outcome categories (e.g. has disease/does not have disease) is fewer than 10 times the number of explanatory variables[1].

Assessing the adequacy of the model

Usually, interest is centred on examining the explanatory variables and their effect on the outcome. This information is routinely available in all advanced statistical computer packages. However, there are inconsistencies between the packages in the way in which the adequacy of the model is assessed, and in the way it is described. The following provides an indication of what your computer output may contain (in one guise or another) for a logistic model with k covariates and a sample size of n (full details may be obtained from more advanced texts[2] and examples are also shown in Appendix C).

Evaluating the model and its fit

• The value of the **deviance** (or **LRS** or **−2log likelihood**) – on its own (i.e. without subtracting the deviance from that of an alternative model), this compares the likelihood of the model with k covariates to that of a saturated (i.e. a perfectly fitting) model. This test statistic approximately follows a Chi-squared distribution with $(n - k - 1)$ degrees of freedom: a significant result suggests the model does not fit the data well. Thus the deviance is a measure of poorness of fit.

• The **model Chi-square**, the **Chi-square for covariates** or **G** – this tests the null hypothesis that all k regression coefficients in the model are zero by subtracting the deviance of the model from that of the null model which contains no explanatory variables (Chapter 32). G approximately follows a Chi-squared distribution with k degrees of freedom; a significant result suggests that at least one covariate is significantly associated with the dependent variable.

• The **Hosmer–Lemeshow test** (recommended only if n is large, say > 400) – this assesses goodness of fit (Chapter 46).

Indices of goodness of fit, such as R_L^2 and the Pseudo R^2, similar to R^2 in linear regression (Chapter 27), may also be determined although they are more difficult to interpret in logistic regression analysis.

Assessing predictive efficiency

• A **2 × 2 classification table** – this illustrates the ability of the model to correctly discriminate between those who do and do not have the outcome of interest (e.g. disease): the rows often represent the predicted outcomes from the model (where an individual is predicted to have or not have the disease according to whether his/her predicted probability is greater or less than the (usual) cut-off of 0.5) and the columns represent the observed outcomes. The entries in all cells of the table are frequencies. If the logistic model is able to classify patients perfectly (i.e. there is no misclassification of patients), the only cells of the table that contain non-zero entries are those lying on the diagonal and the overall percent correct is 100%. Note that it is possible to have a high percent correctly predicted (say 70%) when, at its most extreme, 100% of the individuals are predicted to belong to the more frequently occurring outcome group (e.g. diseased) and 0% to the other group. Terms associated with the classification table are as follows (Chapter 38):

▪ **Sensitivity** – the percent correctly predicted to have the disease.

▪ **Specificity** – the percent correctly predicted to be disease-free.

▪ **False positive rate** – the percent incorrectly predicted to have the disease.

▪ **False negative rate** – the percent incorrectly predicted to be disease-free.

• A **histogram** – this illustrates the observed outcomes (e.g. disease or no disease) of patients according to their predicted probability (p) of belonging to the outcome category of interest, e.g. has disease. The horizontal axis, with a scale from 0 to 1, represents the predicted probability that an individual has the disease. The column (or bar) for a particular predicted probability comprises 1's and/or 0's, each entry representing the observed outcome for one individual (the codes 1 and 0 indicate whether the individual does or does not have the disease, respectively). A good model will separate the symbols into two groups with little or no overlap – i.e. most or all of the 0's will lie on the far left of the histogram and most or all of the 1's will lie on the far right. Any 1's on the left of the histogram (where $p < 0.5$) or 0's on the right (where $p > 0.5$) will indicate individuals who have been misclassified.

- A **receiver operating characteristic (ROC) curve** – this plots the sensitivity of the model against 1 minus the specificity (Chapter 38) for different cut-offs of the predicted probability, *p*. Lowering the cut-off increases the sensitivity and raising the cut-off increases the specificity of the model. The closer the curve is to the upper left corner of the diagram, the better the predictive ability of the model. The greater the area under the curve (upper limit = 1), the better the model is at discriminating between outcomes.

Investigating the assumptions

We explain how to assess the **linearity** assumption in Chapter 33.

A **logistic regression coefficient** with a **large standard error** may indicate:
- **collinearity** (Chapter 33) – the explanatory variables are highly correlated; or
- a **zero cell count** – this occurs when all of the individuals within a particular category for a qualitative explanatory variable have the same outcome (e.g. all have the disease), so that none of them has the other outcome (disease-free). In this situation, we should consider combining categories if the covariate has more than two categories or, if this is not possible, removing the covariate from the model. Similar procedures should be adopted when the data are 'sparse' (e.g. when the expected frequency is < 5) in any category.

Deviance divided by the degrees of freedom ($df = n - k - 1$) is a ratio that has an expected value of 1 when the residual variance corresponds to that expected under a Binomial model. There is **extra-Binomial variation** indicating overdispersion if the ratio is substantially greater than 1 (the regression coefficients have standard errors which are underestimated, perhaps because of lack of independence – Chapters 41 and 42) and underdispersion if the ratio is substantially less than 1 (see also Chapters 31 and 42).

Logistic regression diagnostics

Outliers and influential points in logistic regression are usually identified by constructing appropriate diagrams and looking for points in them that appear to lie apart from the main body of the data. Note that a 'point' in these circumstances relates to individuals with the same covariate pattern, not to a particular individual as in multiple regression (Chapter 29). For example, outliers may be detected by plotting the logistic residual (e.g. the Pearson or deviance residual) against the predicted probability, and influential points may be detected by plotting an influence statistic (e.g. the change in the deviance attributable to deleting an individual from the analysis) against the predicted probability[2].

Comparing the odds ratio and the relative risk

Although the odds ratio is often taken as an estimate of the relative risk, it will only give a similar value if the outcome is rare. Where the outcome is not rare, the odds ratio will be greater than the relative risk if the relative risk is greater than one, and it will be less than the relative risk otherwise. Although the odds ratio is less easily interpreted than the relative risk, it does have attractive statistical properties and thus is usually preferred (and must be used in a case–control study when the relative risk cannot be estimated directly (Chapter 16)).

Multinomial and ordinal logistic regression

Multinomial (also called **polychotomous**) and **ordinal** logistic regression are extensions of logistic regression; we use them when we have a **categorical dependent variable** with more than two categories. When the dependent variable is *nominal* (Chapter 1) (e.g. the patient has one of three back disorders: lumbar disc hernia, chronic low-back pain or acute low-back pain) we use **multinomial logistic regression**. When the dependent variable is *ordinal* or ranked (e.g. mild, moderate or severe pain) we use **ordinal** logistic regression. These methods are complex and so you should refer to more advanced texts[3] and/or seek specialist advice if you want to use them. As a simple alternative, we can combine the categories in some appropriate way to create a new binary outcome variable, and then perform the usual two-category logistic regression analysis (recognizing that this approach may be wasteful of information). The decision on how to combine the categories should be made in advance, before looking at the data, in order to avoid bias.

Conditional logistic regression

We can use **conditional logistic regression** when we have *matched* individuals (as in a **matched case–control study** (Chapter 16)) and we wish to adjust for possible confounding factors. Analysis of a matched case–control study using ordinary logistic regression or the methods described in Chapter 16 is inefficient, may produce biased results and lacks power because neither acknowledges that cases and controls are linked to each other. Conditional logistic regression allows us to compare cases with controls in the same matched 'set' (i.e. each pair in the case of one-to-one matching). In this situation, the 'outcome' is defined by the patient being a case (usually coded 1) or a control (usually coded 0). While advanced statistical packages may sometimes allow us to perform conditional logistic regression directly, it may be necessary to use the **Cox proportional hazards regression model** (Chapter 44).

References

1 Peduzzi, P., Concato, J., Kemper, E., Holford, T.R. and Feinstein, A.R. (1996) A simulation study of the number of events per variable in logistic regression analysis. *Journal of Clinical Epidemiology*, 49, 1373–1379.

2 Hosmer, D.W., Lemeshow, S. and Sturdivant, R.X. (2013) *Applied Logistic Regression*. 3rd edition. Wiley Series in Probability and Statistics. Hoboken, NJ: Wiley.

3 Agresti, A. (2013) *Categorical Data Analysis*. 3rd edition. Wiley Series in Probability and Statistics. Hoboken, NJ: Wiley.

Example

In a study of the relationship between human herpesvirus type 8 (HHV-8) infection (described in Chapter 23) and sexual behaviour, 271 homosexual/bisexual men were asked questions relating to their past histories of a number of sexually transmitted diseases (gonorrhoea, syphilis, herpes simplex type 2 (HSV-2) and HIV). In Chapter 24 we showed that men who had a history of gonorrhoea had a higher seroprevalence of HHV-8 than those without a previous history of gonorrhoea. A **multivariable logistic regression** analysis was performed to investigate whether this effect was simply a reflection of the relationships between HHV-8 and the other infections and/or the man's age. The explanatory variables were the presence of each of the four infections, each coded as '0' if the patient had no history of the particular infection or '1' if he had a history of that infection, and the patient's age in years.

A typical computer output is displayed in Appendix C. It shows that the Chi-square for covariates equals 24.60 on 5 degrees of freedom ($P = 0.0002$), indicating that at least one of the covariates is significantly associated with HHV-8 serostatus. The following table summarizes the information about each variable in the model.

Variable	Parameter estimate	Standard error	Wald test statistic	P-value	Estimated odds ratio	95% CI for odds ratio
Intercept	−2.2242	0.6512	−3.416	0.0006	–	–
Gonorrhoea	0.5093	0.4363	1.167	0.2431	1.664	(0.71–3.91)
Syphilis	1.1924	0.7111	1.677	0.0935	3.295	(0.82–13.28)
HSV-2 positivity	0.7910	0.3871	2.043	0.0410	2.206	(1.03–4.71)
HIV	1.6357	0.6028	2.713	0.0067	5.133	(1.57–16.73)
Age	0.0062	0.0204	0.302	0.7628	1.006	(0.97–1.05)

These results indicate that HSV-2 positivity ($P = 0.04$) and HIV status ($P = 0.007$) are independently associated with HHV-8 infection; individuals who are HSV-2 seropositive have 2.21 times ($= \exp[0.7910]$) the odds of being HHV-8 seropositive as those who are HSV-2 seronegative, after adjusting for the other infections and age. In other words, the odds of HHV-8 seropositivity in these individuals is increased by 121%. The upper limit of the confidence interval for this odds ratio shows that this increased odds could be as much as 371%. HSV-2 infection is a well-documented marker of sexual activity. Thus, rather than HSV-2 being a cause of HHV-8 infection, the association may be a reflection of the sexual activity of the individual.

Furthermore, the multiplicative effect of the model suggests that a man who is both HSV-2 and HIV seropositive is estimated to have $2.206 \times 5.133 = 11.3$ times the odds of HHV-8 infection compared with a man who is seronegative for both, after adjusting for the other infections.

In addition, there is a tendency for a history of syphilis to be associated with HHV-8 serostatus. Although this is marginally nonsignificant ($P = 0.09$), we should note that the confidence interval does include values for the odds ratio as high as 13.28. In contrast, there is no indication of an independent relationship between a history of gonorrhoea and HHV-8 seropositivity, suggesting that this variable appeared, by the univariable Chi-squared test (Chapter 24), to be associated with HHV-8 serostatus because of the fact that many men who had a history of one of the other sexually transmitted diseases in the past also had a history of gonorrhoea. There is no significant relationship between HHV-8 seropositivity and age; the odds ratio indicates that the estimated odds of HHV-8 seropositivity increases by 0.6% for each additional year of age.

The probability that a 51-year-old man has HHV-8 infection if he has gonorrhoea and is HSV-2 positive (but does not have syphilis and is not HIV positive) is estimated as 0.35, i.e. it is $\exp[-0.6077]/[1 + \exp(-0.6077)]$ where $-0.6077 = -2.2242 + 0.5093 + 0.7910 + (0.0062 \times 51)$.

The area under the ROC curve shown in Appendix C is 0.6868, indicating that the model fits moderately well and has reasonably good discriminatory ability. Two different cut-offs for the predictive probability are chosen by examining the ROC curve. It can be seen from the relevant 2×2 classification tables in Appendix C that a cut-off of 0.5 leads to very poor sensitivity (19.15%) and extremely high specificity (97.65%) whereas a cut-off of 0.2 increases the sensitivity to 51.06% but lowers the specificity to 79.81%.

31 Rates and Poisson regression

Learning objectives

By the end of this chapter, you should be able to:
- Define a rate and describe its features
- Distinguish between a rate and a risk, and between an incidence rate and a mortality rate
- Define a relative rate and explain when it is preferred to a relative risk
- Explain when it is appropriate to use Poisson regression
- Define the Poisson regression equation and interpret the exponential of a Poisson regression coefficient
- Calculate, from the Poisson regression equation, the event rate for a particular individual
- Explain the use of an offset in a Poisson regression analysis
- Explain how to perform a Poisson regression analysis with (1) grouped data and (2) variables that change over time
- Explain the meaning and the consequences of extra-Poisson dispersion
- Explain how to identify extra-Poisson dispersion in a Poisson regression analysis

Relevant Workbook questions: MCQs 59, 60, 61, 62 and 63; SQs 16, 17, 18 and 29 available online

Rates

In any longitudinal study (Chapter 12) investigating the occurrence of an event (such as death), we should take into account the fact that individuals are usually followed for different lengths of time. This may be because some individuals drop out of the study or because individuals are entered into the study at different times, and therefore follow-up times from different people may vary at the close of the study. As those with a longer follow-up time are more likely to experience the event than those with shorter follow-up, we consider the **rate** at which the event occurs *per person per period of time*. Often the unit which represents a convenient period of time is a year (but it could be a minute, day, week, etc.). Then the event rate per person per year (i.e. **per person-year of follow-up**) is estimated by

$$\text{Rate} = \frac{\text{Number of events occurring}}{\text{Total number of years of follow-up for all individuals}}$$
$$= \frac{\text{Number of events occurring}}{\text{Person-years of follow-up}}$$

Each individual's length of follow-up is usually defined as the time from when he or she enters the study until the time when the event occurs or the study draws to a close if the event does not occur. The total follow-up time is the sum of all the individuals' follow-up times.

The rate is called an **incidence rate** when the event is a new case (e.g. of disease) or the **mortality rate** when the event is death. When the rate is very small, it is often multiplied by a *convenience factor* such as 1000 and re-expressed as the rate per 1000 person-years of follow-up.

Features of the rate

- When calculating the rate, we do not distinguish between person-years of follow-up that occur in the same individual and those that occur in different individuals. For example, the person-years of follow-up contributed by 10 individuals, each of whom is followed for 1 year, will be the same as that contributed by one person followed for 10 years.
- Whether we also include multiple events from each individual (i.e. when the event occurs on more than one occasion) depends on the hypothesis of interest. If we are only interested in first events, then follow-up must cease at the point at which an individual experiences his or her first event as the individual is no longer at risk of a first event after this time. Where multiple events from the same individual are included in the calculation of the rate, we have a special form of **clustered data** (Chapter 41), and appropriate statistical methods must be used (Chapters 41 and 42).
- A rate cannot be calculated in a cross-sectional study (Chapter 12) since this type of study does not involve time.

Comparing the rate and the risk

The **risk** of an event (Chapter 15) is simply the total number of events divided by the number of individuals included in the study at the start of the investigation, with no allowance for the length of follow-up. As a result, the risk of the event will be greater when individuals are followed for longer, since they will have more opportunity to experience the event. In contrast, the **rate** of the event should remain relatively stable in these circumstances, as the rate takes account of the duration of follow-up.

Relative rates

We may be interested in comparing the rate of disease in a group of individuals exposed to some factor of interest ($\text{Rate}_{exposed}$) with that in a group of individuals not exposed to the factor ($\text{Rate}_{unexposed}$).

$$\text{Relative rate} = \frac{\text{Rate}_{exposed}}{\text{Rate}_{unexposed}}$$

The relative rate (or **rate ratio**, sometimes referred to as the **incidence rate ratio**) is interpreted in a similar way to the **relative risk** (Chapter 15) and to the **odds ratio** (Chapters 16 and 30); a relative rate of 1 (unity) indicates that the rate of disease is the same in the two groups, a relative rate greater than 1 indicates that the rate is higher in those exposed to the factor than in those who are unexposed, and a relative rate less than 1 indicates that the rate is lower in the group exposed to the factor.

Although the relative rate is often taken as an estimate of the relative risk, the relative rate and the relative risk will only be similar if the event (e.g. disease) is rare. When the event is not rare and individuals are followed for varying lengths of time, the rate, and therefore the relative rate, will not be affected by the different follow-up times. This is not the case for the relative risk as the risk, and thus the relative risk, will change as individuals

Medical Statistics at a Glance, Fourth Edition. Aviva Petrie and Caroline Sabin. © 2020 Aviva Petrie and Caroline Sabin. Published 2020 by John Wiley & Sons Ltd.
Companion Website: www.medstatsaag.com

are followed for longer periods. Hence, the relative rate is always preferred when follow-up times vary between individuals in the study.

Poisson regression

What is it?

The Poisson distribution (named after a French mathematician) is a probability distribution (Chapter 8) of the count of the number of rare events that occur randomly over an interval of time (or space) at a constant average rate. This forms the basis of Poisson regression, which is used to analyse the rate of some event (e.g. disease) when individuals have different follow-up times. This contrasts with logistic regression (Chapter 30) which is concerned only with whether or not the event occurs and is used to estimate odds ratios. In Poisson regression, we assume that the rate of the event among individuals with the same explanatory variables (e.g. age and sex) is constant over the whole study period. We generally want to know which explanatory variables influence the rate at which the event occurs, and may wish to compare this rate in different exposure groups and/or predict the rate for groups of individuals with particular characteristics.

The equation and its interpretation

The Poisson regression model takes a very similar form to the logistic regression model (Chapter 30), each having a (usually) linear combination of explanatory variables on the right-hand side of the equation. Poisson regression analysis also mirrors logistic regression analysis in that we transform the outcome variable in order to overcome mathematical difficulties. We use the natural log transformation (ln) of the rate and an iterative process (maximum likelihood, Chapter 32) to produce an estimated regression equation from the sample data of the form

$$\ln(r) = a + b_1 x_1 + b_2 x_2 + \ldots + b_k x_k$$

where:

- x_i is the ith explanatory variable ($i = 1, 2, 3, \ldots, k$);
- r is the estimated value of the mean or expected rate for an individual with a particular set of values for $x_1, \ldots, x_k$;
- a is the estimated constant term providing an estimate of the log rate when all x_i's in the equation take the value zero (the log of the baseline rate);
- $b_1, b_2, \ldots, b_k$ are the estimated **Poisson regression coefficients**.

The exponential of a particular coefficient, for example, e^{b_1}, is the estimated **relative rate** associated with the relevant variable. For a particular value of x_1, it is the estimated rate of disease for $(x_1 + 1)$ relative to the estimated rate of disease for x_1, while adjusting for all other x_i's in the equation. If the relative rate is equal to 1 (unity), then the event rates are the same when x_1 increases by one unit. A value of the relative rate above 1 indicates an increased event rate, and a value below 1 indicates a decreased event rate, as x_1 increases by one unit.

As with logistic regression, Poisson regression models are fitted on the log scale. Thus, the effects of the x_i's are *multiplicative* on the rate of disease.

We can manipulate the Poisson regression equation to estimate the event rate for an individual with a particular combination of values of $x_1, \ldots, x_k$. For each set of covariate values for $x_1, \ldots, x_k$, we calculate

$$z = a + b_1 x_1 + b_2 x_2 + \ldots + b_k x_k$$

Then, the event rate for that individual is estimated as e^z.

Use of an offset

Although we model the rate at which the event occurs (i.e. the number of events divided by the person-years of follow-up), most statistical packages require the number of events occurring to be specified as the dependent variable rather than the rate itself. The log of each individual's person-years of follow-up is then included as an **offset** in the model. Assuming that we are only interested in including a single event per person, the number of events occurring in each individual will either take the value 0 (if the event did not occur) or 1 (if the event did occur). This provides a slightly different formulation of the model which allows the estimates to be generated in a less computationally intensive way. The results from the model, however, are exactly the same as they would be if the rate were modelled.

Entering data for groups

Note that when all of the explanatory variables are categorical, we can simplify the data entry process by making use of the fact that the calculation of the rate does not distinguish between person-years of follow-up that occur in the same individual and those that occur in different individuals. For example, we may be interested in the effect of only two explanatory variables, sex (male or female) and age (< 16, 16–20 and 21–25 years), on the rate of some event. Between them, these two variables define six groups (i.e. males aged < 16 years, females aged < 16 years, ..., females aged 21–25 years). We can simplify the entry of these data by determining the total number of events for all individuals within the same sex/age group and the total person-years of follow-up for these individuals. The estimated rate in each group is then calculated as the total number of events divided by the person-years of follow-up in that group. Using this approach, rather than entering data for the n individuals one by one, we enter the data for each of the six groups, and do so by creating a model in which the explanatory variables are the binary and dummy variables (Chapter 29) for sex and age. Note that when entering data in this way, it is not possible to accommodate numerical covariates to define the groups or include an additional covariate in the model that takes different values for the individuals in a group.

Incorporating variables that change over time

By splitting the follow-up period into shorter intervals, it is possible to incorporate variables that **change over time** into the model. For example, we may be interested in relating the smoking history of middle-aged men to the rate at which they experience lung cancer. Over a long follow-up period, many of these men may give up smoking and their rates of lung cancer may be lowered as a result. Thus, categorizing men according to their smoking status at the start of the study may give a poor representation of the impact of smoking status on lung cancer. Instead, we split each man's follow-up into short time intervals in such a way that his smoking status remains constant in each interval. We then perform a Poisson regression analysis, treating the relevant information in each short time interval for each man (i.e. the occurrence/non-occurrence of the event, his follow-up time and smoking status) as if it came from a different man.

Computer output

Comprehensive computer output for a Poisson regression analysis includes, for each explanatory variable, the estimated Poisson regression coefficient with standard error, the estimated relative rate (i.e. the exponential of the coefficient) with a confidence interval for its true value, and a Wald test statistic (testing the null hypothesis that the regression coefficient is zero or, equivalently, that the relative rate of 'disease' associated with this variable is unity) and associated P-value. As with the output from logistic regression (Chapter 30), we can assess the adequacy of the model using – 2log likelihood (LRS or deviance) and the model Chi-square or the Chi-square for covariates (see also Chapter 32).

Extra-Poisson variation

One concern when fitting a Poisson regression model is the possibility of *extra-Poisson variation*, which usually implies *overdispersion*. This occurs when the residual variance is greater than would be expected from a Poisson model, perhaps because an outlier is present (Chapter 3), because an important explanatory variable has not been included in the model, or because the data are clustered (Chapters 41 and 42) and the clustering has not adequately been taken into account. Then the standard errors are usually underestimated and, consequently, the confidence intervals for the parameters are too narrow and the P-values too small. A way to investigate the possibility of extra-Poisson variation is to divide – 2log likelihood (LRS or deviance) by the degrees of freedom, $n - k - 1$, where n is the number of individuals in the data set and k is the number of explanatory variables in the model. This quotient should be approximately equal to 1 if there is no extra-Poisson variation; values substantially above 1 may indicate overdispersion. If there is overdispersion, then it is possible to use the **scale parameter** (which is usually assumed to equal 1 when there is no extra-Poisson variation) to fit a Poisson regression model that is appropriate for overdispersed data. Alternatively, it may be advisable to fit a regression model based on the negative Binomial distribution (another type of probability distribution that can be used for counts) instead of the Poisson distribution. *Underdispersion*, where the residual variance is less than would be expected from a Poisson model and where the ratio of – 2log likelihood to $n - k - 1$ is substantially less than 1, may also occur (e.g. if high counts cannot be recorded accurately). Underdispersion and overdispersion may also be a concern when performing logistic regression (Chapter 30), when they are referred to as *extra-Binomial variation*.

Alternative to Poisson analysis

When a group of individuals is followed from a natural 'starting point' (e.g. an operation) until the time that the person develops an endpoint of interest, we may use an alternative approach known as **survival analysis**, which, in contrast to Poisson regression, does not assume that the 'hazard' (the rate of the event in a small interval) is constant over time. This approach is described in detail in Chapter 44.

Example

Individuals with HIV infection treated with highly active antiretroviral therapy (HAART) usually experience a decline in HIV viral load to levels below the limit of detection of the assay (an *initial response*). However, some of these individuals may experience virological failure after this stage; this occurs when an individual's viral load becomes detectable again while on therapy. Identification of factors that are associated with an increased rate of virological failure may allow steps to be taken to prevent this occurring. As patients are followed for different lengths of time, a **Poisson regression analysis** is appropriate.

A group of 516 patients who experienced an initial response to therapy were identified and followed until the time of virological failure, or until their last date of follow-up if their viral load remained suppressed at this time. Follow-up started on the first date that their viral load became undetectable. The explanatory variable of primary interest was the duration of time on treatment since an initial response but this was a variable whose values were constantly changing for each patient during the study period. Therefore, to investigate whether the virological failure rate did change over time, the duration of time on treatment since an initial response was split into three time intervals: < 1, 1–2 and > 2 years (this created 988 sets of observations), with the broad assumption that the virological failure rate was approximately constant within each period. Failure rates in the three time periods were then compared. The data (the length of follow-up in that interval, whether or not virological failure was experienced in that interval, and relevant explanatory variables) were entered on to a spreadsheet for each patient in every interval in which he or she was followed up. The explanatory variables considered included demographics, the stage of disease at the time of starting therapy, the year of starting HAART and whether or not the patient had received treatment in the past.

In order to *limit the number of covariates* in the multivariable Poisson regression model, a separate univariable Poisson regression model for each covariate was used to identify the covariates associated with virological failure (see Chapter 33).

Over a total follow-up of 718 person-years, 61 patients experienced virological failure, an unadjusted event rate of 8.50 per 100 person-years (95% confidence interval: 6.61, 10.92). Unadjusted virological failure rates were 8.13 (6.31, 10.95) in the first year after initial response to therapy, 12.22 (7.33, 17.12) in the second year and 3.99 (1.30, 9.31) in later years. Results from a Poisson regression model that incorporated only two dummy variables (Chapter 29) to reflect the categories of 1–2 and > 2 years, each compared with < 1 year, since an initial response to therapy, suggested that time since initial virological response was significantly associated with virological failure ($P = 0.04$). In addition, the patient's sex ($P = 0.03$), his or her baseline CD8 count ($P = 0.01$) and treatment status at the time of starting the current regimen (previously received treatment, never received treatment; $P = 0.008$) were all significantly associated with virological failure in univariable Poisson models. Thus, a multivariable Poisson regression analysis was performed to assess the relationship between virological failure and duration of time on therapy, after adjusting for these other variables. The results are summarized in Table 31.1; full computer output is shown in Appendix C.

The results from this multivariable model suggested that there was a trend towards a higher virological failure rate in the period 1–2 years after initial response compared with that seen in the first year (virological failure rate was increased by 53% in the period 1–2 years), but a *lower* rate after the second year (failure rate was reduced by 44% in this period compared with that seen in the first year after initial response), although neither of these effects was statistically significant. After adjusting for all other variables in the model, patients who were receiving their first treatment had an estimated virological failure rate that was 44% lower than that of patients who had

continued

previously received treatment, the estimated virological failure rate in men was 39% less than that seen in women (this was not statistically significant), and the estimated virological failure rate was reduced by 5% if the CD8 count at baseline was 100 cells/mm³ higher. See also the Examples in Chapters 32 and 33 for additional analyses relating to this Poisson model, including assessments of overdispersion, goodness of fit and linearity of the covariates.

Table 31.1 Results from multivariable Poisson regression analysis of factors associated with virological failure.

Variable*		Parameter estimate	Standard error	Estimated relative rate	95% confidence interval for relative rate	Wald P-value[†]
Time since initial response to therapy (years)						
	<1	reference	–	1	–	–
	1–2	0.4256	0.2702	1.53	0.90–2.60	0.12
	>2	−0.5835	0.4825	0.56	0.22–1.44	0.23
Treatment status						
Previously received treatment (0)		reference	–	1	–	
Never received treatment (1)		−0.5871	0.2587	0.56	0.33–0.92	0.02
Sex						
Female (0)		reference	–	1	–	
Male (1)		−0.4868	0.2664	0.61	0.36–1.04	0.07
CD8 count (per 100 cells/mm³)		−0.0558	0.0267	0.95	0.90–1.00	0.04

* Codes for binary variables (sex and treatment status) are shown in parentheses. Time since initial response to therapy was included by incorporating dummy variables to reflect the periods 1–2 years and >2 years after initial response.
[†] An alternative method of assessing the significance of categorical variables with more than two categories is described in Chapters 32 and 33.

Adapted from work carried out by Ms Colette Smith, Department of Primary Care and Population Sciences, Royal Free and University College Medical School, London, UK.

32 Generalized linear models

Statistical modelling includes the use of simple and multiple linear regression (Chapters 27–29), logistic regression (Chapter 30), Poisson regression (Chapter 31) and some methods that deal with survival data (Chapter 44). All these methods rely on generating a **mathematical model** that best describes the relationship between an outcome and one or more explanatory variables. Generation of such a model allows us to determine the extent to which each explanatory variable is related to the outcome after adjusting for all other explanatory variables in the model and, if desired, to predict the value of the outcome from these explanatory variables.

The **generalized linear model (GLM)** can be expressed in the form

$$g(Y) = a + b_1 x_1 + b_2 x_2 + \ldots + b_k x_k$$

where:
- Y is the estimated value of the predicted, mean or expected value of the dependent variable which follows a known probability distribution (e.g. Normal, Binomial, Poisson);

- $g(Y)$, called the **link function**, is a transformation of Y which produces a linear relationship with $x_1, \ldots, x_k$, the predictor or explanatory variables;
- $b_1, \ldots, b_k$ are estimated regression coefficients that relate to these explanatory variables; and
- a is a constant term.

Each of the regression models described in earlier chapters can be expressed as a particular type of GLM (Table 32.1). The link function is the **logit** of the proportion (i.e. the $\log_e$ of the odds) in logistic regression and the $\log_e$ of the rate in Poisson regression. No transformation of the dependent variable is required in simple and multiple linear regression; the link function is then referred to as the **identity link**. Once we have specified which type of regression we wish to perform, most statistical packages incorporate the link function into the calculations automatically without any need for further specification.

Which type of model do we choose?

The choice of an appropriate statistical model will depend on the outcome of interest (Table 32.1). For example, if our dependent variable is a continuous numerical variable, we may use simple or multiple linear regression to identify factors associated with this variable. If we have a binary outcome (e.g. patient died or did not die) and all patients are followed for the same amount of time, then a logistic regression model would be the appropriate choice.

Note that we may be able to choose a different type of model by modifying the format of our dependent variable. In particular, if we have a continuous numerical outcome but one or more of the assumptions of linear regression are not met, we may choose to categorize our outcome variable into two groups to generate a new binary outcome variable. For example, if our dependent variable is systolic blood pressure (a continuous numerical variable) after a 6-month period of anti-hypertensive therapy, we may choose to dichotomize the systolic blood

Table 32.1 Choice of appropriate types of GLM for use with different types of outcome.

Type of outcome	Type of GLM commonly used	See Chapter
Continuous numerical	Simple or multiple linear	28, 29
Binary		
Incidence of disease in longitudinal study (patients followed for equal periods of time)	Logistic	30
Binary outcome in cross-sectional study	Logistic	30
Unmatched case–control study	Logistic	30
Matched case–control study	Conditional logistic	30
Categorical outcome with more than two categories	Multinomial or ordinal logistic regression	30
Event rate or count	Poisson	31
Time to event*	Exponential, Weibull or Gompertz models	44

*Time to event data may also be analysed using a Cox proportional hazards regression model (Chapter 44).

Medical Statistics at a Glance, Fourth Edition. Aviva Petrie and Caroline Sabin. © 2020 Aviva Petrie and Caroline Sabin. Published 2020 by John Wiley & Sons Ltd.
Companion Website: www.medstatsaag.com

pressure as high or low using a particular cut-off, and then use logistic regression to identify factors associated with this binary outcome. While dichotomizing the dependent variable in this way may simplify the fitting and interpretation of the statistical model, some information about the dependent variable will usually be discarded. Thus the advantages and disadvantages of this approach should always be considered carefully.

Likelihood and maximum likelihood estimation

When fitting a GLM, we generally use the concept of **likelihood** to estimate the parameters of the model. For any GLM characterized by a known probability distribution, a set of explanatory variables and some potential values for each of their regression coefficients, the likelihood of the model (L) is the *probability* that we would have obtained the *observed results* had the regression coefficients taken those values. We estimate the coefficients of the model by selecting the values for the regression coefficients that maximize L (i.e. they are those values that are *most likely* to have produced our observed results); the process is **maximum likelihood estimation (MLE)** and the estimates are **maximum likelihood estimates**. MLE is an iterative process and thus specialized computer software is required. One exception to MLE is in the case of simple and multiple linear regression models (with the identity link function) where we usually estimate the parameters using the **method of least squares** (the estimates are often referred to as **ordinary least squares (OLS)** estimates (Chapter 27)); the OLS and MLE estimates are identical in this situation.

Assessing adequacy of fit

Although MLE maximizes L for a given set of explanatory variables, we can always improve L further by including additional explanatory variables. At its most extreme, a **saturated** model is one that includes a separate variable for each observation (i.e. individual) in the data set. While such a model would explain the data perfectly, it is of limited use in practice as the prediction of future observations from this model is likely to be poor. The saturated model does, however, allow us to calculate the value of L that would be obtained if we could model the data perfectly. Comparison of this value of L with the value obtained after fitting our simpler model with fewer variables provides a way of assessing the **adequacy of the fit** of our model. We consider the **likelihood ratio**, the ratio of the value of L obtained from the saturated model to that obtained from the fitted model, in order to compare these two models. More specifically, we calculate the **likelihood ratio statistic (LRS)** as

$$\text{LRS} = -2 \times \frac{\log(L_{\text{saturated}})}{\log(L_{\text{fitted}})}$$
$$= -2 \times [\log(L_{\text{saturated}}) - \log(L_{\text{fitted}})]$$

The LRS, often referred to as **–2log likelihood** (Chapters 30 and 31) or as the **deviance**, approximately follows a Chi-squared distribution with degrees of freedom equal to the difference in the number of parameters fitted in the two models (i.e. $n - k - 1$, where n is the number of observations in the data set and k is the number of parameters, apart from the intercept, in the simpler model). The null hypothesis is that the extra parameters in the larger saturated model are all zero; a high value of the LRS will give a significant result indicating that the goodness of fit of the model is poor.

The LRS can also be used in other situations. In particular, the LRS can be used to compare two models, neither of which is saturated, when one model is **nested** within another (i.e. the larger model includes all of the explanatory variables that are included in the smaller model, in addition to extra variables). In this situation, the test statistic is the difference between the value of the LRS from the model which includes the extra variables and that from the model which excludes these extra variables. The test statistic follows a Chi-squared distribution with degrees of freedom equal to the number of *additional* parameters included in the larger model, and is used to test the null hypothesis that the extra parameters in the larger model are all zero. The LRS can also be used to test the null hypothesis that all the parameters associated with the covariates of a model are zero by comparing the LRS of the model which includes the covariates with that of the model which excludes them. This is often referred to as the **model Chi-square** or **the Chi-square for covariates** (Chapters 30 and 31).

Regression diagnostics

When performing any form of regression analysis, it is important to consider a series of regression diagnostics. These allow us to examine our fitted regression model and look for flaws that may affect our parameter estimates and their standard errors. In particular, we must consider whether the assumptions underlying the model are violated and whether our results are heavily affected by influential observations (Chapter 28).

Example

In the Example in Chapter 31, we used Wald tests to identify individual factors associated with virological rebound in a group of 516 HIV-positive patients (with 988 sets of observations) who had been treated with highly active antiretroviral therapy (HAART). In particular, we were interested in whether the rate of virological failure increased over time, after controlling for other potentially confounding variables that were related to virological failure. Although the outcome of primary interest was binary (patient experienced virological failure, patient did not experience virological failure), a Poisson regression model rather than a logistic model was chosen as individual patients were followed for different lengths of time. Thus, the outcome variable for the analysis performed was an event rate. In this chapter, P-values for the variables have been calculated using **likelihood ratio statistics**. In particular, to calculate the single P-value associated with both dummy variables representing the time since initial response to therapy, two models were fitted. The first included the variables relating to treatment status (previously received treatment, never received treatment), sex and baseline CD8 count (Model 1); the second included these variables as well as the two time dummy variables (Model 2). The difference between the values obtained for **−2log likelihood**

(i.e. the LRS or deviance) from each of the models was then considered (Table 32.2). A full computer output is shown in Appendix C.

The inclusion of the two dummy variables was associated with a reduction in the value of −2log likelihood of 5.53 (= 393.12 − 387.59). This test statistic follows the Chi-squared distribution with 2 degrees of freedom (as two additional parameters were included in the larger model); the P-value associated with this test statistic was 0.06 indicating that the relationship between virological failure and time since initial response is marginally non-significant. The value of −2log likelihood for Model 2 also allowed us to assess the adequacy of fit of this model by comparing its value of −2log likelihood to a Chi-squared distribution with 982 degrees of freedom. The P-value obtained for this comparison was > 0.99, suggesting that the goodness of fit of the model is acceptable. However, it should be noted that after including these five variables in the model, there was some evidence of **underdispersion**, as the ratio of −2log likelihood to its degrees of freedom was 0.39, which is substantially less than 1, suggesting that the amount of residual variation was less than would be expected from a Poisson model (Chapter 31).

Table 32.2 − 2log likelihood values, degrees of freedom and number of parameters fitted in models that exclude and include the time since initial response to therapy.

Model	Variables included	−2log likelihood	Degrees of freedom for the model	Number of parameters fitted in the model, including the intercept
1	Treatment status, sex and baseline CD8 count	393.12	984	4
2	Treatment status, sex, baseline CD8 count and two dummy variables for time since initial response to therapy	387.59	982	6

33 Explanatory variables in statistical models

Whichever type of statistical model we choose, we have to make decisions about which explanatory variables to include in the model and the most appropriate way in which they should be incorporated. These decisions will depend on the type of explanatory variable (either nominal categorical, ordinal categorical or numerical) and the relationship between these variables and the dependent variable.

Nominal explanatory variables

It is usually necessary to create **dummy** or **indicator** variables (Chapter 29) to investigate the effect of a nominal categorical explanatory variable in a regression analysis. Note that when assessing the adequacy of fit of a model that includes a nominal variable with more than two categories, or when assessing the significance of that variable, it is important to include *all* of the dummy variables in the model *at the same time*; if we do not do this (i.e. if we only include one of the dummy variables for a particular level of the categorical variable), then we would only partially assess the impact of that variable on the outcome. For this reason, it is preferable to judge the significance of the variable using the likelihood ratio test statistic (LRS – Chapter 32), rather than by considering individual *P*-values for each of the dummy variables.

Ordinal explanatory variables

In the situation where we have an ordinal variable with more than two categories, we may take one of two approaches.
- Treat the categorical variable as a continuous numerical measurement by allocating a numerical value to each category of the variable. This approach makes full use of the ordering of the categories but it usually assumes a linear relationship (when the numerical values are equally spaced) between the explanatory variable and the dependent variable (or a transformation of it) and this should be validated.
- Treat the categorical variable as a nominal explanatory variable and create a series of dummy or indicator variables for it (Chapter 29). This approach does not take account of the ordering of the categories and is therefore wasteful of information. However, it does not assume a linear relationship with the dependent variable and so may be preferred.

The difference in the values of the LRS from these two models provides a test statistic for a **test of linear trend** (i.e. an assessment of whether the model assuming a linear relationship gives a better fitting model than one for which no linear relationship is assumed). This test statistic follows a Chi-squared distribution with degrees of freedom equal to the difference in the number of parameters in the two models; a significant result suggests non-linearity. See also Chapter 25 for a test of a linear trend in proportions.

Numerical explanatory variables

When we include a numerical explanatory variable in the model, the estimate of its regression coefficient provides an indication of the impact of a one-unit increase in the explanatory variable on the outcome. Thus, for simple and multiple linear regression, the relationship between each explanatory variable and the dependent variable is assumed to be linear. For Poisson and logistic regression, the parameter estimate provides a measure of the impact of a one-unit increase in the explanatory variable on the $\log_e$ of the dependent variable (i.e. the model assumes an exponential relationship with the actual rate or odds). It is important to check the appropriateness of the assumption of linearity (see next section) before including numerical explanatory variables in regression models.

Assessing the assumption of linearity

To check the linearity assumption in a simple or multiple linear regression model, we plot the numerical dependent variable, *y*, against the numerical explanatory variable, *x*, or plot the residuals of the model against *x* (Chapter 28). The raw data should approximate a straight line and there should be no discernible pattern in the residuals. We may assess the assumption of linearity in logistic regression (Chapter 30) or Poisson regression

(Chapter 31) by categorizing individuals into a small number (5–10) of equally sized subgroups according to their values of x. In Poisson regression, we calculate the log (to any base) of the rate of the outcome in each subgroup and plot this against the mid-point of the range of values for x for the corresponding subgroup (Fig. 33.1). For logistic regression, we similarly calculate the log odds for each subgroup and plot this against the mid-point. In each case, if the assumption of linearity is reasonable, we would expect to see a similarly sized step-wise increase (or decrease) in the log of the rate or odds when moving between adjacent categories of x. Another approach to checking for linearity in a regression model is to give consideration to higher order models (see polynomial regression in the next section).

Dealing with non-linearity

If non-linearity is detected in any of these plots, there are a number of approaches that can be taken.

• Replace x by a set of dummy variables created by categorizing the individuals into three or four subgroups according to the magnitude of x (often defined using the tertiles or quartiles of the distribution). This set of dummy variables can be incorporated into the multivariable regression model as categorical explanatory variables (see Example).

• Transform the x variable in some way (e.g. by taking a logarithmic or square root transformation of x; Chapter 9) so that the resulting relationship between the transformed value of x and the dependent variable (or its $\log_e$ for Poisson or its logit for logistic regression) *is* linear.

• Find some algebraic description that approximates the non-linear relationship using higher orders of x (e.g. a quadratic or cubic relationship). This is known as **polynomial regression**. We just introduce terms that represent the relevant higher orders of x into the equation. So, for example, if we have a cubic relationship, our estimated multiple linear regression equation is $Y = a + b_1x + b_2x^2 + b_3x^3$. We fit this model, and proceed with the analysis in exactly the same way as if the quadratic and cubic terms represented different variables (x_2 and x_3, say) in a multiple regression analysis. For example, we may fit a quadratic model that comprises the explanatory 'variables' height and height^2. We can **test for linearity** by comparing the LRS in the linear and quadratic models (Chapter 32), or by testing the coefficient of the quadratic term.

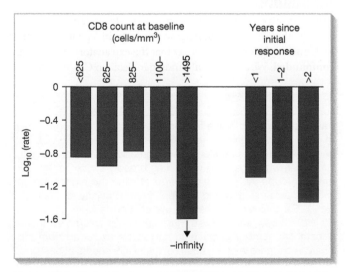

Figure 33.1 Plot of the $\log_{10}$ (rate) according to the baseline CD8 count and the time since initial response to HAART. Neither variable exhibits linearity.

Selecting explanatory variables

Even if not saturated (Chapter 32), there is always the danger of **overfitting** models by including a very large number of explanatory variables; this may lead to spurious results that are inconsistent with expectations, especially if the variables are highly correlated. For a multiple linear regression model, a usual rule of thumb is to ensure that there are *at least 10 times as many individuals as explanatory variables*. For logistic and Poisson regression, there should be at least 10 times as many *responses* or *events* in each of the two outcome categories as explanatory variables.

Often, we have a large number of explanatory variables that we believe may be related to the dependent variable. For example, many factors may appear to be related to systolic blood pressure, including age, dietary and other lifestyle factors. We should only include explanatory variables in a model if there is reason to suppose, from a biological or clinical standpoint, that they are related to the dependent variable. We can eliminate some variables by performing a *univariable* analysis (perhaps with a less stringent significance level of 0.10 rather than the more conventional 0.05) for each explanatory variable to assess whether it is likely to be related to the dependent variable, e.g. if we have a numerical dependent variable, we may perform a simple regression analysis if the explanatory variable is numerical or an unpaired t-test if it is binary. We then consider only those explanatory variables that were significant at this first stage for our multivariable model (see Example in Chapter 31).

Automatic selection procedures

When we have a large number of potential explanatory variables and are particularly interested in using the model for prediction, rather than in gaining insight into whether an explanatory variable influences the outcome or in estimating its effect, computer-intensive **automatic selection procedures** provide a means of identifying the optimal model by selecting some of these variables.

• **All subsets** – every combination of explanatory variables is considered; that which provides the best fit, as described by the model R^2 (Chapter 27) or LRS (Chapter 32), is selected.

• **Backward selection** – all possible variables are included; those that are judged by the model to be least important (where this decision is based on the change in R^2 or the LRS) are progressively removed until none of the remaining variables can be removed without significantly affecting the fit of the model.

• **Forward selection** – variables that contribute most to the fit of the model (based on the change in R^2 or the LRS) are progressively added until no further variable significantly improves the fit of the model.

• **Stepwise selection** – a combination of forward and backward selection that starts by progressing forward and then, at the end of each 'step', checks backward to ensure that all of the included variables are still required.

Disadvantages

Although these automatic procedures remove much of the manual aspect of model selection, they have some disadvantages.

• It is possible that two or more models will fit the data equally well, or that changes in the data set will produce different models.

• Because of the multiple testing that occurs when repeatedly comparing one model to another within an automatic selection procedure, the Type I error rate (Chapter 18) is particularly high. Thus, some significant findings may arise by chance. This problem may be alleviated by choosing a more stringent significance level (say 0.01 rather than 0.05).

- If the model is refitted to the data set using the *m*, say, variables remaining in the final automatic selection model, its estimated parameters may differ from those of the automatic selection model. This is because the automatic selection procedure uses in its analysis only those individuals who have complete information on *all* the explanatory variables, but the sample size may be greater when individuals are included if they have no missing values only for the relevant *m* variables.

- The resulting models, although mathematically justifiable, may not be sensible. In particular, when including a series of dummy variables to represent a single categorical variable (Chapter 29), automatic models may include only some of the dummy variables, leading to problems in interpretation.

Therefore, a combination of these procedures and common sense should be applied when selecting the best-fitting model. Models that are generated using automatic selection procedures should be validated on other external data sets where possible (Chapter 46).

Interaction

What is it?

Statistical **interaction** (also known as **effect modification**, Chapter 13) between two explanatory variables in a regression analysis occurs where the relationship between one of the explanatory variables and the dependent variable *is not the same for different levels* of the other explanatory variables, i.e. the two explanatory variables do not act independently on the dependent variable. For example, suppose that we want to assess the association between an individual's body weight (the explanatory variable) and the amount of a particular drug in his or her blood (the dependent variable). If we believe that this association is different for men and women in the study, we may wish to investigate whether there is an interaction between body weight and sex. If statistical testing reveals that there is evidence of a significant interaction, we may be advised to describe the association between body weight and the amount of the drug in the blood separately in men and women.

Testing for interaction

Testing for statistical interaction in a regression model is usually straightforward and many statistical packages allow you to request the inclusion of interaction terms. If the package does not provide this facility then an interaction term may be created manually by including the product of the relevant variables as an additional explanatory variable. Thus, to obtain the value of the variable that represents the interaction between two variables (both binary, both numerical or one binary and one numerical), we multiply the individual's values of these two variables. If both variables are numerical, interpretation may be easier if we create an interaction term from the two binary variables obtained by dichotomizing each numerical variable. If one of the two variables is categorical with more than two categories, we create a series of dummy variables from it (Chapter 29) and use each of them, together with the second binary or numerical variable of interest, to generate a series of interaction terms. This procedure can be extended if both variables are categorical and each has more than two categories.

Interaction terms should only be included in the regression model after the **main effects** (the effects of the variables without any interaction) have been included. Note that statistical tests of interaction are usually of **low power** (Chapter 18). This is of particular concern when both explanatory variables are categorical and few events occur in the subgroups formed by combining each level of one variable with every level of the other, or if these subgroups include very few individuals.

Collinearity

When two explanatory variables are highly correlated, it may be difficult to evaluate their individual effects in a multivariable regression model. As a consequence, while each variable may be significantly associated with the dependent variable in a univariable model (i.e. when there is a single explanatory variable), neither may be significantly associated with it when both explanatory variables are included in a multivariable model. This **collinearity** (also called **multi-collinearity**) can be detected by examining the correlation coefficients between each pair of explanatory variables (commonly displayed in a correlation matrix and of particular concern if the coefficient, ignoring its sign, is greater than 0.8) or by visual impression of the standard errors of the regression coefficients in the multivariable model (these will be substantially larger than those in the separate univariable models if collinearity is present). The easiest solution, if collinearity is detected between two variables, is to include only one of the variables in the model. In situations where many of the variables are highly correlated, it may be necessary to seek statistical advice.

Confounding

When two explanatory variables are both related to the outcome and to each other so that it is difficult to assess the independent effect of each one on the outcome, we say that the explanatory variables are **confounded**. We discuss confounding in detail in Chapter 34.

Example

In Chapters 31 and 32 we studied the factors associated with virological failure in HIV-positive patients receiving highly active antiretroviral therapy (HAART). In this multivariable Poisson regression analysis, the individual's CD8 count at baseline was included as a continuous explanatory variable (it was divided by 100 so that each unit increase in the scaled variable reflected a 100 cell/mm^3 increase in the CD8 count); the results indicated that a higher baseline CD8 count was associated with a significantly reduced rate of virological failure. In order to assess the validity of the **linearity assumption** associated with this variable, five groups were defined on the basis of the quintiles of the CD8 distribution, and the failure rate was calculated in each of the five groups. A plot of the $\log_{10}$ (rate) in each of these groups revealed that the relationship was *not* linear as there was no stepwise progression (see Fig. 33.1). In particular, while the $\log_{10}$ (rate) was broadly similar in the four lowest groups, no events occurred at all in the highest group (> 1495 cells/mm^3), giving a value of minus infinity for the $\log_{10}$ (rate). For this reason, the two upper groups were combined for the subsequent analysis. Furthermore, it was noted that a substantial number of patients had to be excluded from this analysis as there was no record of their CD8 counts at baseline.

Thus, because of the lack of linearity between the log of the virological failure rate and the actual CD8 count, the continuous

continued

explanatory variable representing the CD8 count in the Poisson regression model was replaced by a series of four dummy variables (Chapter 29). Individuals with baseline CD8 counts in the range 825 < CD8 < 1100 cells/mm^3 were treated as the reference group for these indicator variables. Each of three dummy variables provided a comparison of one of the remaining CD8 groups with the reference group, and the fourth dummy provided a comparison of those with missing CD8 counts with the reference group. The results are summarized in Table 33.1; a full computer output is shown in Appendix C. A comparison of the value for − 2log likelihood (i.e. the LRS or deviance) from the model that included the four dummy variables for the CD8 count (387.15) with that from the model that included the same variables apart from these dummy variables (392.50) gave a P-value of 0.25 (test statistic of 5.35 on 4 degrees of freedom). Thus, after incorporating it in this way, the CD8 count no longer had a statistically significant relationship with virological failure in contrast to the model which, inappropriately, incorporated the CD8 count as a continuous explanatory variable. The relationships between virological failure and treatment status, sex and time since initial response to therapy, however, remained similar.

Table 33.1 Results from multivariable Poisson regression analysis of factors associated with virological failure, after including the CD8 count as a categorical variable in the model.

Variable*	Parameter estimate	Standard error	Estimated relative rate	95% confidence interval for relative rate	P-value[†]
Time since initial response to therapy (years)					
<1	reference	−	1	−	
1–2	0.4550	0.2715	1.58	0.93–2.68	
>2	−0.5386	0.4849	0.58	0.23–1.51	0.06
Treatment status					
Previously received treatment (0)	reference	−	1	−	
Never received treatment (1)	−0.5580	0.2600	0.57	0.34–0.95	0.03
Sex					
Female (0)	reference	−	1	−	
Male (1)	−0.4970	0.2675	0.61	0.36–1.03	0.07
CD8 count (cells/mm^3)					
<625	−0.2150	0.6221	0.81	0.24–2.73	
≥625, < 825	−0.3646	0.7648	0.63	0.16–3.11	
≥825, <1100	reference	−	1	−	
≥1100	−0.3270	1.1595	0.78	0.07–7.00	
Missing	−0.8264	0.6057	0.44	0.13–1.43	0.25

* Codes for binary variables (sex and treatment status) are shown in parentheses. Time since initial response to therapy was included by incorporating two dummy variables to reflect the periods 1–2 years and > 2 years after initial response. The baseline CD8 count was incorporated as described in the text.

[†] P-values were obtained using LRS (Chapter 32); where dummy variables were used to incorporate more than two categories of the variable, the P-value reflects the combined effect of these dummies.

34 Bias and confounding

In many cases, despite all of our efforts to design a robust study and perform appropriate statistical analyses, the results from our study may not accurately reflect the true situation. This may be due to the presence of bias which can be introduced at any stage of the study, perhaps resulting from a failure to take account of important exposure (explanatory) variables.

Bias

What is it?

Bias is said to have occurred when there is a systematic difference between the results from a study and the true state of affairs. Bias may be introduced at all stages of the research process, from study design, through to analysis and publication. Bias can create a spurious association (i.e. overestimation of an effect) or mask a real one (underestimation of an effect). While appropriate statistical methods can reduce the effect of bias, they may not be able to eliminate it entirely. It is thus preferable to design a study so that bias is minimized (e.g. by taking steps to reduce recall bias in a case–control study, or by attempting to minimize loss to follow-up in a longitudinal study). It should be noted that increasing the sample size *does not* reduce bias – if anything, increasing the sample size might actually increase the impact of bias.

We have already described the biases that are most commonly encountered in clinical trials (Chapter 14), case–control studies (Chapter 15) and cohort studies (Chapter 16). However, there are many forms of bias[1] which may broadly be categorized as forms of either selection or information bias. A third type of bias, caused by confounding, is discussed in the next section. Even if obvious sources of bias have been addressed, **funding bias**, whereby there is a tendency to report findings in the direction favoured by the funding body (such as a pharmaceutical company), and **publication bias**, whereby there is a tendency to publish only those papers that report positive or topical results, may mean that the results from publicly available studies are still misleading.

Selection bias

Selection bias occurs when patients included in the study are not representative of the population to which the results will be applied, e.g. patients who agree to participate in a study may differ from those who do not agree to participate (this form of bias is a particular problem in retrospective studies when patients who have died are not included in the study). Selection bias includes the following:

- **Ascertainment bias** may occur when the sample included in a study is not randomly selected from the population and differs in some important respects from that population, e.g. when doctors interested in the genetics of a particular medical condition collect information on the patients in their clinic, rather than using a random sample from the population.
- **Attrition bias** arises when those who are lost to follow-up in a longitudinal study (Chapter 12) differ in a systematic way from those who are not lost to follow-up.
- The **healthy entrant effect** occurs where mortality and morbidity rates are lower in the initial stages of a longitudinal study than in the general population because the individuals included in the study are disease-free at its outset (Chapter 15).
- **Response bias** is caused by differences in characteristics between those who choose or volunteer to participate in a study and those who do not.
- **Survivorship bias** occurs when survival is compared in patients who do or who do not receive a particular intervention where this intervention only became available at some point after the start of the study so that patients have to survive long enough to be eligible to receive the intervention.

Information bias

Information bias occurs during data collection when measurements on exposure and/or disease outcome are incorrectly recorded in a systematic manner. Information bias includes the following:

- **Central tendency bias** often arises when using a Likert scale (comprising a small number of graded alternative responses such as very poor, poor, no opinion, good, excellent) where responders tend to move towards the mid-point of the scale (usually 'no opinion' or 'just right').
- **Lead-time bias** occurs particularly in studies assessing changes in survival over time where the development of more accurate diagnostic procedures may mean that patients entered later into the study are diagnosed at an earlier stage in their disease, resulting in an apparent increase in survival from the time of diagnosis.
- **Measurement bias** arises when a systematic error is introduced by an inaccurate measurement tool (e.g. a set of poorly calibrated scales); it may also be introduced by **digit preference** or **rounding error**.
- **Misclassification bias** occurs when we incorrectly classify a categorical exposure and/or outcome variable. This may dilute or exaggerate the effect of interest, depending on whether the misclassification occurs equally in all groups or varies according to exposure group.

Medical Statistics at a Glance, Fourth Edition. Aviva Petrie and Caroline Sabin © 2020 Aviva Petrie and Caroline Sabin. Published 2020 by John Wiley & Sons Ltd.
Companion Website: www.medstatsaag.com

- **Observer bias** occurs when one observer tends to under-report (or over-report) a particular variable; also called **assessment bias**.
- **Regression dilution bias** may occur when fitting a regression model to describe the association between an outcome variable and one or more exposure variable(s). If there is substantial measurement error (Chapter 39) around one of the exposure variables, the associated regression parameter from the model may be attenuated.
- **Reporting bias** occurs when participants give answers in the direction they perceive are of interest to the researcher or under-report socially unacceptable or embarrassing behaviours or disorders (e.g. alcohol consumption or sexually transmitted disease).
- **Regression to the mean** occurs where measurements that follow particularly low measurements tend to be higher than those recorded previously, and those that follow particularly high measurements tend to be lower (Chapter 27).

The **ecological fallacy** results in a bias which sometimes occurs when we reach conclusions based solely on aggregate statistics for groups within a population. We believe mistakenly that an association that we observe between variables at an aggregate level reflects the corresponding association at an individual level in the same population. This is particularly relevant when we do not have the necessary information about a variable at the patient level but only at the study level (e.g. in a meta-analysis, Chapter 43), and is common in ecological studies where we note associations between the level of disease in a population (often an entire country) which are not apparent when we consider the association at the individual level. For example, living in a more deprived area has been shown[2] to be associated with an increased likelihood of being diagnosed with Stage III or IV breast cancer, but since the study used an area-based measure of low socioeconomic background, these results cannot be extended to individual women living in the area. The ecological fallacy is particularly true in meta-regression (Chapter 43).

Confounding

What is it?

Confounding occurs when we find a spurious association between a potential risk factor and a disease outcome or miss a real association between them because we have failed to adjust for any confounding variables. A **confounding variable** or **confounder** is an exposure variable that is related to both the outcome variable (e.g. disease) and to one or more of the other exposure variables. For example, we may be interested in studying the effect of smoking status on the incidence of coronary heart disease (CHD) in a cohort of middle-aged men. However, we know that alcohol consumption is associated with the development of CHD, and that alcohol consumption and smoking are also related to each other (i.e. men who consume alcohol are more likely to smoke than men who do not consume alcohol). Thus, in this study, unless we adjust for it, the effect of alcohol consumption may confound an apparent relationship between smoking and the incidence of CHD. Any analysis that considers the effect of an exposure variable on the outcome but does not take into account the confounder may misrepresent the true role of the exposure variable. Failure to adjust for confounding factors in a regression analysis will lead to biased estimates of the parameters of the model.

We should be aware that **Simpson's paradox** (Chapter 24) may arise when the effect of confounding is very strong.

Dealing with confounding

Confounding may be dealt with at the design stage of an experimental study (e.g. by matching or randomization) or at the analysis stage of an observational study in one of a number of ways. A brief description of each approach follows and their advantages and disadvantages are summarized in Table 34.1.

- Create **subgroups** by stratifying the data set by the levels of the confounding variable (e.g. create two subgroups, drinkers and non-drinkers) and then perform an analysis separately in each subgroup. While this approach is simple and has much to recommend it when there are few confounders,
  - the subgroups may be small, and thus the analyses will have reduced power to detect a significant effect;
  - spurious significant results may arise because of multiple testing (Chapter 18) if a hypothesis test is performed in each subgroup; and
  - it may be difficult to combine the separate estimates of the effect of interest for each subgroup (although this is sometimes achieved by the **Mantel–Haenszel** method[3]).
- Identify pairs of individuals, one of whom falls into each category of the exposure variable (e.g. a smoker and a non-smoker), who are **matched** on the basis of all confounding variables. By performing an appropriate paired analysis (e.g. McNemar's test or a paired t-test) of the association between the exposure variable and the dependent variable, the effects of any potential confounding variables will be removed. However, if there are many confounders, it may be difficult to identify sufficient pairs of matched individuals to ensure an adequately powered analysis.
- Adjust for each confounding variable by including it as an explanatory variable in a **multivariable regression model**, e.g. multiple linear (Chapter 29), logistic (Chapter 30) or Poisson (Chapter 31) regression models. This approach, which is particularly useful when there are many confounders in the study, provides an estimate of the relationship between the explanatory and dependent variables *that cannot be explained* by the relationship between the dependent variable and the confounding variables. In order to obtain meaningful results, however, there must be reasonable overlap between the distributions of the confounding variables in the groups defined by the exposure variable (i.e. smokers and non-smokers should have fairly similar demographic profiles if these comprise the confounding variables).
- Use a **propensity score**[4] approach. This method is most useful when the exposure variable of interest (smoking status) has two levels (categories) and is specified at the start of the study, and where there are many potential confounders. A score is calculated for each individual, often using a logistic regression model (Chapter 30) that describes his/her *propensity* (or probability) to fall into one particular category of the exposure variable as opposed to the other (i.e. to be a smoker or a non-smoker). This propensity score is generated using the data on all variables that may be associated with smoking, some of which may also be associated with the outcome and will therefore be confounders (e.g. alcohol status). We then use this propensity score in one of the following ways:
  - Adjust for this propensity score, rather than the variables used to generate the score (including the confounders), in a multivariable regression analysis that aims to investigate the association between the exposure variable (smoking) and the dependent variable (CHD). As well as distributional advantages, this approach has the advantage of reducing the number of covariates in the model.

Table 34.1 Advantages and disadvantages of various methods to remove confounding during the analytical stage of a study.

Method	Advantages	Disadvantages
Stratification by confounding variable	• Simple to visualize findings and interpret results • Straightforward • Provides a means of checking that there is sufficient overlap in the confounders between the different exposure groups • Results are not affected by any assumptions about the form of the relationship between the confounder and the outcome (e.g. linearity)	• Only suitable if there are a small number of confounders • May result in very small strata and hence a low power within specific strata (Chapter 18) • Multiple testing may lead to spurious significant findings (Chapter 18) • May be difficult to provide a single estimate of the treatment effect
Direct matching confounders	• Intuitively simple and simple to interpret findings • Can deal with more than one confounder • Results are not affected by any assumptions about the form of the relationship between the confounder and the outcome (e.g. linearity)	• May not be possible to find a match for each patient; exclusion of unmatched patients from the analysis may result in loss of power • Cannot estimate the effects of the confounders on the outcome • May be computationally difficult to match patients if there are many confounders
Statistical adjustment in multivariable regression model	• Suitable if there are many confounders, provided the sample size is adequate • Can estimate the effects of the confounders on the outcome • Computationally straightforward	• If there are a large number of confounders, study power may be reduced • Only provides meaningful results if the groups defined by the exposure variable are reasonably well balanced in terms of the confounders • Can only adjust for confounders for which data have been collected
Calculation of propensity scores	• Relatively easy to calculate when the exposure variable has two levels • Even if there is insufficient overlap of specific confounders across exposure groups, the distribution of propensity scores should be similar across the groups	• Difficult to calculate when the exposure variable has more than two levels • Only suitable when the exposure variable does not change over time • Most efficient when the sample size is large
Use of propensity scores		
• Statistical adjustment for propensity score in multivariable regression model	• Reduces the number of covariates in the model	• If confounders are also included in the model (i.e. there is interest in their associations with the outcome), there may be collinearity (Chapter 33) between them and the propensity score
• Stratification by propensity score	• Removes the effect of potential confounding variables in each stratum	• May be difficult to combine estimates from the different propensity score strata
• Matching on propensity score	• Removes the effect of potential confounding variables without the need to adjust for them in the analysis	• May be difficult to match patients

▪ Use the propensity score as a stratification variable, with the effect of the exposure variable on which it was based (smoking) estimated separately for those in different propensity score strata (often using a multivariable regression analysis) – the argument being that individuals in the same propensity score stratum should have similar levels of the potential confounding variables. We can use Mantel–Haenszel methods to obtain a combined estimate of the effect of interest from the different strata.

▪ Identify pairs of individuals, one of whom falls into each category of the exposure variable (e.g. a smoker and a non-smoker) but who are *matched* on the basis of the *propensity scores* (i.e. the likelihood of being a smoker is similar in the two members of a pair, even though one of them is not a smoker). As when matching on the confounding variables, this matched analysis of the association between the exposure variable and the dependent variable will remove the effects of any potential confounding variables without the need to adjust for these variables in the analysis. The disadvantage of this approach is that some individuals may have to be excluded from the analysis if a suitable matched pair cannot be identified, although matching on the propensity scores should result in exclusion of a smaller number of individuals than a similar analysis that matches on the confounding variables.

▪ Use double-robust estimation (beyond the scope of this book).

Note that neither a multivariable regression model nor a propensity score approach can remove the effects of unmeasured or unknown confounders.

Confounding in non-randomized studies

Confounding is a particular concern in cohort studies (Chapter 15) when risk factors are not distributed randomly in the population. In particular, when we are interested in the effect of a specific intervention (e.g. a treatment) on an outcome in a cohort study, we have to be aware that individuals may be selected for this intervention on the basis of disease history or demographic or lifestyle factors, some of which may also be related to the outcome. If the characteristics of patients receiving this intervention differ from those of patients receiving other types of interventions, then **allocation** or **channelling bias** has occurred. Suppose, for example, we are interested in comparing the effect of treatment on the incidence of cardiovascular disease in a cohort of middle-aged men, when the men are receiving either statins or fibrates at the time of cohort enrolment. The choice of whether a man receives a statin or a fibrate will be based on a number of factors (e.g. their lipid measurements), many of which will also be associated with the development of cardiovascular disease. While multivariable regression models and/or propensity score methods (using the choice of treatment as the exposure variable of interest for which a propensity score is determined) can be used to adjust for any differences in the distribution of the factors in the different treatment groups, this is only possible if the study investigators are aware of the confounding factors and have recorded them in the data set. Randomized controlled trials (Chapter 14) rarely suffer from confounding as patients are randomly allocated to treatment groups and therefore all covariates, both confounders and other explanatory variables, should be evenly distributed in the different treatment groups.

The causal pathway and confounding

The **causal pathway** is the chain of events or factors leading in sequence to an outcome when the effect of any step in the sequence is caused by the event at the previous step(s). The causal pathway is particularly useful in helping us consider opportunities for disease prevention and is sometimes represented by a path diagram on which the causal relationship is shown by arrows (e.g. multiple birth → preterm delivery → neonatal cerebral damage in cerebral palsy). Where a variable (B) is known to lie on the causal pathway between an exposure (A) and the outcome of interest (C), it is known as an **intermediate variable** and it should not be treated as a confounder.

Consider the situation where we are conducting a randomized placebo-controlled trial of the effect of a new cholesterol-lowering drug on the incidence of CHD (the outcome, C) and our exposure variable (A) is a binary variable that indicates whether or not each individual is receiving the new drug. An elevated cholesterol is one of the known risk factors for CHD, and we expect levels to decline in treated individuals but remain unchanged or increase in untreated individuals. Although we may adjust for any discrepancies between the cholesterol levels of patients in the two treatment groups at the *start* of the trial (although this should not be necessary if randomization has been successful), we should be careful about adjusting for any *changes* in cholesterol (B) that occur during the trial period. If we were to do so, the observed treatment effect would only estimate any residual benefit that remains after effects of cholesterol have been removed; it would not estimate the total benefit of the new drug. Indeed, if the drug acts solely through changes in cholesterol, it is likely that there will be no residual effects – this does not mean that the drug does not work, simply that it does not have any effects over and above those it has on cholesterol.

Time-varying confounding

A particular problem arises if a variable is both a potential confounder for an exposure of interest and also lies on the causal pathway between that exposure and the study outcome. Where the exposure itself may change over time, the confounder is known as a **time-varying confounder**. Suppose, for example, that we wish to use data from a cohort study to describe the effect of antiretroviral treatment on survival in individuals infected with HIV. HIV acts by gradually depressing an individual's immune system; this is measured through the CD4 cell count, which will decline over time in an HIV-positive person. Currently, antiretroviral treatment in the developed world is generally offered to an HIV-positive individual whose CD4 cell count has already fallen to a low level (usually below 350 cells/mm^3). However, once treatment is initiated, most individuals will experience a rapid increase in their CD4 cell count and this increase is associated with prolonged survival. In this situation, the CD4 count (which may be measured regularly over the period of infection) is a time-varying confounder, as it is both a predictor of the initiation of treatment and it lies on the causal pathway between initiation of antiretroviral treatment and death. In such circumstances, the usual approach to analysing the data using standard regression models with time-dependent covariates (Chapter 31) will not provide a meaningful estimate of the effect of treatment. Complex analytical methods (*causal modelling, marginal structural models, G-estimation*) provide a more appropriate estimate of this treatment effect[5] but they should only be used in discussion with a statistician.

References

1 Delgado-Rodriguez, M. and Llorca, J. (2004) Bias. *Journal of Epidemiology and Community Health*, **58**, 635–641.

2 Downing, A., Prakash, K., Gilthorpe, M.S., Mikeljevic, J.S. and Forman, D. (2007) Socioeconomic background in relation to stage at diagnosis, treatment and survival in women with breast cancer. *British Journal of Cancer*, **96**, 836–840.

3 Fleiss, J.L., Levin, B. and Paik, M.C. (2003). *Statistical Methods for Rates and Proportions*. 3rd edition. New York: Wiley.

4 Austin, P.C. (2011) A tutorial and case study in propensity score analysis: an application to estimating the effect of in-hospital smoking cessation counseling on mortality. *Multivariate Behavioral Research*, **46**, 119–151.

5 Hernán, M.A. and Robins, J.M. (2006) Estimating causal effects from epidemiological data. *Journal of Epidemiology and Community Health*, **60**, 578–586.

35 Checking assumptions

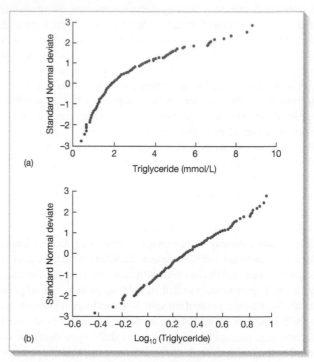

Figure 35.1 (a) Normal plot of untransformed triglyceride levels described in Chapter 19. These are skewed and the resulting Normal plot shows a distinct curve. (b) Normal plot of $\log_{10}$ (triglyceride levels). The approximately straight line indicates that the log transformation has been successful at removing the skewness in the data.

Why bother?

Computer analysis of data offers the opportunity of handling large data sets that might otherwise be beyond our capabilities. However, do not be tempted to 'have a go' at statistical analyses simply because they are available on the computer. The validity of the conclusions drawn relies on the appropriate analysis being conducted in any given circumstance, and a requirement that the underlying assumptions inherent in the proposed statistical analysis are satisfied.

Are the data Normally distributed?

Many analyses make assumptions about the underlying distribution of the data. The following procedures verify approximate Normality, the most common of the distributional assumptions.
• We produce a dot plot (for small samples) or a histogram, stem-and-leaf plot (Fig. 4.2) or box plot (Fig. 6.1) to show the empirical frequency distribution of the data (Chapter 4). We conclude that the distribution is approximately Normal if it is bell-shaped and symmetrical. The median in a box plot should cut the rectangle defining the first and third quartiles in half, and the two whiskers should be of equal length if the data are Normally distributed.
• Alternatively, we can produce a **Normal plot** (preferably on the computer) which plots the Standard Normal deviate for the cumulative distribution against the sample values. Lack of Normality is indicated by the resulting plot producing a curve that deviates from a straight line (Fig. 35.1).

Although both approaches are subjective, the Normal plot is more effective for smaller samples. The **Kolmogorov–Smirnov** and **Shapiro–Wilk tests**, both performed on the computer, can be used to assess Normality more objectively.

Are two or more variances equal?

We explained how to use the t-test (Chapter 21) to compare two means and ANOVA (Chapter 22) to compare more than two

means. Underlying these analyses is the assumption that the variability of the observations in each group is the same, i.e. we require equal variances, described as **homogeneity of variance** or **homoscedasticity**. We have **heterogeneity of variance** if the variances are unequal.
• We can use **Levene's test**, using a computer program, to test for homogeneity of variance in two or more groups. The null hypothesis is that all the variances are equal. Levene's test has the advantage that it is not strongly dependent on the assumption of Normality. **Bartlett's test** can also be used to compare more than two variances, but it is non-robust to departures from Normality.
• We can use the **F-test (variance ratio test)** described in the following box to compare two variances, provided the data in each group are approximately Normally distributed (the test is non-robust to a violation of this assumption). The two estimated variances are s_1^2 and s_2^2, calculated from n_1 and n_2 observations, respectively. By convention, we choose s_1^2 to be the larger of the two variances, if they differ.
• We also assume homogeneity of variance of the *residuals* in simple and multiple regression (Chapters 28 and 29) and in random effects models (Chapter 42). We explained how to check this assumption in Chapters 28 and 29.

---

1 **Define the null and alternative hypotheses under study**
   H_0: the two population variances are equal
   H_1: the two population variances are unequal.
2 **Collect relevant data from a sample of individuals**
3 **Calculate the value of the test statistic specific to H_0**

$$F = s_1^2 / s_2^2$$

which follows an F-distribution with $n_1 - 1$ df in the numerator, and $n_2 - 1$ df in the denominator. Since $s_1^2 \geq s_2^2$, the F-ratio ≥ 1. This allows us to use the tables of the F-distribution that are tabulated only for values ≥ 1.
4 **Compare the value of the test statistic to values from a known probability distribution**
   Refer F to Appendix A5. Our two-sided alternative hypothesis leads to a two-tailed test.
5 **Interpret the P-value and results**
   Note that we are rarely interested in the variances *per se*, so we do not usually calculate confidence intervals for them[1].

Are variables linearly related?

Most of the techniques discussed in Chapters 26–31 and described in Chapter 42 assume that there is a **linear** (straight line) relationship between two variables. We explained how to check for linearity and how to deal with non-linearity in regression analysis in Chapters 28 and 29 (for simple and multiple regression) and in Chapter 33 (for other generalized linear models, e.g. logistic and Poisson).

What if the assumptions are not satisfied?

We have various options.

• Proceed as planned, recognizing that this may result in a non-robust analysis. Be aware of the implications if you do this. Do not be fooled into an inappropriate analysis just because others, in similar circumstances, have done one in the past!

• Take an appropriate transformation of the raw data so that the transformed data satisfy the assumptions of the proposed analysis (Chapter 9). In regression analysis, this usually means transforming an x variable although other approaches are possible (Chapter 32).

• If feasible, perform a **non-parametric test** (Chapter 17) that does not make any assumptions about the distribution of the data (e.g. Normality). You may also come across the term *non-parametric regression analysis*[2]; its purpose is to estimate the functional form (rather than the parameters) of the relationship between a response variable and one or more explanatory variables. Using non-parametric regression, we relax the linearity assumption of the model and fit a smooth curve to the data so that we can visualize trends without specifying a parametric model.

Sensitivity analysis

An analysis is robust if it is not very sensitive to a departure from its assumptions, i.e. the P-value and power (Chapter 18) and, if relevant, parameter estimates are not appreciably affected by violations of the assumptions. Thus, the conclusions drawn from the study are likely to be correct even though the assumptions are violated. However, a non-robust analysis could result in misleading conclusions being drawn. After any analysis, it is thus always wise to consider performing one or more **sensitivity analyses** to investigate the robustness of the findings. To do this, we use a slightly different approach to analysing the data (e.g. by omitting data, varying the assumptions or using a different method of analysis) and measure the impact of any changes on our estimates and conclusions. Note that sensitivity analyses should always be described as such when presenting results – it is inappropriate, for example, to perform multiple different statistical tests that essentially investigate the same or similar hypotheses and display all their results without identifying which was the primary analysis and which were sensitivity analyses. Furthermore, if sensitivity analyses are to be presented, it is inappropriate to show only the most favourable results (i.e. those that most strongly support the primary aims). The following are examples of different sensitivity analyses:

• Rather than assuming a linear relationship between the dependent variable and a continuous explanatory variable in a regression analysis (Chapter 29), we re-fit the regression model after creating a new nominal explanatory variable based on categories of the original explanatory variable (Chapter 33). If there are two categories of interest then we have one binary nominal variable but if there are more than two categories we would create dummy binary variables (Chapter 29).

• Having performed a parametric analysis of the data (e.g. an unpaired t-test), we repeat the analysis using a non-parametric approach (e.g. the Mann–Whitney U test).

• After identifying influential points (Chapter 29) in a multiple regression analysis, we re-fit the model excluding these points.

• Having performed a meta-analysis (Chapter 43) using the data from all studies, we repeat it but exclude poorer quality studies.

• We undertake both a fixed and a random effects meta-analysis to assess how robust the results are to the method used.

• We assess the effect of the approach taken to deal with any missing data (Chapter 3) by repeating the analysis after using a different approach.

References

1 Armitage, P., Berry, G. and Matthews, J.N.S. (2002) *Statistical Methods in Medical Research*. 4th edition. Oxford: Blackwell Science.
2 Eubank, R.L. (1999) *Nonparametric Regression and Spline Smoothing*. New York: Marcel Dekker

Example

In Example 1 in Chapter 21, 98 school-age children were randomly assigned to receive either inhaled beclomethasone dipropionate or a placebo to determine their effects on wheezing. We used the unpaired t-test to compare the mean forced expiratory volume in 1 second (FEV1) in each group over the 6 months, but need assurance that the underlying assumptions (Normality and constant variance) are satisfied. The stem-and-leaf plot in Fig. 4.2 shows that the data in each group are approximately Normally distributed. We performed the **F-test** to investigate the assumption of equal variances.

1 H_0: the variance of FEV1 measurements in the population of school-age children is the same in the two groups

H_1: the variance of FEV1 measurements in the population of school-age children is not the same in the two groups.

2 Treated group: sample size, $n_1 = 50$, standard deviation, $s_1 = 0.29$ litres

Placebo group: sample size, $n_2 = 48$, standard deviation, $s_2 = 0.25$ litres.

3 The test statistic $F = \dfrac{s_1^2}{s_2^2} = \dfrac{0.29^2}{0.25^2} = \dfrac{0.0841}{0.0625} = 1.346$

follows an F-distribution with $50 - 1 = 49$ and $48 - 1 = 47$ df in the numerator and denominator, respectively.

4 We refer $F = 1.35$ to Appendix A5 for a two-sided test at the 5% level of significance. Because Appendix A5 is restricted to entries of 25 and infinity df in the numerator, and 30 and 50 df in the denominator, we have to interpolate (Chapter 21). The required tabulated value at the 5% level of significance lies between 1.57 and 2.12; thus $P > 0.05$ because 1.35 is less than the minimum of these values (computer output gives $P = 0.31$).

5 There is insufficient evidence to reject the null hypothesis that the variances are equal. It is reasonable to use the unpaired t-test, which assumes Normality and homogeneity of variance, to compare the mean FEV1 in the two groups.

36 Sample size calculations

The importance of sample size

If the number of patients in our study is small, we may have inadequate power (Chapter 18) to detect an important existing effect, and we shall have wasted all our resources. On the other hand, if the sample size is unduly large, the study may be unnecessarily time-consuming, expensive and unethical, depriving some of the patients of the superior treatment. We therefore have to choose the optimal sample size that strikes a balance between the implications of making a Type I or Type II error (Chapter 18). Unfortunately, in order to calculate the sample size required, we have to have some idea of the results we expect in the study.

Requirements

We shall explain how to calculate the optimal sample size in simple situations; often more complex designs can be simplified for the purpose of calculating the sample size. If our investigation involves a number of tests, we concentrate on the most important or evaluate the sample size required for each and choose the largest.

Our focus is the calculation of the optimal sample size in relation to a proposed hypothesis test. However, it is possible to base the sample size calculation on other aspects of the study, such as on the precision of an estimate or on the width of a confidence interval (the process usually adopted in equivalence and non-inferiority studies, Chapter 17).

To calculate the optimal sample size for a test, we need to specify the following quantities *at the design stage of the investigation*.

- **Power** (Chapter 18) – the chance of detecting, as statistically significant, a specified effect if it exists. We usually choose a power of at least 80%.
- **Significance level**, α (Chapter 17) – the cut-off level below which we will reject the null hypothesis, i.e. it is the maximum probability of incorrectly concluding that there is an effect. We usually fix this as 0.05 or, occasionally, as 0.01, and reject the null hypothesis if the *P*-value is less than this value.
- **Variability** of the observations, e.g. the standard deviation, if we have a numerical variable.
- **Smallest effect of interest** – the magnitude of the effect that is clinically important and which we do not want to overlook. This is often a *difference* (e.g. difference in means or proportions). Sometimes it is expressed as a multiple of the standard deviation of the observations (the **standardized difference**).

It is relatively simple to choose the power and significance level of the test that suit the requirements of our study. The choice is usually governed by the implications of a Type I and a Type II error, but may be specified by the regulatory bodies in some drug licensing studies. Given a particular clinical scenario, it is possible to specify the effect we regard as clinically important. The real difficulty lies in providing an estimate of the variation in a numerical variable before we have collected the data. We may be able to obtain this information from published studies with similar outcomes or we may need to carry out a **pilot study**. Although a pilot study is usually a distinct preliminary investigation, we may incorporate the data gathered in the pilot study into the main study using an **internal pilot study**[1], provided all details of it are documented in the protocol. We determine the optimal sample size on the best, although perhaps limited, information available at the design stage of the study. We then use the relevant information from a pilot study (the size of which is pre-specified, may be relatively large and is usually determined through practical considerations) to revise our estimated sample size for the main study. (Note: the calculation must be based on the originally defined smallest effect of interest, *not* on the effect observed in the pilot study, and the revised sample size estimate utilized only if it exceeds the original estimate.) In such situations, the information gathered in the internal pilot study may be used in the final analysis of the data.

Methodology

We can calculate sample size in a number of ways, each of which requires essentially the same information (described in 'Requirements') in order to proceed:

- **General formulae**[2]– these can be complex but may be necessary in some situations (e.g. to retain power in a cluster randomized trial (Chapters 14 and 41), we multiply the sample size that would be required if we were carrying out individual randomization by the design effect equal to $[1 + (m - 1)\rho]$, where m is the average cluster size and ρ is the intraclass correlation coefficient (Chapter 42)).
- **Quick formulae** – these exist for particular power values and significance levels for some hypothesis tests (e.g. Lehr's formulae[3], see later in this chapter).
- **Special tables**[2]– these exist for different situations (e.g. for *t*-tests, Chi-squared tests, tests of the correlation coefficient, comparing two survival curves, and equivalence studies).

Medical Statistics at a Glance, Fourth Edition. Aviva Petrie and Caroline Sabin. © 2020 Aviva Petrie and Caroline Sabin. Published 2020 by John Wiley & Sons Ltd.
Companion Website: www.medstatsaag.com

- **Altman's nomogram** – this is an easy-to-use diagram which is appropriate for various tests. Details are given in the next section.
- **Computer software** – this has the advantage that results can be presented graphically or in tables to show the effect of changing the factors (e.g. power, size of effect) on the required sample size.

Altman's nomogram

Notation

We show in Table 36.1 the notation for using Altman's nomogram (Appendix B) to estimate the sample size of two *equally sized* groups of observations for three frequently used hypothesis tests of means and proportions.

Method

For each test, we calculate the standardized difference and join its value on the left-hand axis of the nomogram to the power we have specified on the right-hand vertical axis. The required sample size is indicated at the point at which the resulting line and sample size axis meet.

Note that we can also use the nomogram to evaluate the power of a hypothesis test for a given sample size. Occasionally, this is useful if we wish to know, retrospectively, whether we can attribute lack of significance in a hypothesis test to an inadequately sized sample. In such *post hoc* power calculations, the clinically important treatment difference must be that which was decided *a priori*; it is not the observed treatment effect. Remember, also, that a wide confidence interval for the effect of interest indicates an imprecise estimate, often due to an insufficiently sized study (Chapter 11).

Quick formulae

For the unpaired *t*-test and Chi-squared test, we can use **Lehr's formula**[3] for calculating the sample size for a power of 80% and a two-sided significance level of 0.05. The required sample size in each group is

$$\frac{16}{(\text{Standardized difference})^2}$$

If the standardized difference is small, this formula overestimates the sample size. Note that a numerator of 21 (instead of 16) relates to a power of 90%.

Power statement

It is often essential and always useful to include a power statement in a study protocol or in the methods section of a paper (see Appendix D, Table D1) to show that careful thought has been given to sample size at the design stage of the investigation. A typical statement might be '110 patients in the early physical therapy and 110 patients in the usual care group are required, using the unpaired *t*-test, to have a 90% chance of detecting a difference of 7 points in the mean change in ODI at 3 months between the two groups (SD = 16 points) at the 5% level of significance' (see Example 1).

Adjustments

We may wish to adjust the sample size:
- to allow for **losses to follow-up** by recruiting more patients into the study at the outset. If we believe that the drop-out rate will be *r*%, then the adjusted sample size is obtained by multiplying the unadjusted sample size by $100/(100 - r)$;
- to have independent **groups of different sizes**. This may be desirable when one group is restricted in size, perhaps because the disease is rare in a case–control study (Chapter 16) or because the novel drug treatment is in short supply. Note, however, that the imbalance in numbers usually results in a larger overall sample size when compared with a balanced design if a similar level of power is to be maintained. If the ratio of the sample sizes in the two groups is *k* (e.g. *k* = 3 if we require one

Table 36.1 Information for using Altman's nomogram

Hypothesis test	Standardized difference	Explanation of *N* in nomogram	Terminology
Unpaired *t*-test (Chapter 21)	$\dfrac{\delta}{\sigma}$	*N*/2 observations in each group	δ: the smallest difference in means that is clinically important σ: the assumed equal standard deviation of the observations in each of the two groups. You can estimate it using results from a similar study conducted previously or from published information. Alternatively, you could perform a pilot study to estimate it. Another approach is to express δ as a multiple of the standard deviation (e.g. the ability to detect a difference of two standard deviations)
Paired *t*-test (Chapter 20)	$\dfrac{2\delta}{\sigma_d}$	*N* pairs of observations	δ: the smallest mean difference that is clinically important σ_d: the standard deviation of the *differences* in response, usually estimated from a pilot study
Chi-squared test (Chapter 24)	$\dfrac{p_1 - p_2}{\sqrt{\overline{p}(1 - \overline{p})}}$	*N*/2 observations in each group	$p_1 - p_2$: the smallest difference in the proportions of 'success' in the two groups that is clinically important. One of these proportions is often known, and the relevant difference evaluated by considering what value the other proportion must take in order to constitute a noteworthy change $\overline{p} = \dfrac{p_1 + p_2}{2}$

group to be three times the size of the other), then the adjusted overall sample size is

$$N' = N(1+k)^2/(4k)$$

where N is the unadjusted overall sample size calculated for equally sized groups. Then $N'/(1+k)$ of these patients will be in the smaller group and the remaining patients will be in the larger group.

Increasing the power for a fixed sample size

If we regard the significance level and important treatment difference defined by a particular variable as fixed (we can rarely justify increasing either of them) and assume that our test is two-tailed (a one-tailed test has greater power but is usually inappropriate (Chapter 17)), we can increase the power for a fixed sample size in a number of ways. For example we might:

- use a more informative response variable (e.g. a numerical variable such as systolic blood pressure instead of the binary responses normal/hypertensive);
- perform a different form of analysis (e.g. parametric instead of non-parametric);
- reduce the random variation when collecting the data (e.g. by standardizing conditions or training observers (Chapter 39));
- modify the original study design in such a way that the variability in measurements is reduced (e.g. by incorporating stratification or using matched pairs instead of two independent groups (Chapter 13)).

References

1 Birkett, M.A. and Day, S.J. (1994) Internal pilot studies for estimating sample size. *Statistics in Medicine*, 13, 2455–2463.
2 Machin, D., Campbell, Tan, S.B. and Tan, S.H. (2018) *Sample Size Tables for Clinical, Laboratory and Epidemiological Studies*. 4th edition. Oxford: Wiley-Blackwell.
3 Lehr, R. (1992) Sixteen S-squared over D-squared: a relation for crude sample size estimates. *Statistics in Medicine*, 11, 1099–1102.

Example 1

Comparing means in independent groups using the unpaired *t*-test

Objective – to examine the effectiveness of early physical therapy compared with usual care in improving disability for patients with lower back pain (LBP). At baseline, all eligible participants were advised to remain as active as possible and were given documentation which provided messages consistent with LBP guidelines, and these were reviewed with the researcher. Those receiving early physical therapy (manipulation and an exercise regimen) had four timetabled sessions given by a physical therapist within the first 4 weeks after enrolment. Usual care involved no additional interventions during the first 4 weeks.

Design – randomized single-blind parallel group clinical trial.

Main outcome measure for the determination of sample size – change from baseline in the Oswestry Disability Index (ODI) score (range: 0–100; higher scores indicate greater disability) at 3 months.

Sample size question – how many patients are required in order to have a 90% power, at the 5% level of significance, of detecting a difference of 7 points in the change in ODI at 3 months between the early physical therapy and the usual care groups? This is with a view to performing a two-tailed unpaired *t*-test to compare the mean changes in ODI if we believe that the standard deviation of the change is approximately 16 points.

Using the nomogram
$\delta = 7$ and $\sigma = 16$. Thus the standardized difference equals

$$\frac{\delta}{\sigma} = \frac{7}{16} = 0.44$$

The line connecting a standardized difference of 0.44 and a power of 90% cuts the sample size axis at approximately 220. Therefore about 110 patients are required in each group. (Note: (i) if δ were lowered to 6, then the standardized difference equals 0.38 and the required sample size would increase to approximately 300 in total, i.e. 150 in each group; and (ii) if, using the original specification, the investigators wanted twice as many patients receiving early physical therapy compared with those with usual care (i.e. $k = 2$), then the adjusted sample size would be

$$N' = \frac{N(1+k)^2}{4k} = 220\frac{(1+2)^2}{4 \times 2} = 247.5$$

Thus there would be $247.5/3 \cong 83$ patients receiving early physical therapy and the remaining 137 patients would receive usual care. Fig. 18.1 shows power curves for this example.

Quick formula
If the power is 90%, then the required sample size in each group, assuming the original specification, is

$$\frac{21}{(\text{standardized difference})^2} = \frac{21}{(0.44)^2} = 109 \text{ (rounded up from 108.5)}$$

Based on Fritz, J.M., Magel, J.S., McFadden, M., *et al.* (2015) Early physical therapy vs usual care in patients with recent-onset low back pain: a randomized clinical trial. *JAMA*, **314(14)**, 1459–1467.

Example 2

Comparing two proportions in independent groups using the Chi-squared test

Objective – to compare strategies of peanut consumption and avoidance to determine which strategy is most effective in preventing the development of peanut allergy in infants at high risk for the allergy.

Design – randomized controlled trial (RCT) in which infants aged between 4 and 11 months at randomization with severe eczema, egg allergy or both, and a wheal measuring 1–4 mm in diameter after testing, are randomly allocated to consume or avoid peanuts until 60 months of age.

Main outcome measure for determining sample – the proportion of infants with peanut allergy at 60 months of age, determined by an oral food challenge.

Sample size question – how many infants are required in order to have, using a two-tailed Chi-squared test, an 80% power of detecting a clinically important difference of 30 percentage points (50% in the consumption group *vs* 20% in the avoidance group) in the proportion with peanut allergy at 60 months of age if the significance level is 5%?

Using the nomogram

$$p_1 = 0.5 \text{ and } p_2 = 0.2 \text{ so } \bar{p} = \frac{0.5 + 0.2}{2} = 0.35$$

Therefore the standardized difference

$$= \frac{p_1 - p_2}{\sqrt{\bar{p}(1 - \bar{p})}} = \frac{0.5 - 0.2}{\sqrt{0.35 \times 0.65}} = 0.63$$

The line connecting a standardized difference of 0.63 and a power of 80% cuts the sample sizes axis at about 80. Hence approximately 40 infants are required in each group. (Note: (i) if the power were increased to 90%, then the required sample size would increase to approximately 102 in total, i.e. 51 infants would be required in each group; and (ii) if the drop-out rate was expected to be around 10%, the adjusted overall sample size (with a power of 80%) would be 80 × 100/(100 – 10) = 90 (rounded from 88.9), with 45 infants in each group.) Figure 18.2 shows power curves for this example.

Quick formula

If the power is 80%, then the required sample size in each group is

$$\frac{16}{(\text{standardized difference})^2} = \frac{16}{0.63^2} = 40.3$$

which, when rounded up, indicates that each group should comprise 41 infants.

Du Toit, G., Roberts, G., Sayre, P.H., *et al.* (2015) Randomised trial of peanut consumption in infants at risk for peanut allergy. *New England Journal of Medicine*, **372(8)**, 803–812.

37 Presenting results

An essential facet of statistics is the ability to summarize the important attributes of the analysis. We must know what to include and how to display our results in a manner that enables others to obtain relevant and important information easily and draw correct conclusions[1]. This chapter describes the key features of presentation.

Numerical results

- Give figures only to the degree of accuracy that is appropriate (as a guideline, one significant figure more than the raw data). If analysing the data by hand, only round up or down at the end of the calculations.
- Give the number of items on which any summary measure (e.g. a percentage) is based.
- Report total sample and group sizes for each analysis.
- Describe any outliers and explain how they are handled (Chapter 3).
- Include the units of measurement.
- When interest is focused on a parameter (e.g. the mean, regression coefficient), always indicate the precision of its estimate. We recommend using a confidence interval. *Avoid* using the ± symbol, as in mean ± SEM (Chapter 10), because by adding and subtracting the SEM, we create a 67% confidence interval that can be misleading for those used to 95% confidence intervals. If absolutely necessary, it is better to show the standard error in brackets (making it clear that this is the SEM) after the parameter estimate, e.g. mean = 16.6 g (SEM 0.5 g).
- When interest is focused on the distribution of observations, always indicate a measure of the 'spread' of the data. The range of values that excludes outliers (typically, the range of values containing the central 95% of the observations (Chapter 6)) is a useful descriptor provided the minimum and maximum values of the range are provided. If the data are Normally distributed, this range is approximated by the sample mean $\pm 1.96 \times$ SD (Chapter 7). The mean and SD can be quoted instead, e.g. mean = 35.9 mm (SD 2.8 mm), but this leaves the reader to evaluate the range.

Tables

- Do not give too much information in a table.
- Include a concise, informative and unambiguous title.
- Label each row and column.
- Remember that it is easier to scan information down columns rather than across rows.

Diagrams

- Keep a diagram simple and avoid unnecessary frills (e.g. making a pie chart three-dimensional).
- Include a concise, informative and unambiguous title.
- Label all axes, segments and bars, and explain the meaning of symbols.
- Avoid distorting results by exaggerating the scale on an axis.
- Indicate where two or more observations lie in the same position on a scatter diagram, e.g. by using a different symbol.
- Ensure that all the relevant information is contained in the diagram (e.g. link paired observations).

Presenting results in a paper

When presenting results in a paper, we should ensure that the paper contains enough information for the reader to understand what has been done. He or she should be able to reproduce the results, given the data. All aspects of the design of the study and the statistical methodology must be fully described. This implies stating the primary aim of the study, summarizing each of the variables used in the analysis with descriptive statistics, fully describing the statistical methods for the primary and any secondary analyses (rather than listing all the methods in one place), indicating, if relevant, how any allowances were made for multiple comparisons, reporting the significance level used for hypothesis tests and naming the statistical package used for the analysis.

The EQUATOR Network (Appendix D) provides resources and training for the reporting of health research. Its website (www.equator-network.org) provides links to guidelines for the presentation of study results: these are available for many types of study design[2], including randomized trials (CONSORT, Chapter 14), clinical trial protocols (SPIRIT, Chapter 14), observational studies (STROBE, Chapters 15 and 16), diagnostic accuracy (STARD, Chapter 38), reliability and agreement studies (GRRAS, Chapter 39), systematic reviews and meta-analyses (PRISMA and MOOSE, Chapter 43) and model development and validation (TRIPOD, Chapter 46). In addition, the SAMPL guidelines (www.equator-network.org/reporting-guidelines/sampl/) explain how to report basic statistical methods and results.

In the sections that follow, we provide a summary of how to report common types of statistical analysis.

Medical Statistics at a Glance, Fourth Edition. Aviva Petrie and Caroline Sabin. © 2020 Aviva Petrie and Caroline Sabin. Published 2020 by John Wiley & Sons Ltd.
Companion Website: www.medstatsaag.com

Results of a hypothesis test
- Include a relevant diagram, if appropriate.
- Indicate the hypotheses of interest.
- Name the test and state whether it is one- or two-tailed.
- Justify the assumptions (if any) underlying the test (e.g. Normality, constant variance (Chapter 35)), and describe any transformations (Chapter 9) required to meet these assumptions (e.g. taking logarithms).
- Specify the observed value of the test statistic, its distribution (and degrees of freedom, if relevant) and, if possible, the *exact* P-value (e.g. $P = 0.03$) rather than an interval estimate of it (e.g. $0.01 < P < 0.05$) or a star system (e.g. *, **, *** for increasing levels of significance). Avoid writing 'n.s.' when $P > 0.05$; an exact P-value is preferable even when the result is non-significant.
- Include an estimate of the *relevant* effect of interest (e.g. the difference in means for the two-sample t-test, or the mean difference for the paired t-test) with a confidence interval (preferably) or standard error.
- Draw conclusions from the results (e.g. reject the null hypothesis), interpret any confidence intervals and explain their implications.

Results of a regression analysis
Here we include simple (Chapters 27 and 28) and multiple linear regression (Chapter 29), logistic regression (Chapter 30), Poisson regression (Chapter 31), Cox proportional hazards regression (Chapter 44) and regression methods for clustered data (Chapter 42). Full details of these analyses are explained in the associated chapters.
- Include relevant diagrams (e.g. a scatter plot with the fitted line for simple regression taking care not to extend the regression line beyond the minimum and maximum values of the data).
- Describe the purpose of the analysis, clearly stating which is the dependent variable and which is (are) the explanatory variable(s).
- Justify underlying assumptions and explain the results of regression diagnostics, if appropriate.
- Describe any transformations, and explain their purpose.
- Report how outlying values and missing values were treated in the analysis
- Where appropriate, describe the possible numerical values taken by any categorical variable (e.g. male = 0, female = 1), how

dummy variables were created (Chapter 29), and the units of numerical variables.
- Give an indication of the goodness of fit of the model (e.g. quote R^2 (Chapter 29) or likelihood ratio statistic (Chapter 32)).
- If appropriate (e.g. in multiple regression), give the results of the overall F-test from the analysis of variance table.
- For multivariable regression, report whether the variables were assessed for collinearity and interaction, and describe the variable selection process by which the final model was developed (e.g. forward stepwise).
- Provide estimates of *all* the coefficients in the model (including those that are not significant, if applicable) together with the confidence intervals for the coefficients or standard errors of their estimates. In logistic regression (Chapter 30), Poisson regression (Chapter 31) and Cox proportional hazards regression (Chapter 44), convert the coefficients to estimated odds ratios, relative rates or relative hazards (with confidence intervals). Interpret the relevant coefficients.
- Show the results of the hypothesis tests on the coefficients (i.e. include the test statistics and the P-values). Draw appropriate conclusions from these tests.

Complex analyses
There are no simple rules for the presentation of the more complex forms of statistical analysis. Be sure to describe the design of the study fully (e.g. the factors in the analysis of variance and whether there is a hierarchical arrangement), and include a validation of underlying assumptions, relevant descriptive statistics (with confidence intervals), test statistics and P-values. A brief description of what the analysis is doing helps the uninitiated; this should be accompanied by a reference for further details.

References
1 Lang, T.A. and Secic, M. (2006) *How to Report Statistics in Medicine: Annotated Guidelines for Authors, Editors and Reviewers*. 2nd edition. Philadelphia: American College of Physicians.
2 Moher, D., Altman, D.G., Schulz, K., Simera, I. and Wager, E. (eds) (2014) *Guidelines for Reporting Health Research: A User's Manual*. Oxford: Wiley-Blackwell.

Example

Table 37.1 and Fig. 37.1 provide examples indicating how important features of the relevant data sets may be displayed.

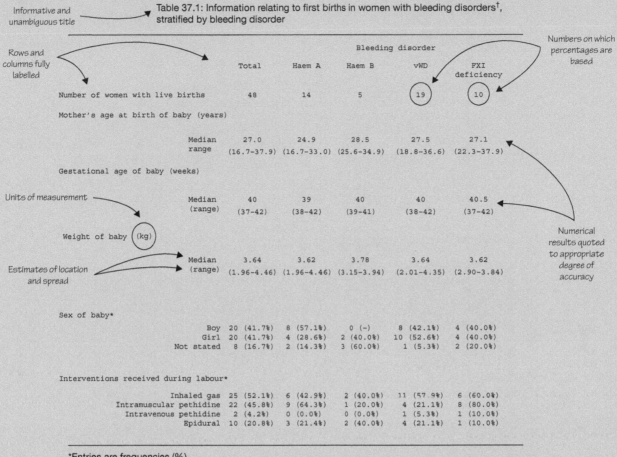

Informative and unambiguous title

Table 37.1: Information relating to first births in women with bleeding disorders[†], stratified by bleeding disorder

Rows and columns fully labelled

Numbers on which percentages are based

	Total	Haem A	Haem B	vWD	FXI deficiency
Number of women with live births	48	14	5	19	10

Mother's age at birth of baby (years)

	Total	Haem A	Haem B	vWD	FXI deficiency
Median	27.0	24.9	28.5	27.5	27.1
range	(16.7–37.9)	(16.7–33.0)	(25.6–34.9)	(18.8–36.6)	(22.3–37.9)

Gestational age of baby (weeks)

Units of measurement

	Total	Haem A	Haem B	vWD	FXI deficiency
Median (range)	40 (37–42)	39 (38–42)	40 (39–41)	40 (38–42)	40.5 (37–42)

Numerical results quoted to appropriate degree of accuracy

Weight of baby (kg)

Estimates of location and spread

	Total	Haem A	Haem B	vWD	FXI deficiency
Median (range)	3.64 (1.96–4.46)	3.62 (1.96–4.46)	3.78 (3.15–3.94)	3.64 (2.01–4.35)	3.62 (2.90–3.84)

Sex of baby*

	Total	Haem A	Haem B	vWD	FXI deficiency
Boy	20 (41.7%)	8 (57.1%)	0 (–)	8 (42.1%)	4 (40.0%)
Girl	20 (41.7%)	4 (28.6%)	2 (40.0%)	10 (52.6%)	4 (40.0%)
Not stated	8 (16.7%)	2 (14.3%)	3 (60.0%)	1 (5.3%)	2 (20.0%)

Interventions received during labour*

	Total	Haem A	Haem B	vWD	FXI deficiency
Inhaled gas	25 (52.1%)	6 (42.9%)	2 (40.0%)	11 (57.9%)	6 (60.0%)
Intramuscular pethidine	22 (45.8%)	9 (64.3%)	1 (20.0%)	4 (21.1%)	8 (80.0%)
Intravenous pethidine	2 (4.2%)	0 (0.0%)	0 (0.0%)	1 (5.3%)	1 (10.0%)
Epidural	10 (20.8%)	3 (21.4%)	2 (40.0%)	4 (21.1%)	1 (10.0%)

*Entries are frequencies (%).
[†]The study is described in Chapter 2.

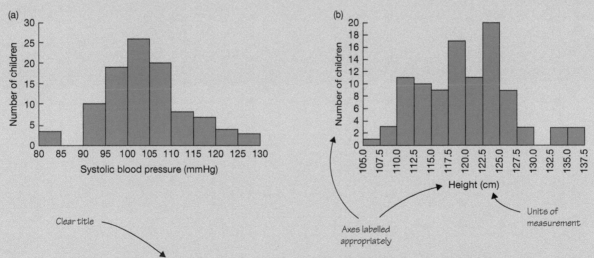

Clear title

Axes labelled appropriately

Units of measurement

Figure 37.1 Histograms showing the distribution of (a) systolic blood pressure and (b) height in a sample of 100 children (Chapter 26).

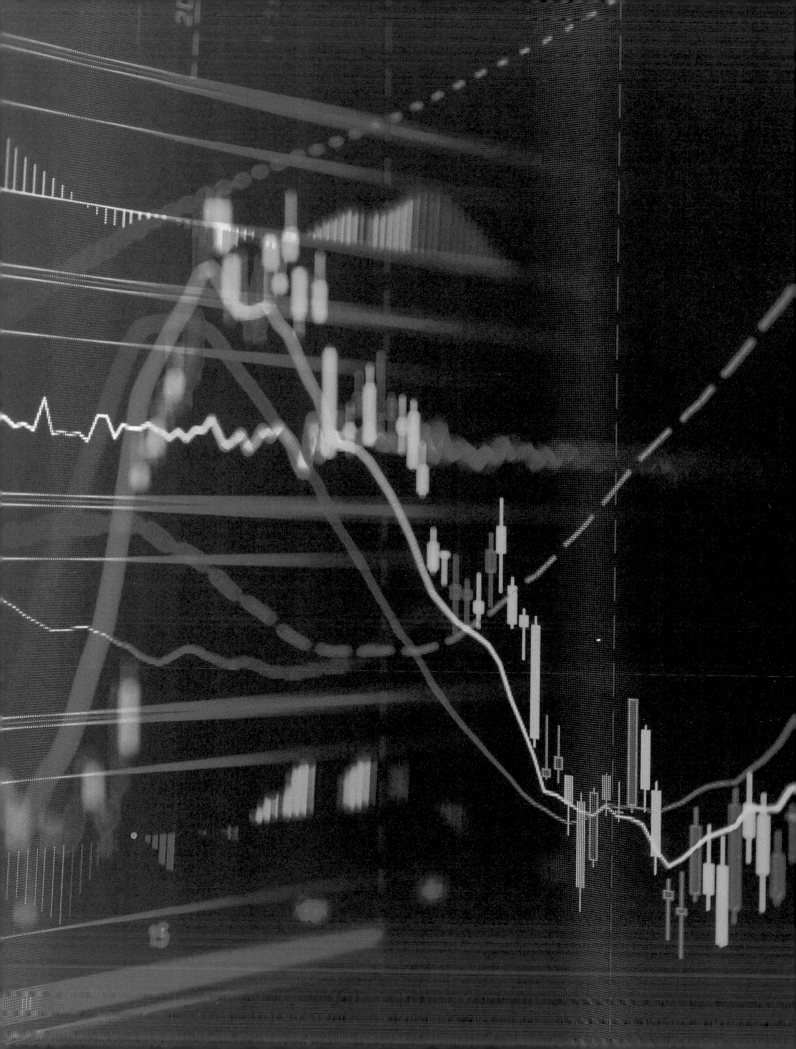

Additional chapters

Part 6

Chapters

38 Diagnostic tools

An individual's state of health is often characterized by a number of numerical or categorical measures. In this context, an appropriate **reference interval** (Chapters 6 and 7) and/or **diagnostic test** may be used:

• by the clinician, together with a clinical examination, to **diagnose** or exclude a particular disorder in his or her patient;

• as a **screening** device to ascertain which individuals in an apparently healthy population are likely to have (or sometimes, not have) the disease of interest. Individuals flagged in this way will then usually be subjected to more rigorous investigations in order to have their diagnosis confirmed. It is only sensible to screen for a disease if there are adequate facilities for treating the disease at the pre-symptomatic stages, this treatment being less costly and/or more effective than when given at a later stage (or, occasionally, if it is believed that individuals who are diagnosed with the disease will modify their behaviour to prevent the disease spreading).

A diagnostic test may also be used:

• as one of an array of **routine** tests (e.g. blood tests) that may identify a disorder unrelated to the condition under investigation;

• as a **staging** test (e.g. for cancer);

• as a **monitoring** test to track a patient's progress over time (e.g. blood pressure).

This chapter describes some of the methods that are used to develop these diagnostic tools for clinical use and explains how to interpret their results. STARD, another component of the EQUATOR network (see Appendix D and Chapter 37), provides reporting guidelines for studies of diagnostic accuracy (www.equator-network.org/reporting-guidelines/stard/ and http://www.equator-network.org/reporting-guidelines/stard/).

Reference intervals

A **reference interval** (often referred to as a **normal range**) for a single numerical variable, calculated from a very large sample, provides a range of values that are typically seen in healthy individuals. If an individual's value is above the upper limit, or below the lower limit, we consider it to be unusually high (or low) relative to healthy individuals.

Calculating reference intervals

Two approaches can be taken.

• We make the assumption that the data are Normally distributed. Approximately 95% of the data values lie within 1.96 standard deviations of the mean (Chapter 7). We use our data to calculate these two limits (mean ± 1.96 × standard deviation).

• An alternative approach, which does not make any assumptions about the distribution of the measurement, is to use a central range that encompasses 95% of the data values (Chapter 6). We put our values in order of magnitude and use the 2.5th and 97.5th percentiles as our limits.

The effect of other factors on reference intervals

Sometimes the values of a numerical variable depend on other factors, such as age or sex. It is important to interpret a particular value only after considering these other factors. For example, we generate reference intervals for systolic blood pressure separately for men and women.

Diagnostic tests

The **gold standard test** that provides a definitive diagnosis of a particular condition may sometimes be impractical or not routinely available. We would like a simple test, depending on the presence or absence of some marker, which provides a reasonable guide to whether or not the patient has the condition.

To evaluate a diagnostic test, we apply this test to a group of individuals whose true disease status is known from the gold standard test. We can draw up the 2 × 2 table of frequencies (Table 38.1).

Table 38.1 Table of frequencies.

Test result	Gold standard test		
	Disease	**No disease**	**Total**
Positive	a	b	$a + b$
Negative	c	d	$c + d$
Total	$a + c$	$b + d$	$n = a + b + c + d$

Medical Statistics at a Glance, Fourth Edition. Aviva Petrie and Caroline Sabin. © 2020 Aviva Petrie and Caroline Sabin. Published 2020 by John Wiley & Sons Ltd.
Companion Website: www.medstatsaag.com

Of the n individuals studied, $a + c$ individuals have the disease. The **prevalence** (Chapter 12) of the disease in this sample is

$$\frac{(a+c)}{n}$$

Of the $a + c$ individuals who have the disease, a have positive test results (**true positives**) and c have negative test results (**false negatives**). Of the $b + d$ individuals who do not have the disease, d have negative test results (**true negatives**) and b have positive test results (**false positives**).

Assessing the effectiveness of the test: sensitivity and specificity

Sensitivity = proportion of individuals with the disease who are correctly identified by the test

$$= \frac{a}{(a+c)}$$

Specificity = proportion of individuals without the disease who are correctly identified by the test

$$= \frac{d}{(b+d)}$$

These are usually expressed as percentages. As with all estimates, we should calculate confidence intervals for these measures (Chapter 11).

We would like our test to have a sensitivity and specificity that are both as close to 1 (or 100%) as possible. However, in practice, we may gain sensitivity at the expense of specificity, and *vice versa*. Whether we aim for a high sensitivity or high specificity depends on the condition we are trying to detect, along with the implications for the patient and/or the population of either a false negative or false positive test result. For conditions that are easily treatable, we prefer a high sensitivity; for those that are serious and untreatable, we prefer a high specificity in order to avoid making a false positive diagnosis. It is important that, before screening is undertaken, subjects should understand the implications of a positive diagnosis, as well as having an appreciation of the false positive and false negative rates of the test.

Using the test result for diagnosis: predictive values

Positive predictive value = proportion of individuals with a positive test result who have the disease, calculated as

$$= \frac{a}{(a+b)}$$

Negative predictive value = proportion of individuals with a negative test result who do not have the disease, calculated as

$$= \frac{d}{(c+d)}$$

We calculate confidence intervals for these predictive values, often expressed as percentages, using the methods described in Chapter 11.

The sensitivity and specificity quantify the diagnostic ability of the test but it is the predictive values that indicate how likely it is that the individual has or does not have the disease, given his or her test result. Predictive values are dependent on the prevalence of the disease in the population being studied.

In populations where the disease is common, the positive predictive value of a given test will be much higher than in populations where the disease is rare. The converse is true for negative predictive values. Therefore, predictive values can rarely be generalized beyond the study.

The use of a cut-off value

Sometimes we wish to make a diagnosis on the basis of a numerical or ordinal measurement. Often there is no threshold above (or below) which disease definitely occurs. In these situations, we need to define a cut-off value ourselves above (or below) which we believe an individual has a very high chance of having the disease.

A useful approach is to use the upper (or lower) limit of the reference interval. We can evaluate this cut-off value by calculating its associated sensitivity, specificity and predictive values. If we choose a different cut-off, these values may change as we become more or less stringent. We choose the cut-off to optimize these measures as desired.

The receiver operating characteristic (ROC) curve

This provides a way of assessing whether a particular type of test provides useful information, and can be used to compare two different tests, and to select an optimal cut-off value for a test.

To draw the **receiver operating characteristic (ROC) curve** for a given test, we consider all cut-off points that give a unique pair of values for sensitivity and specificity, and plot the *sensitivity* against *one minus the specificity* (thus comparing the probabilities of a positive test result in those with and without disease) and connect these points by lines (Fig. 38.1).

The ROC curve for a test that has some use will lie to the left of the diagonal (i.e. the 45° line) of the graph. Depending on the implications of false positive and false negative results, and the prevalence of the condition, we can choose the optimal cut-off for a test from this graph. The overall accuracy of two or more tests for the same condition can be compared by considering the area under each curve (sometimes referred to as AUROC);

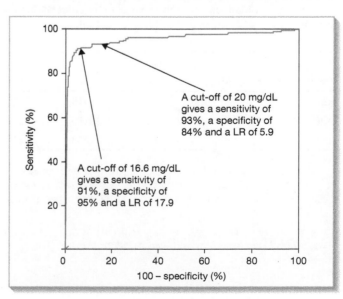

Figure 38.1 Receiver operating characteristic (ROC) curve, highlighting the results with two cut-off values of ceruloplasmin level: 16.6 and 20 mg/dL.

this area can be calculated manually or is given by the *c* **statistic**. *c* can be interpreted as the probability that a randomly chosen subject from the disease group has a higher predicted probability of having the disease than a randomly chosen subject from the disease-free group. The test with the greater area (i.e. the higher *c* statistic) is better at discriminating between disease outcomes. A test that is perfect at discriminating between the disease outcomes has *c* = 1 and a non-discriminating test that performs no better than chance has *c* = 0.5.

We also discuss the area under the ROC curve in Chapter 46 in the context of prognostic scores.

Is a test useful?

The **likelihood ratio (LR)** for a positive test result is the ratio of the chance of a positive result if the patient has the disease to the chance of a positive result if he or she does not have the disease (see also Chapter 32). For example, a LR of 2 for a positive result indicates that a positive result is twice as likely to occur in an individual with disease than in one without it.

It can be shown that

$$LR \text{ for a positive result} = \frac{sensitivity}{(1-specificity)}$$

A LR can also be generated for a negative test result and is most easily calculated as (1 – sensitivity)/specificity. A high LR (e.g. >10) for a positive test result suggests that the test is useful and provides evidence to support the diagnosis. Similarly, a LR close to 0 (e.g. <0.01) for a negative result allows us to rule out the diagnosis. We discuss the LR in the context of diagnostic tests in a Bayesian framework in Chapter 45.

Example

Wilson's disease (WD) is a genetic disorder with copper metabolism disturbances leading to copper accumulation in many organs, inducing secondary damage. Early diagnosis and treatment are important to prevent permanent damage to the liver and to avoid disease progression in the brain. In addition, WD can progress to severe haemolytic anaemia or fulminant hepatic failure, which can lead to death if diagnosis is delayed. For the initial screening of WD in the general population, measurement of serum ceruloplasmin levels is the first-line diagnostic test due to its rapidity and low cost. Although it is conventional to use a ceruloplasmin concentration <20 mg/dL as the cut-off, this level may not be optimal for children and young adults with hepatitis who tend to have lower ceruloplasmin concentrations than older patients. Jung Ah Kim *et al.* evaluated the diagnostic value of ceruloplasmin concentration for the diagnosis of WD among children and young adults with hepatitis in a medical centre in Korea. All 2834 patients, reviewed retrospectively, were under 20 years of age, and 181 of them were diagnosed as having WD, confirmed by the identification of pathogenic variants in the *ATP7B* gene. No differences were seen in the distributions of the basic characteristics of those with and without WD, including age. The table of frequencies shows the results the investigators obtained using a ceruloplasmin concentration <20 mg/dL as their cut-off; the box contains calculations of estimates of measures of interest for this cut-off.

	Wilson's disease		
Ceruloplasmin (mg/dL)	**Yes**	**No**	**Total**
<20	169	418	587
≥20	12	2235	2247
Total	181	2653	2834

Therefore for a cut-off of <20 mg/dL, there is high sensitivity and relatively high specificity. The false positive rate is (418)/(2653) × 100 = 15.8% (95% CI 14.4% to 17.1%). The LR of a

positive test result of 5.9 indicates that this test could be useful, in that a ceruloplasmin concentration <20 mg/dL is nearly six times more likely in an individual (i.e. a child or young adult with hepatitis) with WD than in one without WD. However, in order to investigate other cut-off values, a ROC curve was plotted (Fig 38.1). The area under the ROC curve is 0.96 (95% CI 0.94 to 0.98), indicating that using ceruloplasmin concentration as a diagnostic tool is very accurate at discriminating between those who do and do not have WD. Further investigation of the ROC curve shows that the most useful cut-off is 16.6 mg/dL, which gives a sensitivity of 91.2% (95% CI 87.0% to 95.3%), a specificity of 94.9% (95% CI 94.1% to 95.8%), a false positive rate of 5.1% (95% CI 4.2% to 5.9%) and a LR of 17.9 (95% CI 15.0 to 21.0). Thus, if clinicians were to use the test with the lower cut-off value in those aged <20 years with hepatitis, a ceruloplasmin concentration <16.6 mg/dL would indicate that the individual would be very likely to have WD. Clearly, the diagnostic value of ceruloplasmin concentration appears to be strengthened by using the revised cut-off value in those with hepatitis aged <20 years.

Prevalence = (181/2834) × 100 = 6.4% (95% CI 5.5% to 7.3%)

Sensitivity = (169/181) × 100 = 93.4% (95% CI 89.7% to 97.0%)

Specificity = (2235/2653) × 100 = 84.2% (95% CI 82.9% to 85.6%)

Positive predictive value = (169/587) × 100 = 28.8% (95% CI 25.1% to 32.5%)

Negative predictive value = (2235/2247) × 100 = 99.5% (95% CI 99.2% to 99.8%)

Likelihood ratio for positive result = (0.934)/(1 – 0.842) = 5.9 (95% CI 5.4 to 6.5, obtained from computer output)

Likelihood ratio for negative result = (1 – 0.934)/(0.842) = 0.08 (95% CI 0.05 to 0.14, obtained from computer output)

Jung Ah Kim, Hyun Jin Kim, Jin Min Cho, *et al*. (2015) Diagnostic value of ceruloplasmin in the diagnosis of pediatric Wilson's disease. *Pediatric Gastroenterology, Hepatology and Nutrition*, **18(3)**, 187–192.

39 Assessing agreement

Measurement variability and error

A biological variable measured on each of a number of individuals will always exhibit a certain amount of variability. The measurements are likely to vary *between* individuals (**inter-individual** variation) as well as *within* the same individual (**intra-individual** variation) if the measurement on that individual is repeated, either immediately or some time later. Much of this variability arises because of differences in associated factors, e.g. genetic, environmental or lifestyle factors. For example, blood pressure measurements may vary between individuals if these individuals differ in terms of their sex, age, weight or smoking status and within an individual at different times of the day. We refer to this type of variability as **measurement variability**. We define **measurement error** as that which arises when there is a difference between the observed (or 'measured') values and true values of a variable (note that although we refer to the 'true' measurement here, it is rarely possible to obtain this value). Measurement error may be:
- **Systematic** – the observed values tend to be too high (or too low) because of some known or unknown extraneous factor affecting the measurements in the same way (e.g. an observer overestimating the values). Systematic errors lead to biased estimates, raising concerns about validity, and should be reduced as far as possible by, for example, standardizing conditions, training observers and/or calibrating the instrument (i.e. verification by comparison with a known standard).
- **Random** – the observed values are sometimes greater and sometimes less than the true values but they tend to balance out on average. For example, random errors may occur because of a lack of sensitivity of the measuring instrument. Random error is governed by chance although the degree of error may be affected by external factors (e.g. the pH in fresh blood samples may exhibit greater random error when these samples are at room temperature rather than on ice).

Both measurement variability and error are important when assessing a measurement technique. Although the description of error in this section has focused on laboratory measurements, the same concepts apply even if we are interested in other forms of measurement, such as an individual's state of health on a particular day, as assessed by a questionnaire.

Reliability

There are many occasions when we wish to compare results that should concur. In particular, we may want to assess and, if possible, quantify the following two types of **agreement** or **reliability**.
- **Reproducibility (method/observer agreement)** – do two techniques used to measure a particular variable, in otherwise identical circumstances, produce the same result? Do two or more observers using the same method of measurement obtain the same results?
- **Repeatability** – does a single observer obtain the same results when she or he takes repeated measurements in identical circumstances?

Reproducibility and repeatability can be approached in the same way. In each case, the method of analysis depends on whether the variable is **categorical** (e.g. poor/average/good) or **numerical** (e.g. systolic blood pressure). For simplicity, we shall restrict the problem to that of comparing only **paired** results (e.g. two methods/two observers/duplicate measurements).

Categorical variables

Suppose we wish to gauge the extent to which there is agreement between two methods of assessing a disease using a categorical scale of measurement, after previously showing each method to be repeatable.

Is there a systematic effect?

If there is a systematic effect then one of the two methods produces a greater proportion of patients in one disease category than the other method. We may assess this if there are only two disease categories by using McNemar's test comparing proportions in related groups (Chapter 24). If there are more than two disease categories, the McNemar–Bowker test may be used, but this is beyond the scope of this book. A non-significant result suggests that there is no evidence of a systematic effect. If one set of results represents the 'gold standard', as is likely in a method comparison study, this implies that **bias** is not indicated.

The kappa measure of agreement

We present the results in a two-way contingency table of frequencies with the rows and columns indicating the categories of response for each method (see Table 39.1, which shows the assessments of two different methods of testing for human papillomavirus (HPV) DNA). The frequencies with which there is agreement between the methods are shown along the **diagonal** of the table. We calculate the corresponding frequencies that would be **expected** if the categorizations were made at random, in the same way as we calculated expected frequencies in the Chi-squared test of association (Chapter 24), i.e. each expected frequency is the product of the relevant row and column totals divided by the overall total. Then we measure agreement by

$$\text{Cohen's kappa, } \kappa = \frac{\left(\dfrac{O_d}{m} - \dfrac{E_d}{m} \right)}{\left(1 - \dfrac{E_d}{m} \right)}$$

which represents the chance corrected proportional agreement, where:

- m = total observed frequency (e.g. total number of patients)
- O_d = sum of observed frequencies *along the diagonal*
- E_d = sum of expected frequencies *along the diagonal*
- 1 in the denominator represents maximum agreement.

$\kappa = 1$ implies perfect agreement and $\kappa = 0$ suggests that the agreement is no better than that which would be obtained by chance. There are no objective criteria for judging intermediate values. However, kappa is often judged as providing agreement[1] which is:

- poor if $\kappa < 0.00$
- slight if $0.00 \leq \kappa \leq 0.20$
- fair if $0.21 \leq \kappa \leq 0.40$
- moderate if $0.41 \leq \kappa \leq 0.60$
- substantial if $0.61 \leq \kappa \leq 0.80$
- almost perfect if $\kappa > 0.80$.

Although it is possible to estimate a standard error and confidence interval[2] for kappa, we do not usually test the hypothesis that kappa is zero since this is not really pertinent or realistic in a reliability study.

Note that kappa is dependent both on the number of categories (i.e. its value is greater if there are fewer categories) and the prevalence of the condition, so care must be taken when comparing kappas from different studies. For ordinal data, we can also calculate a **weighted kappa**[3] which takes into account the extent to which the methods **disagree** (the non-diagonal frequencies) as well as the frequencies of agreement (along the diagonal). The weighted kappa is very similar to the **intraclass correlation coefficient** (see next section and Chapter 42).

Numerical variables

Suppose an observer takes duplicate measurements of a numerical variable on n individuals (just replace the word 'repeatability' by 'reproducibility' in the text which follows if considering the similar problem of method agreement, but remember to assess the repeatability of each method before carrying out the method agreement study).

Is there a systematic effect?

If we calculate the difference between each pair of measurements and find that the average difference is zero (this is usually assessed by the paired t-test but we might use the sign test or signed ranks test (Chapters 19 and 20)), then we can infer that there is *no systematic difference* between the pairs of results, i.e *on average*, the duplicate readings agree. If one set of readings represents the true values, as is likely in a method comparison study, this means that there is no evidence of bias.

Measures of repeatability and the Bland and Altman diagram

The estimated standard deviation of the differences (s_d) provides a measure of agreement for an *individual*. However, it is more usual to calculate the **British Standards Institution repeatability coefficient** = $2s_d$. This is the maximum difference that is likely to occur between two measurements. Assuming a Normal distribution of differences, we expect approximately 95% of the differences in the population to lie between $\bar{d} \pm 2s_d$ where $\bar{d}$ is the mean of the observed differences. The upper and lower limits of this interval are called the **limits of agreement**; from them, we can decide (subjectively) whether the agreement between pairs of readings in a given situation is acceptable. The limits are usually indicated on a **Bland and Altman diagram** which is obtained by calculating the mean of and the difference between each pair of readings, and plotting the n differences against their corresponding means[4] (Fig. 39.1). The diagram can also be used to detect outliers (Chapter 3).

It makes no sense to calculate a *single* measure of repeatability if the extent to which the observations in a pair disagree depends on the magnitude of the measurement. We can check this using the Bland and Altman diagram (Fig 39.1). If we observe a random scatter of points (evenly distributed above and below zero if there is no systematic difference between the pairs), then a single measure of repeatability is acceptable. If, however, we observe a funnel effect, with the variation in the differences being greater (say) for larger mean values, then we must reassess the problem. We may be able to find an appropriate transformation of the raw data (Chapter 9) so that, when we repeat the process on the transformed observations, the required condition is satisfied.

Indices of reliability

Intraclass correlation coefficient

An index of reliability commonly used to measure repeatability and reproducibility is the **intraclass correlation coefficient** (ICC, Chapter 42), which takes a value from 0 (no agreement) to 1 (perfect agreement). When measuring the agreement between pairs of observations, the ICC is the proportion of the variability in the observations that is due to the differences between pairs, i.e. it is the between-pair variance expressed as a proportion of the total variance of the observations.

When there is no evidence of a systematic difference between the pairs, we may calculate the ICC as the Pearson correlation coefficient (Chapter 26) between the $2n$ pairs of observations obtained by including each pair twice, once when its values are as observed and once when they are interchanged (see Example 2).

If we wish to take the systematic difference between the observations in a pair into account, we estimate the ICC as

$$\frac{s_a^2 - s_d^2}{s_a^2 + s_d^2 + \dfrac{2}{n}(n\bar{d}^2 - s_d^2)}$$

where we determine the difference between and the sum of the observations in each of the n pairs and:

- s_a^2 is the estimated variance of the n sums
- s_d^2 is the estimated variance of the n differences
- $\bar{d}$ is the estimated mean of the differences (an estimate of the systematic difference).

We usually carry out a reliability study as part of a larger investigative study. The sample used for the reliability study should be a reflection of that used for the investigative study. We should not compare values of the ICC in different data sets as the ICC is influenced by features of the data, such as its variability (the ICC will be greater if the observations are more variable). Note that the ICC is not related to the actual scale of measurement nor to the size of error which is clinically acceptable.

Lin's concordance correlation coefficient

It is *inappropriate* to calculate the Pearson correlation coefficient (Chapter 26) between the n pairs of readings (e.g. from the first and second occasions or from two methods/observers) as a measure of reliability. We are not really interested in whether the points in the scatter diagram (e.g. of the results from the first occasion plotted against those from the second occasion) lie on a straight line; we want to know whether they conform to the line of equality (i.e. the 45° line through the origin when the two scales are the same). This will not be established by testing the null hypothesis that the true Pearson correlation coefficient is 0. It would, in any case, be very surprising if the pairs of measurements were not related, given the nature of the investigation. Instead, we may calculate **Lin's concordance correlation coefficient**[5] as an index of reliability which is almost identical to the ICC. Lin's coefficient modifies the Pearson correlation coefficient which assesses the closeness of the data about the line of best fit (Chapters 28 and 29) in the scatter plot by taking into account how far the line of best fit is from the 45° line through the origin. The maximum value of Lin's coefficient is 1, achieved when there is perfect concordance, with all the points lying on the 45° line drawn through the origin. The coefficient can be calculated as

$$r_c = \frac{2rs_x s_y}{s_x^2 + s_y^2 + (\overline{x} - \overline{y})}$$

where r is the estimated Pearson correlation coefficient (Chapter 26) between the n pairs of results (x_i, y_i), and $\overline{x}$ and $\overline{y}$ are the sample means of x and y, respectively.

$$s_x^2 = \frac{\sum (x_i - \overline{x})^2}{n} = \frac{n-1}{n} \text{ times the estimated variance of } x$$

$$s_y^2 = \frac{\sum (y_i - \overline{y})^2}{n} = \frac{n-1}{n} \text{ times the estimated variance of } y$$

More complex situations

Sometimes you may come across more complex problems when assessing agreement. For example, there may be more than two replicates, or more than two observers, or each of a number of observers may have replicate observations. You can find details of the analysis of such problems in Streiner and Norman[6].

Reporting guidelines

GRRAS, another component of the EQUATOR network (Appendix D and Chapter 37), proposes a checklist for the reporting of reliability and agreement studies (www.equator-network.org/reporting-guidelines/guidelines-for-reporting-reliability-and-agreement-studies-grras-were-proposed/).

References

1 Landis, J.R. and Koch, G.G. (1977) The measurement of observer agreement for categorical data. *Biometrics*, **33**, 159–174.
2 Altman, D.G. (1991) *Medical Statistics for Medical Research*. London: Chapman and Hall/CRC.
3 Cohen, J. (1968). Weighted kappa: nominal scale agreement with provision for scale disagreement or partial credit. *Psychological Bulletin*, **70**, 213–220.
4 Bland, J.M. and Altman, D.G. (1986). Statistical methods for assessing agreement between two pairs of clinical measurement. *Lancet*, **I**, 307–310.
5 Lin L.I.-K. (1989) A concordance correlation coefficient to evaluate reproducibility. *Biometrics*, **45**, 255–268.
6 Streiner, D.R. and Norman, G.L. (2003) *Health Measurement Scales: a Practical Guide to Their Development and Use*. 3rd edition. Oxford: Oxford University Press.

Example 1

Assessing agreement – categorical variable

Investigators studied whether a dry cervical sample taken with a flocked swab is a valid alternative for human papillomavirus (HPV) DNA testing compared with the standard practice of a wet sample taken with a cyto-broom placed directly into liquid media. Samples from 209 women attending a dysplasia clinic in Melbourne were compared; the order of the sampling method (wet or dry) had been randomized. HPV results were classified as being HPV16 positive (HPV16+), HPV18 positive (HPV18+), positive for another HPV type (Other HPV+) or negative (HPV–). The observed frequencies are shown in Table 39.1. The bold figures along the diagonal show the observed frequencies of agreement; the corresponding expected frequencies are in brackets. We calculated **Cohen's kappa** to assess the agreement between the two observers.

We estimate Cohen's kappa as

$$\kappa = \frac{[(19 + 2 + 56 + 117)/209] - [(1.73 + 0.04 + 18.66 + 74.13)/209]}{1 - [(1.73 + 0.04 + 18.66 + 74.13)/209]}$$

$$= \frac{(0.9282 - 0.4524)}{1 - 0.4524} = 0.87$$

Since $\kappa = 0.87$ (95% CI 0.80 to 0.93, from computer output) there appears to be almost perfect agreement between the two collection methods for the detection of different HPV types.

Thus, it is reasonable to use the dry sampling method as a valid alternative to the wet sampling method for HPV DNA testing.

continued

Table 39.1 Observed (and expected) frequencies of HPV detection from dry and wet collection methods.

| Wet collection | Dry collection | | | | |
	HPV16+	HPV18+	Other HPV+	HPV−	Total
HPV16+	**19** (1.73)	0	0	0	19
HPV18+	0	**2** (0.04)	0	1	3
Other HPV+	0	0	**56** (18.66)	9	65
HPV−	0	1	4	**117** (74.13)	122
Total	19	3	60	127	209

Data extracted from Sultana, F., Gertig, D.M., Wrede, C.D., *et al.* (2015) A pilot study to compare dry cervical sample collection with standard practice of wet cervical samples for human papillomavirus testing. *Journal of Clinical Virology*, **69**, 210–213.

Example 2

Assessing agreement – numerical variables

In order to plan facial jaw surgery (orthognathic surgery), vertical measurements of plaster models of the patient's upper jaw are measured in millimetres using an electronic caliper set into a granite platform known as an Erickson model platform. These measurements are usually carried out by the Chief Orthodontic Technician, very experienced in using this piece of measuring equipment. A clinician (Operator 1), inexperienced in the Erickson model platform, wished to test whether, using the Erickson technique on the same plaster models under identical conditions, her 50 readings agreed with those of the experienced technician (Operator 2) whose measurements could be taken as the 'gold standard'. The results are shown in Table 39.2. The differences (Operator 1 – Operator 2) can be shown to be approximately Normally distributed: they have a mean of $\bar{d}$ = 0.0112 mm and a standard deviation s_d = 0.0498 mm. The test statistic for the paired t-test is equal to 1.59 (degrees of freedom = 49), giving P = 0.119. This non-significant result indicates that there is no evidence of any systematic difference (i.e. bias) between the results measured by the two operators.

The British Standards Institution repeatability coefficient is $2s_d$ = 2 × 0.0498 = 0.0996 mm. Approximately 95% of the differences in the population of such patients would be expected to lie between $\bar{d} \pm 2s_d$, i.e. between −0.089 and 0.111 mm. These limits are indicated by the red lines in Fig. 39.1, which shows that the differences are randomly scattered around a mean of approximately zero.

The index of reliability is estimated as

$$\frac{16.1532 - 0.00248}{16.1532 + 0.00248 + \frac{2}{50}\left(50(0.0012)^2 - 0.00248\right)} = 0.9997$$

Because the systematic difference is negligible, this value for the ICC is the same as the one we get by calculating the Pearson correlation coefficient for the 50 pairs of results obtained by using each pair of results twice, once with the order reversed. As an illustration of the technique, consider the first five pairs of pre-treatment values: (92.38, 92.39), (91.79, 91.84), (88.84, 88.82), (86.84, 86.78) and (92.80, 92.70). If we reverse the order of each pair, we obtain a second set of five pairs: (92.39, 92.38), (91.84, 91.79), (88.82, 88.84), (86.78, 86.84) and (92.70, 92.80). By repeating this process for the remaining 45 pairs, and combining the second set of pairs with the first set, we obtain a total of 100 pairs, which we use to calculate the correlation coefficient, an estimate of the ICC. The

Table 39.2 Vertical measurements (mm) of the plaster models of 50 jaws taken by Operator 1 (clinician) and Operator 2 (experienced technician).

1	2	1	2	1	2	1	2	1	2
92.38	92.39	93.36	93.40	92.01	91.90	93.60	93.63	91.58	91.57
91.79	91.84	93.37	93.31	91.37	91.32	91.46	91.44	92.73	92.75
88.84	88.82	94.91	94.87	90.57	90.54	89.76	89.69	92.57	92.64
86.84	86.78	94.79	94.80	92.09	92.03	93.32	93.32	90.04	90.07
92.80	92.70	92.22	92.17	92.07	92.15	93.28	93.29	88.12	88.06
92.69	92.67	89.83	89.85	90.06	90.00	95.09	95.09	90.59	90.58
94.80	94.73	93.77	93.71	88.76	88.63	95.19	95.23	89.71	89.70
95.05	95.11	93.56	93.52	92.42	92.43	93.44	93.44	90.88	90.88
93.22	93.14	95.38	95.38	92.25	92.29	91.91	91.94	90.73	90.81
91.49	91.57	93.60	93.57	93.75	93.75	92.23	92.21	88.38	88.38

continued

estimate produced this way is identical to the estimate of Lin's concordance correlation coefficient, which is calculated as

$$\frac{2(0.9997)(2.0047)(2.0147)}{4.0188 + 4.0590 + (92.0930 - 92.0818)^2} = 0.9997$$

Since the maximum likely difference between measurements taken by the clinician and the experienced technician is around 0.0996 mm, which is clinically acceptable, and since virtually all (i.e. 99.97%) of the variability in the results can be attributed to differences between patients, the clinician (Operator 1) felt that her results were reproducible when compared to those of the experienced technician (Operator 2). Having previously confirmed that her results were repeatable (by investigating duplicate measurements, taken 1 week apart, of each model), the clinician was confident to use her own vertical measurements when planning orthognathic surgery.

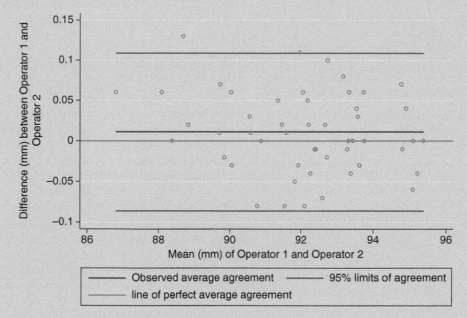

Figure 39.1 Difference between vertical measurements (mm) of plaster models of 50 jaws taken by Operator 1 and Operator 2 plotted against their mean.

Data kindly provided by Dr Helen Moss of the UCL Eastman Dental Institute, London, UK

40 Evidence-based medicine

Straus et al.[1] describe **evidence-based medicine (EBM)** as 'the conscientious, explicit and judicious use of current best evidence in making decisions about the care of individual patients'. To practice EBM, you must be able to locate the research relevant to the care of your patients, and judge its quality. Only then can you think about applying the findings in clinical practice.

In order to assess the strength of the findings about any particular topic, it is important to recognize that different study designs provide varying **levels of evidence** relating to the answers obtained from the question posed. These levels may be specified in the following hierarchy (starting with the strongest and leading to the weakest evidence): systematic review or meta-analysis of a randomized controlled trial (RCT) → RCT → cohort study → case–control study → cross-sectional survey → case reports → expert opinion → anecdotal information. Note that the hierarchy is not set in stone, as its arrangement depends partly on the problem at hand and partly on the quality of the individual studies themselves. For example, we would choose to perform an RCT to investigate a novel treatment; if, on the other hand, we wish to identify risk factors for a disease outcome, an RCT would not necessarily be appropriate and a cohort or case–control study would provide stronger evidence.

In Appendix D, in addition to the CONSORT checklist and flow chart (Table D1 and Fig. D1) for reporting RCTs (Chapter 14) and the STROBE checklist (Table D2) for reporting observational studies (Chapters 15 and 16), we also include templates that you may find helpful when critically appraising or evaluating the evidence in published papers on RCTs (Template D1) and observational studies (Template D2). You may find it useful to refer to AMSTAR 2[2] when critically appraising systematic reviews containing randomized and non-randomized studies.

Straus et al. suggest the following approach to EBM that provides more generic instructions than those in the templates, which focus on two particular types of study. However, for convenience, we have phrased the third and fourth points below

in terms of clinical trials and observational studies; they can be modified to suit other forms of investigations (e.g. diagnostic tests, Chapter 38).

1 Formulate the clinical question (PICO)

The four main elements of a clinical question may be remembered by the mnemonic PICO:

- **P** (*Patient population*) – what are the important characteristics of the patient population about which you are asking the clinical question? In the example in this chapter, the population comprises English speaking patients aged over 18 years with proven coronary heart disease (CHD) in Sydney, Australia.
- **I** (*Intervention*) – which main diagnostic or therapeutic intervention, prognostic factor or exposure are you considering? In the example, the therapeutic intervention is that of mobile phone text messages (four per week for 6 months) in addition to usual care.
- **C** (*Comparison*) – what is the alternative to compare to the intervention? This is an optional component of PICO as there may be no alternative or it is not required. In the example, the alternative is usual care alone.
- **O** (*Outcome*) – what do you hope to accomplish in a specified time frame in terms of a measureable effect? In the example, it is a greater mean reduction in the text messaging group in low-density lipoprotein cholesterol (LDL-C) at 6 months.

2 Locate the relevant information (e.g. on diagnosis, prognosis or therapy)

Often the relevant information will be found in published papers, but you should also consider other possibilities, such as conference abstracts. You must know what databases (e.g. Medline) and other sources of evidence are available, how they are organized, which search terms to use, and how to operate the searching software.

3 Critically appraise the methods in order to assess the validity (closeness to the truth) of the evidence

The following questions should be asked.

- Have all **important** *outcomes* been considered?
- Was the study conducted using an **appropriate spectrum of patients**?
- Do the results make **biological sense**?
- Was the study designed to eliminate **bias** (Chapter 34)? For example, in a clinical trial, was the study **controlled**, was **randomization** used in the assignment of patients, was the assessment of response 'blind', were any patients lost to follow-up, were the groups treated in a similar fashion aside from the fact that they received different treatments, and was an '**intention-to-treat**' (ITT) analysis performed (Chapter 14)?

- Are the statistical methods appropriate (e.g. have underlying assumptions been verified, have dependencies in the data such as pairing been taken into account in the analysis)?

4 Extract the most useful results and determine whether they are important

Extracting the most useful results

You should ask the following questions.

(a) What is the **main outcome variable** (i.e. that which relates to the major objective)?

(b) How **large** is the **effect of interest**, expressed in terms of the main outcome variable? If this variable is:
- **Binary** (e.g. died/survived):
  (i) What are the rates/risks/odds of occurrence of this event (e.g. death) in the (two) comparison groups?
  (ii) The effect of interest may be the difference in rates or risks (the absolute reduction) or a ratio (the relative rate or risk or odds ratio) – what is its magnitude?
- **Numerical** (e.g. systolic blood pressure):
  (i) What is the mean (or median) value of the variable in each of the comparison groups?
  (ii) What is the effect of interest, i.e. the difference in means (medians)?

- How **precise** is the **effect of interest**? Ideally, the research being scrutinized should include the confidence interval for the true effect (a wide confidence interval is an indication of poor precision). Is this confidence interval quoted? If not, is sufficient information (e.g. the standard error of the effect of interest) provided so that the confidence interval can be determined?

Deciding whether the results are important

- Consider the **confidence interval** for the effect of interest (e.g. the difference in treatment means):
  (i) Would you regard the observed effect to be clinically important (irrespective of whether or not the result of the relevant hypothesis test is statistically significant) if the lower limit of the confidence interval represented the true value of the effect?

  (ii) Would you regard the observed effect to be clinically important if the upper limit of the confidence interval represented the true value of the effect?
  (iii) Are your answers to the above two points sufficiently similar to declare the results of the study unambiguous and important?

- To assess therapy in a randomized controlled trial, evaluate the **number of patients you need to treat** (NNT) with the experimental treatment rather than the control treatment in order to prevent one of them developing the 'bad' outcome. The NNT can be determined in various ways depending on the information available. It is, for example, the reciprocal of the difference in the proportions of individuals with the bad outcome in the control and experimental groups.

5 Apply the results in clinical practice

If the results are to help you in caring for your patients, you must ensure that:

- your patient is similar to those on whom the results were obtained;
- the results can be applied to your patient;
- all clinically important outcomes have been considered;
- the likely benefits are worth the potential harms and costs.

6 Evaluate your performance

Self-evaluation involves questioning your abilities to complete tasks 1 to 5 successfully. Are you then able to integrate the critical appraisal into clinical practice, and have you audited your performance? You should also ask yourself whether you have learnt from past experience so that you are now more efficient and are finding the whole process of EBM easier.

References

1 Straus, S.E., Richardson, W.S., Glasziou, P. and Haynes, R.B. (2005) *Evidence-based Medicine: How to Practice and Teach EBM.* 3rd edition. London: Churchill-Livingstone.
2 Shea, B.J., Reeves, B.C., Wells, G., et al (2017) AMSTAR 2: a critical appraisal tool for systematic reviews that include randomised or non-randomised studies of healthcare interventions, or both. *BMJ*, **358**, j4008.

Example

Primary aim specified

Objective To examine the effect of a mobile phone text message-based intervention to encourage lifestyle change on objective measures of cardiovascular risk in individuals with coronary heart disease (CHD). The primary end point was <u>low-density lipoprotein cholesterol (LDL-C) level at 6 months.</u> The <u>secondary end points</u> were systolic blood pressure, body mass index (BMI), total cholesterol level, waist circumference, heart rate, total physical activity, smoking status and the proportion achieving at least 3, at least 4 or all 5 guideline levels of modifiable risk factors ((LDL- C < 77mg/dL, blood pressure < 140/90 mm Hg, exercising regularly [≥ 5 d/wk x 30 minutes exercise per session], non-smoker status and BMI < 25 kg/m^2).

Main outcome variable

All clinically important outcomes considered

Spectrum of patients

Subjects 710 patients with proven coronary heart disease (prior myocardial infarction or proven angiographically) were recruited between September 2011 and November 2013 from a large tertiary hospital in Sydney, Australia. Patients were eligible if they were older than 18 years and were able to provide informed consent. Patients were excluded if they did not have an active mobile phone or sufficient English language proficiency to read text messages.

Avoids bias. Patients could not be blind

Control group included

Avoids bias

Design A <u>parallel group, single-blind, randomized</u> clinical trial. The random allocation sequence was in a uniform 1:1 allocation ratio with a block size of 8 and was <u>concealed from study personnel.</u> Patients in the control group (n=358) received usual care which generally involved community follow-up, with the majority referred to inpatient cardiac rehabilitation. Patients in the intervention group (n = 352) received 4 text messages per week for 6 months in addition to usual care. Text messages provided advice, motivational reminders, and support to change lifestyle behaviours. Messages for each participant were selected from a bank of messages according to baseline characteristics (e.g., smoking) and delivered via an automated computerized message management system. The program was not interactive. All statistical tests were 2-tailed at the 5% level of significance and intervention evaluations were performed on the principle of <u>intention to treat.</u> Analyses were conducted using SAS version 9.3 (SAS Institute Inc.)

Avoids bias

Avoids bias

All secondary endpoints, apart from HDL-C, statistically significant in the direction that favours the intervention

Mean value of primary outcome given for each group

Findings At 6 months, levels of LDL-C were significantly lower in intervention participants. The estimated mean LDL-C was <u>79</u> (95% CI 76 to 82)mg/dL and <u>84</u> (95%CI 76 to 82) mg/dL in the intervention and control groups, respectively. The estimated difference in means was <u>-5 (95% CI-9 to 0)</u> mg/dL, P = 0.04. All individual <u>secondary endpoints</u> were significantly better (P ≤ 0.01) at 6 months in the intervention group compared to the control group, apart from mean HDL-C levels which were not significantly different. A significantly greater proportion (P < 0.001) in the intervention group achieved at least 3, as well as at least 4, of the guideline levels of risk factors. The majority reported the text messages to be useful (91%), easy to understand (97%), and appropriate in frequency (86%).

Magnitude of main effect of interest

Precision of main effect. Mean LDL-C is at worst the same or could be 9 mg/dL lower in the intervention group at 6 months.

Conclusion and relevance Among patients with coronary heart disease, the use of a lifestyle-focused text messaging service compared with usual care resulted in a modest improvement in LDL-C level and greater improvement in other cardiovascular disease risk factors. The duration of these effects and hence <u>whether they result in improved clinical outcomes remains to be determined.</u>

Long-term benefit given consideration

Trial registration anzctr.org.au Identifier: ACTRN12611000161921

[1]Trial profile shown in Fig 14.1

Losses to follow-up documented

Adapted from Chow, C.K., Redfern, J., Hills, G.S., *et al.* (2015) Effect of lifestyle-focused text messaging on risk factor modification in patients with coronary heart disease. A randomized clinical trial. *JAMA*, **314(12)**, 1255–1263.

41 Methods for clustered data

Clustered data conform to a hierarchical or nested structure in which, in its simplest form (the univariable **two-level structure**), the value of a single response variable is measured on a number of *level 1 units* contained in different groups or clusters (*level 2 units*). For example, the level 1 and level 2 units, respectively, may be teeth in a mouth, knees in a patient, patients in a hospital, clinics in a region, children in a class, successive visit times for a patient (i.e. *longitudinal* data, Fig. 41.1), etc. The statistical analysis of such **repeated measures** data should take into account the fact that the observations in a cluster tend to be correlated, i.e. they are *not independent*. Failure to acknowledge this usually results in underestimation of the standard errors of the estimates of interest and, consequently, confidence intervals that are too narrow and *P*-values that are too small, leading to increased Type I error rates.

For the purposes of illustration, we shall assume, in this chapter, that we have longitudinal data and our repeated measures data comprise each patient's values of the variable at different time points, i.e. the patient is the cluster. We summarize the data by describing the patterns in individual patients, and, if relevant, assess whether these patterns differ between two or more groups of patients.

Displaying the data

A plot of the measurement against time for each patient in the study provides a visual impression of the pattern over time. When we are studying only a small group of patients, it may be possible to show all the individual plots in one diagram. However, when we are studying large groups this becomes difficult, and we may illustrate just a selection of 'representative' individual plots (see Fig. 41.3), perhaps in a grid for each treatment group. Note that the average pattern generated by plotting the means over all patients at each time point may be very different from the patterns seen in individual patients.

Comparing groups: inappropriate analyses

Suppose we are interested in comparing treatments that have been randomly assigned to patients, each of whom provides measurements at successive time points. It is *inappropriate* to use all the values in a treatment group to fit a *single* linear regression line (Chapters 27 and 28) or to perform a one-way analysis of variance (ANOVA, Chapter 22) to compare treatment groups because these methods do not take account of the repeated measurements on the same patient. Furthermore, it is also *incorrect* to compare the means in the groups *at each time point separately* using unpaired *t*-tests if there are two treatment groups (Chapter 21) or one-way ANOVA if there are more than two groups for a number of reasons:

- The measurements in a patient from one time point to the next are not independent, so interpretation of the results is difficult. For example, if a comparison is significant at one time point, then it is likely to be significant at other time points, irrespective of any changes in the values in the interim period.
- The large number of tests carried out implies that we are likely to obtain significant results purely by chance (Chapter 18).
- We lose information about within-patient changes.

Comparing groups: appropriate analyses

Using summary measures

We can base our analysis on a **summary measure** that captures the important aspects of the data, and calculate this summary measure *for each patient*. Typical summary measures are:
- change from baseline at a predetermined time point;
- maximum (peak) or minimum (nadir) value reached;

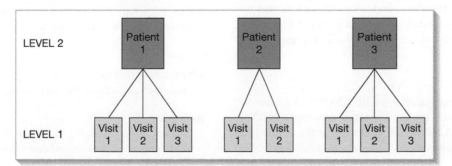

Figure 41.1 Diagrammatic representation of a two-level hierarchical structure for longitudinal data.

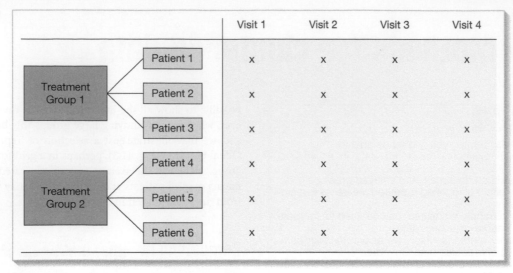

Figure 41.2 Diagrammatic representation of the structure of a hierarchical repeated measures ANOVA.

- time to reach the maximum (or minimum) value;
- time to reach some other pre-specified value;
- average value (e.g. mean);
- area under the curve (AUC, see Fig. 41.4);
- slope or intercept of the patient's regression line (describing the relationship between the measurement and time).

If the parameter (e.g. the mean or slope) is estimated more precisely in some patients than others (perhaps because there are more observations for these patients), we should take account of this in the analysis by giving more weight to those measures that are estimated more precisely.

The choice of summary measure depends on the main question of interest and should be made in advance of collecting the data. For example, if we are considering drug concentrations following treatment with two therapies, we may consider time to maximum drug concentration (C_{max}) or AUC. However, if we are interested in antibody titres following vaccination, then we may be interested in the time it takes the antibody titre to drop below a particular protective level.

We compare the values of the summary measure in the different groups using standard hypothesis tests, such as the Wilcoxon rank sum (Chapter 21) or Kruskal–Wallis tests (Chapter 22). Because we have reduced a number of dependent measurements on each individual to a single quantity, the values included in the analysis are now independent.

While analyses based on summary measures are simple to perform, it may be difficult to find a suitable measure that adequately describes the data, and we may need to use two or more summary measures. In addition, these approaches suffer from the disadvantage that they do not use all data values fully.

Hierarchical repeated measures ANOVA

We can perform a particular type of ANOVA (Chapter 22) called a **hierarchical or nested repeated measures ANOVA**. A repeated measures ANOVA (an extension of the paired t-test when we have more than two related observations) may be performed when every patient provides measurements at three or more successive visits (these are the repeated measures). If, in addition, each patient belongs to (i.e. is nested in) one of two or more treatment groups (Fig. 41.2), then hierarchical repeated measures ANOVA allows us to investigate whether the group means are equal and whether the visit means are equal. In addition, we can assess any interactions (Chapter 33), e.g. the interaction between treatment groups and visits, where a significant interaction would imply that any differences between the group means is not the same for all visits, and *vice versa*. If the ANOVA indicates that there is a significant difference between the treatment groups, provided there is no significant interaction and there are more than two groups, *post hoc* tests, which have P-values adjusted for multiple testing (Chapter 18), can be performed to identify where the differences lie[1].

However, hierarchical repeated measures ANOVA has several disadvantages:

- It may be difficult to perform.
- The results may be difficult to interpret.
- It generally assumes that values are measured at regular time intervals and that there are no missing data, i.e. the design of the study is assumed to be *balanced*. In reality, values are rarely measured at all time points because patients often miss appointments or come at different times to those planned.

Regression methods

Various regression methods, such as those that provide parameter estimates with robust standard errors or use generalized estimating equations (GEE) or random effects models, may be used to analyse clustered data (Chapter 42).

Caution

We must take care to avoid the ecological fallacy when interpreting the results of studies that involve clustered data (Chapter 34).

Reference

1 Mickey, R.M., Dunn, O.J. and Clark, V.A. (2004) *Applied Statistics: Analysis of Variance and Regression*. 3rd edition. Chichester: Wiley.

Example

As part of a practical class designed to assess the effects of two inhaled bronchodilator drugs, fenoterol hydrobromide and ipratropium bromide, 99 medical students were randomized to receive one of these drugs (n = 33 for each drug) or placebo (n = 33). Each student inhaled four times in quick succession. Tremor was assessed by measuring the total time (in seconds) taken to thread five sewing needles mounted on a cork; measurements were made at baseline before inhalation and at 5, 15, 30, 45 and 60 minutes afterwards. The measurements of a representative sample of the students in each treatment group are shown in Fig. 41.3.

It was decided to compare the values in the three groups using the 'area under the curve' (AUC) as a summary measure. The calculation of AUC for one student is illustrated in Fig. 41.4.

The median (range) AUC was 1552.5 (417.5–3875), 1215 (457.5–2500) and 1130 (547.5–2625) seconds[2] in those receiving fenoterol hydrobromide, ipratropium bromide and placebo, respectively. The values in the three groups were compared using the Kruskal–Wallis test, which gave $P = 0.008$. There was thus strong evidence that the distribution of AUC measures was not the same in all three groups. Non-parametric *post hoc* comparisons, adjusted for multiple testing, indicated that values were significantly greater in the group receiving fenoterol hydrobromide, confirming pharmacological knowledge that this drug, as a β_2-adrenoceptor agonist, induces tremor by the stimulation of β_2-adrenoceptors in skeletal muscle.

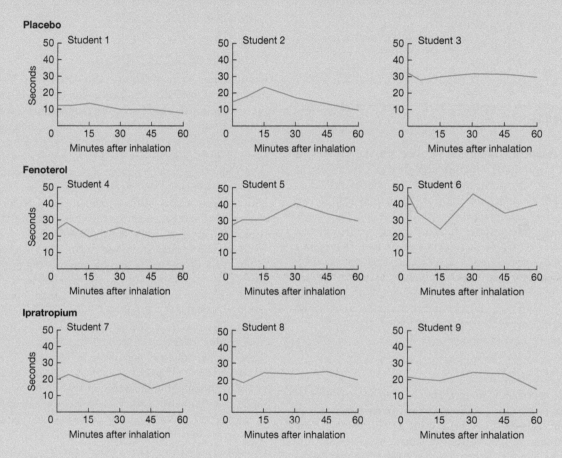

Figure 41.3 Time taken to thread five sewing needles for three representative students in each treatment group.

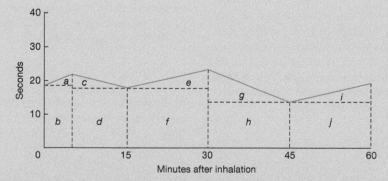

Figure 41.4 Calculation of the AUC for a single student. The total area under the line can be divided into a number of rectangles and triangles (marked *a* to *j*). The area of each can easily be calculated. Total AUC = Area (*a*) + Area (*b*) + … + Area (*j*).

Data kindly provided by Dr R. Morris, Department of Primary Care and Population Sciences, and were collected as part of a student practical class organized by Dr T.J. Allen, Department of Pharmacology, Royal Free and University College Medical School, London, UK.

42 Regression methods for clustered data

Various **regression methods** can be used for the analysis of the two-level hierarchical structure described in Chapter 41, in which each cluster (level 2 unit) contains a number of individual level 1 units. For example, in a study of rheumatoid arthritis, we may measure the flexion angle on both the left and right knees (level 1) of every patient (level 2). Alternatively, we may have a longitudinal data set with a measurement (e.g. total cholesterol) observed at successive times (level 1) on each patient (level 2). The main advantages and disadvantages of each method are summarized in Table 42.1. Most of these methods are unreliable unless there are sufficient clusters, and they can be complicated to perform and interpret correctly; we therefore suggest you consult a specialist statistician for advice.

Aggregate level analysis

A very simple approach is to *aggregate* the data and perform an analysis using an appropriate numerical **summary measure** (e.g. the mean) for each cluster (e.g. the patient) (Chapter 41). The choice of this summary measure will depend on features of the data and on the hypotheses being studied. We perform an ordinary least squares (OLS) multiple regression analysis using the *cluster as the unit of investigation* and the *summary measure as the outcome variable*. If each cluster has been allocated a particular treatment (in the knee example, the patient may be randomly allocated one of two treatments – an exercise regimen or no exercise), then, together with other cluster level covariates (e.g. sex, age), we can incorporate 'treatment' in the regression model as a dummy variable using codes such as 0 and 1 (or as a series of dummy variables if we have more than two treatments (Chapter 29)).

Robust standard errors

If the clustering is ignored in the regression analysis of a two-level structure, an important assumption underlying the linear regression model – that of independence between the observations (Chapters 27 and 28) – is violated. As a consequence, the standard errors of the parameter estimates are likely to be too small and, hence, results may be spuriously significant.

To overcome this problem, we may determine **robust standard errors** of the parameter estimates, basing our calculation of them on the variability in the data (evaluated by appropriate residuals) rather than on that assumed by the regression model. In a multiple regression analysis with robust standard errors, the estimates of the regression coefficients are the same as in OLS linear regression but the standard errors are more robust to violations of the underlying assumptions, our particular concern being lack of independence when we have clustered data.

Random effects models

Random effects models[1] are also known as (for example) **hierarchical**, **multilevel**, **mixed** or **cluster-specific** models, and as **cross-sectional time series**, **panel** or **repeated measures models** when the data are longitudinal. They can be fitted using various comprehensive statistical computer packages, such as R, SAS and Stata, or specialist software such as MLwiN (www.cmm.bristol.ac.uk), all of which use a version of maximum likelihood estimation. The estimate of the effect for each cluster is derived using both the individual cluster information as well as that of the other clusters so that it benefits from the 'shared' information. In particular, *shrinkage* estimates are commonly determined whereby, using an appropriate shrinkage factor, each cluster's estimate of the effect of interest is 'shrunk' towards the estimated overall mean. The amount of shrinkage depends on the cluster size (smaller clusters have greater shrinkage) and on the variation in the data (shrinkage is greater for estimates where the variation within clusters is large when compared to that between clusters).

A random effects model regards the clusters as a sample from a real or hypothetical population of clusters. The individual clusters are not of primary interest; they are assumed to be broadly similar with differences between them attributed to random variation or to other 'fixed' factors such as sex, age, etc. The two-level random effects model differs from the model which takes no account of clustering in that, although both incorporate random or unexplained error due to the variation between level 1 units (the *within*-cluster variance, σ^2), the random effects model also includes random error which is due to the variation *between* clusters, σ_c^2. The variance of an individual observation in this random effects model is therefore the sum of the two components of variance, i.e. it is $\sigma^2 + \sigma_c^2$.

Particular models

When the outcome variable, y, is numerical and there is a single explanatory variable, x, of interest, the simple **random intercepts** linear two-level model assumes that there is a linear relationship between y and x in each cluster, with all the cluster regression lines having a common slope, β, but different intercepts (Fig. 42.1a). The mean regression line has a slope equal to β and an intercept equal to α, which is the mean intercept averaged over all the clusters. The random error (residual) for each cluster is the amount by which the intercept for that cluster regression line differs, in the vertical direction, from the overall mean intercept, α (Fig. 42.1a). The cluster residuals are assumed to follow a Nor-

Table 42.1 Main advantages and disadvantages of regression methods for analysing clustered data.

Method	Advantages	Disadvantages
Aggregate level analysis	• Simple • Easy to perform with basic software	• Does not allow for effects of covariates for level 1 units • Ignores differences in cluster sizes and in precision of the estimate of each cluster summary measure • May not be able to find an appropriate summary measure
Robust standard errors that allow for clustering	• Relatively simple • Can include covariates that vary for level 1 units • Adjusts standard errors, confidence intervals and P-values to take account of clustering • Allows for different numbers of level 1 units per cluster	• Unreliable unless number of clusters large, say >30 • Does not adjust parameter estimates for clustering
Random effects model	• Explicitly allows for clustering by including both inter- and intra-cluster variation in model • Cluster estimates benefit from shared information from all clusters • Adjusts parameter estimates, standard errors, confidence intervals and P-values to take account of clustering • Can include covariates that vary for level 1 units • Allows for different numbers of level 1 units per cluster • Can extend hierarchy from two levels to multi-levels • Can accommodate various forms of a generalized linear model (GLM), e.g. Poisson	• Unreliable unless there are sufficient clusters • Parameter estimates often biased • Complex modelling skills required for extended models • Estimation and interpretation of random effects logistic model not straightforward
Generalized estimating equations (GEE)	• Relatively simple • No distributional assumptions of random effects (due to clusters) required • Can include covariates that vary for level 1 units • Allows for different numbers of level 1 units per cluster • Adjusts parameter estimates, standard errors, confidence intervals and P-values to take account of clustering	• Unreliable unless number of clusters large, say >30 • Treats clustering as a nuisance of no intrinsic interest* • Requires specification of working correlation structure* • Parameter estimates are cluster averages and do not relate to individuals in population*

*These points may sometimes be regarded as advantages, depending on the question of interest.

mal distribution with zero mean and variance = σ_c^2. Within each cluster, the residuals for the level 1 units are assumed to follow a Normal distribution with zero mean and the same variance, σ^2. If the cluster sizes are similar, a simple approach to checking for Normality and constant variance of the residuals for both the level 1 units and clusters is to look for Normality in a histogram of the residuals, and to plot the residuals against the predicted values (Chapter 28).

The random effects model can be *modified* in a number of ways (see also Table 42.1), e.g. by allowing the slope, β, to vary randomly between clusters. The model is then called a **random slopes model**, in which case the cluster-specific regression lines are not parallel to the mean regression line (Fig. 42.1b). See also meta-regression in Chapter 43.

Assessing the clustering effect

The effect of clustering can be assessed by:
• Calculating the **intraclass correlation coefficient** (ICC, sometimes denoted by ρ – see also Chapter 39), which, in the two-level structure, represents the correlation between two randomly chosen level 1 units in one randomly chosen cluster.

$$\text{ICC} = \frac{\sigma_c^2}{\sigma^2 + \sigma_c^2}$$

The ICC expresses the variation between the clusters as a proportion of the total variation; it is often presented as a percentage. ICC = 1 when there is no variation *within* the clusters and all the variation is attributed to differences *between* clusters; ICC = 0 when there is no variation between the clusters. We can use the ICC to make a subjective decision about the importance of clustering.

• Comparing two models where one model is the full random effects model and the other is a regression model with the same explanatory variable(s) but which does not take clustering into account. The relevant *likelihood ratio test* has a test statistic equal to the *difference* in the likelihood ratio statistics of the two models (Chapter 32) and it follows the Chi-squared distribution with 1 degree of freedom.

Generalized estimating equations (GEE)

In the GEE approach[2] to estimation, we adjust both the parameter estimates of a generalized linear model (GLM) and their standard errors to take into account the clustering of the data in a two-level structure. We make distributional assumptions about the dependent variable but, in contrast to the random effects model, do not assume that the between cluster residuals are Normally distributed. We regard the clustering as a nuisance rather than of intrinsic interest, and proceed by postulating a 'working' structure

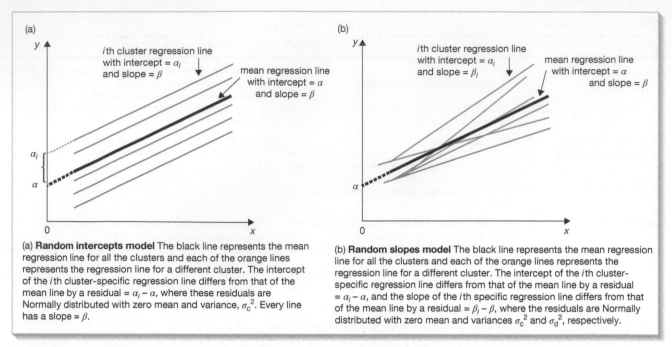

(a) **Random intercepts model** The black line represents the mean regression line for all the clusters and each of the orange lines represents the regression line for a different cluster. The intercept of the ith cluster-specific regression line differs from that of the mean line by a residual $= \alpha_i - \alpha$, where these residuals are Normally distributed with zero mean and variance, σ_c^2. Every line has a slope $= \beta$.

(b) **Random slopes model** The black line represents the mean regression line for all the clusters and each of the orange lines represents the regression line for a different cluster. The intercept of the ith cluster-specific regression line differs from that of the mean line by a residual $= \alpha_i - \alpha$, and the slope of the ith specific regression line differs from that of the mean line by a residual $= \beta_i - \beta$, where the residuals are Normally distributed with zero mean and variances σ_c^2 and σ_d^2, respectively.

Figure 42.1 Two-level random effects linear regression models with a single covariate, x.

for the correlation between the observations within each cluster. This does not have to be correct since, provided there are enough clusters, the robust standard errors and parameter estimates will be acceptable. However, we will obtain better parameter estimates if the structure is plausible. We commonly adopt an *exchangeable* correlation structure which assumes that exchanging two level 1 units within a cluster will not affect the estimation.

The GEE approach is sometimes called **population-averaged** (referring to the population of clusters) or **marginal** because the parameter estimates represent the effects averaged across the clusters (even though all level 1 unit information is included in

the analysis). The GEE approach is often preferred to the more complex random effects model analysis for logistic (Chapter 30) and, sometimes, Poisson (Chapter 31) regression, even though the exchangeable correlation structure is known to be incorrect in these situations.

References

1 Goldstein, H. (2010) *Multilevel Statistical Models*. 4th edition. Wiley Series in Probability and Statistics. Chichester: Wiley.
2 Liang, K.-Y. and Zeger, S.L. (1986) Longitudinal data analysis using generalized linear models. *Biometrika*, **73**, 13–22.

Example

Data relating to periodontal disease were obtained on 96 white male trainee engineers aged between 16 and 20 years entering the apprentice training school at Royal Air Force Halton, England. Each of the possible 28 teeth (excluding wisdom teeth) in every trainee's mouth was examined at four sites (the mesiobuccal, mesiolingual, distobuccal and distolingual). To simplify the analysis, we have considered a subset of the data, namely: (i) the mesiobuccal site in each tooth – this leads to a two-level structure of teeth within subjects (each subject corresponds to a cluster); and (ii) two variables of interest – loss of attachment (LOA, measured in mm) between the tooth and the jawbone evaluated at the mesiobuccal site, and the current cigarette smoking status of the trainee (yes = 1, no = 0). We wish to assess whether smoking is a risk factor for gum disease (where greater loss of attachment indicates worse disease).

Table 42.2 shows extracts of the results from various regression analyses in which the outcome variable is loss of attachment (mm) and the covariate is smoking. Full computer output is given in Appendix C. The estimates of the regression coefficients for

smoking and/or their standard errors vary according to the type of analysis performed. The two OLS analyses have identical estimated regression coefficients (which are larger than those of the other three analyses) but their standard errors are different. The standard error of the estimated regression coefficient in the OLS analysis that ignores clustering is substantially smaller than the standard errors in the other four analyses, i.e. *ignoring clustering results in an underestimation of the standard error of the regression coefficient and, consequently, a confidence interval that is too narrow and a P-value that is too small*. The intracluster correlation coefficient from the random effects model is estimated as 0.224. Thus approximately 22% of the variation in loss of attachment, after taking account of smoking, was between trainees rather than within trainees.

In this particular example, we conclude from all five analyses that smoking is not significantly associated with loss of attachment. This lack of significance for smoking is an unexpected finding and may be explained by the fact that these trainees were very young and so the smokers amongst them would not have smoked for a long period.

continued

Table 42.2 Summary of results of regression analyses in which LOA (mm) is the outcome variable.

Analysis	Estimated coefficient (smoking)	Standard error (SE)	95% CI for coefficient	Test statistic*	P-value
OLS regression ignoring clustering	−0.0105	0.0235	−0.057 to 0.036	$t = -0.45$	0.655
OLS regression with robust SEs	−0.0105	0.0526	−0.115 to 0.094	$t = -0.20$	0.842
Aggregate analysis (OLS regression on group means)	−0.0046	0.0612	−0.126 to 0.117	$t = -0.07$	0.941
Random effects model	−0.0053	0.0607	−0.124 to 0.114	$z = -0.09$	0.930
GEE with robust SEs and exchangeable correlation structure	−0.0053	0.0527	−0.108 to 0.098	$z = -0.10$	0.920

*t = test statistic following t-distribution; z = Wald test statistic following Standard Normal distribution.

Data kindly provided by Dr Gareth Griffiths, Department of Periodontology, UCL Eastman Dental Institute, UK.

43 Systematic reviews and meta-analysis

The systematic review

What is it?

A **systematic review**[1] is a formalized and stringent process of combining the information from *all* relevant studies (both published and unpublished) of the same health condition; these studies are usually clinical trials (Chapter 14) of the same or similar treatments but may be observational studies (Chapters 15 and 16). A systematic review is an integral part of **evidence-based medicine** (EBM, Chapter 40) which applies the results of the best available evidence, together with clinical expertise, to the care of patients. So important is its role in EBM that it has become the focus of an international network of clinicians, methodologists and consumers who have formed the **Cochrane Collaboration**. This has produced the Cochrane Library containing regularly updated evidence-based healthcare databases including the Cochrane Database of Systematic Reviews; full access to these reviews requires subscription but the abstracts are freely available on the internet (community-archive.cochrane.org/Cochrane-reviews).

PRISMA, another component of the EQUATOR network (Chapter 37), provides reporting guidelines for systematic reviews and meta-analyses of healthcare interventions (www.equator-network.org/reporting-guidelines/prisma/ and www.prisma-statement.org); the MOOSE checklist is specifically for the meta-analysis of observational studies in epidemiology (Appendix D).

What does it achieve?

- **Refinement and reduction** – large quantities of information are refined and reduced to a manageable size.
- **Efficiency** – the systematic review is usually quicker and less costly to perform than a new study. It may prevent others embarking on unnecessary studies, and can shorten the time lag between medical developments and their implementation.
- **Generalizability and consistency** – results can often be generalized to a wider patient population in a broader setting than

would be possible from a single study. Consistencies in the results from different studies can be assessed, and any inconsistencies determined.
- **Reliability** – the systematic review aims to reduce errors, and so tends to improve the reliability and accuracy of recommendations when compared with haphazard reviews or single studies.
- **Power and precision** – the quantitative systematic review (see meta-analysis below) has greater power (Chapter 18) to detect effects of interest and provides more precise estimates of them than a single study.

Meta-analysis

What is it?

A **meta-analysis** or **overview** is a particular type of systematic review that focuses on the numerical results. The main aim of a meta-analysis is to combine the results from several independent studies to produce, if appropriate, an estimate of the overall or average effect of interest (e.g. the relative risk, RR; Chapter 15). The direction and magnitude of this average effect, together with a consideration of the associated confidence interval and hypothesis test result, may be used to make decisions about the therapy under investigation, the management of patients and/or the role of the factor of interest, as appropriate.

Statistical approach

1 Decide on the effect of interest and, if the raw data are available, evaluate it for each study. However, in practice, we may have to extract these effects from published results. If the outcome in a clinical trial comparing two treatments is:

- **numerical**, the effect may be the difference in treatment means. A zero difference implies no treatment effect;
- **binary** (e.g. died/survived), we consider the risks, say, of the outcome (e.g. death) in the treatment groups. The effect may be the difference in risks or their ratio, the RR. If the difference in risks equals zero or RR = 1, then there is no treatment effect.

2 Check for statistical homogeneity and obtain an estimate of statistical heterogeneity – we have **statistical heterogeneity** when there is genuine variation between the effects of interest from the different studies.

- We can perform a hypothesis **test of homogeneity** to investigate whether the variation in the individual effects is compatible with chance alone. However, this test has low power (Chapter 18) to detect heterogeneity if there are few studies in the meta-analysis and may, conversely, give a highly significant result if it comprises many large studies, even when the heterogeneity is unlikely to affect the conclusions.
- An **index**, I^2, which does not depend on the number of studies, the type of outcome data or the choice of treatment effect (e.g. RR), can be used to quantify the impact of heterogeneity and assess inconsistency[2] (see Example). The index, I^2, represents the percentage of the total variation across studies due to heterogeneity; it takes values from 0% to 100%, with a

Medical Statistics at a Glance, Fourth Edition. Aviva Petrie and Caroline Sabin. © 2020 Aviva Petrie and Caroline Sabin. Published 2020 by John Wiley & Sons Ltd.
Companion Website: www.medstatsaag.com

value of 0% indicating no observed heterogeneity. If there is evidence of statistical heterogeneity, we should proceed cautiously, investigate the reasons for its presence and modify our approach accordingly (see Point 3).

3 Estimate the average effect of interest (with a confidence interval), and perform the appropriate hypothesis test on the effect (e.g. that the true RR = 1). The average estimate is usually a weighted mean (Chapter 5) of the estimated effects from all the studies, where the weight for each study is the inverse of the variance of the estimate. If there is no evidence of statistical heterogeneity, we generally perform a fixed effects meta-analysis which assumes the true treatment effect is the same in every study and any observed variation in the estimates from different studies is solely due to sampling error. In this case, the within-study variability is the only component of the variance of the average effect of interest. If there is evidence of statistical heterogeneity, it may not be sensible to provide an average effect of interest. However, if one is required, there are various approaches to obtaining it:

- Perform a random effects meta-analysis. This assumes that the separate studies represent a random sample from a population of studies that has a mean treatment effect about which the individual study effects vary. The variance of the average effect of interest incorporates both within- and between-study variability and therefore the standard error of the estimate is greater, the confidence interval for the true average effect wider and its *P*-value larger (i.e. it is less likely to be statistically significant) than the comparable quantities obtained from a fixed effects meta-analysis.

- Stratify the studies into subgroups of those with similar characteristics and perform a separate (usually fixed effects) meta-analysis in each stratum.

- Perform a **meta-regression**[3] that aims to estimate the effect of interest, after adjusting for differences between studies, and to determine which covariates account for the heterogeneity. The dependent variable is the estimated effect of interest for a study (e.g. the RR) and the explanatory variables are one or more study-level characteristics (e.g. the average age of the population, the average duration of treatment, whether the hospital is in an urban or rural setting). The most usual form of meta-regression is a random effects meta-regression which takes account of the between-study variability by including it as a component of error in the model (this is a form of random effects model – see Chapter 42). Unfortunately, because the 'sample size' for the meta-regression is the number of studies (rather than the number of patients in each study), many analyses are insufficiently powered to detect important effects. Furthermore, it may be impossible to separate the effects of different covariates if collinearity is present (Chapter 34), as is often the case, resulting in misleading conclusions. We should also be aware of the *ecological fallacy* (Chapter 34) which may lead us to believe mistakenly that an association that we observe between variables at an aggregate level reflects the corresponding association at an individual level in the same population.

4 Interpret the results and present the findings. It is helpful to summarize the results from each trial (e.g. the sample size, baseline characteristics, effect of interest such as the RR, and related confidence interval, CI) in a table (see Example). The most common graphical display is a **forest plot** (see Fig. 43.2) in which the estimated effect (with CI) for each trial and their average are marked along the length of a vertical line that represents

'no treatment effect' (e.g. this line corresponds to the value 'one' if the effect is a RR). The plotting symbol for the estimated effect for each study is often a box which has an area proportional to the size of that study. Initially, we examine whether the estimated effects from the different studies are on the same side of the line. Then we can use the CIs to judge whether the results are compatible (if the CIs overlap), to determine whether incompatible results can be explained by small sample sizes (if CIs are wide) and to assess the significance of the individual and overall effects (by observing whether the vertical line crosses some or all of the CIs).

Advantages and disadvantages

As a meta-analysis is a particular form of systematic review, it offers all the **advantages** of the latter (see 'What does it achieve?'). In particular, a meta-analysis, because of its inflated sample size, is able to detect treatment effects with *greater power* and estimate these effects with *greater precision* than any single study. Its advantages, together with the introduction of meta-analysis software, have led meta-analyses to proliferate. However, improper use can lead to erroneous conclusions regarding treatment efficacy. The following principal problems should be thoroughly investigated and resolved before a meta-analysis is performed.

- **Publication bias** – the tendency to include in the analysis only the results from published papers; these favour statistically significant findings. We may be able to decide whether publication bias is an issue by drawing a **funnel plot** (Fig 43.1), a scatter diagram that usually has some measure of study size on the vertical axis and the treatment effect (e.g. odds ratio) on the horizontal axis. In the absence of publication bias, the scatter of points (each point representing one study) in the funnel plot will be substantial at the bottom where the study size is small, and will narrow (in the shape of a funnel) towards the top where the study size is large. If publication bias is present, the funnel plot will probably be skewed and asymmetrical, with a gap towards the bottom left-hand corner where both the treatment effect and study size are small (i.e. when the study has low power to detect a small effect).

- **Clinical heterogeneity** – in which differences in the patient population, outcome measures, definition of variables, and/or duration of follow-up of the studies included in the analysis create problems of non-compatibility.

- **Quality differences** – the design and conduct of the studies may vary in their quality. Although giving more weight to the better studies is one solution to this dilemma, any weighting system can be criticized on the grounds that it is arbitrary.

- **Dependence** – the results from studies included in the analysis may not be independent, e.g. when results from a study are published on more than one occasion.

Sensitivity analysis

Sensitivity analysis in a meta-analysis assesses the robustness (Chapter 35) of the common estimate. As in regression analysis, it is important to determine whether any particular study in a meta-analysis strongly influences the average measure of the effect of interest. This may be achieved by deleting each of the *k* studies in turn, using a meta-analysis to estimate the effect of interest from the remaining *k* – 1 studies, and plotting these estimates with their confidence intervals in an **influence plot**. This is similar to a forest plot but the different studies on the vertical axis are replaced by the revised meta-analyses, one for each study omitted. Any estimate that appears on visual inspection to differ substantially from the others may enable the omitted study to be flagged as influential. An alternative approach to assessing the impact of each study is to perform a **cumulative meta-analysis** in which we add the studies one by one in a specified order (usually according to date of publication) and perform a separate meta-analysis on the accumulated studies after each addition. We generally present the results in a cumulative meta-analysis diagram: this looks similar to a forest plot but each of the time-ordered entries on it indicates the overall average estimated effect of interest at the relevant point in time rather than the estimated effect from a single study. An examination of this diagram can help determine whether the pooled estimate has been robust over time.

References

1 Egger, M., Davey Smith, G. and Altman, D. (eds) (2001) *Systematic Reviews in Health Care: Meta-analysis in Context.* 2nd edition. London: BMJ Books.

2 Higgins, P.T., Thompson, S.G., Deeks, J.J. and Altman, D.G. (2003) Measuring inconsistency in meta-analysis. *British Medical Journal,* **237**, 557–560.

3 Morton, S.C., Adams, J.L., Suttorp, M.J. and Shekelle, P.G. (2004) *Meta Regression Approaches: What, Why, When, and How?* Technical Review 8 (Prepared by Southern California–RAND Evidence-based Practice Center, under Contract No. 290-97-0001). AHRQ Publication No. 04-0033. Rockville, MD: Agency for Healthcare Research and Quality.

Example

Anxiety disorders are the most prevalent mental disorders worldwide and are associated with immense healthcare costs and a high burden of disease. Stroke is the second most common cause of death and the third most common cause of reduced disability-adjusted life-years. A better understanding of the association between anxiety disorders and stroke would strengthen the evidence for causality and, since anxiety disorders are modifiable conditions, it could also inform the development of clinical and public health interventions for the management of anxiety and the prevention of stroke. To this end, a meta-analysis of eight observational studies was undertaken to obtain a pooled estimate of the risk of stroke amongst patients with anxiety disorders. All studies were considered to be of high quality and were population-based. The total sample comprised 950,759 patients. The main features of the included studies are shown in Table 43.1 – the effect of interest was the hazard ratio (HR). A funnel plot (Fig. 43.1) demonstrated reasonable symmetry, suggesting that publication bias was unlikely. The estimated HR obtained from each study was graphically presented in a forest plot (Fig. 43.2). Although the individual estimates of the HR vary quite considerably, from demonstrating a reduction in the

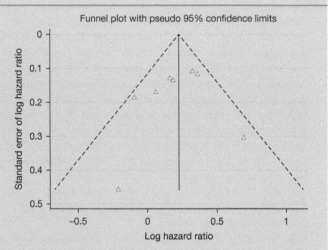

Figure 43.1 Funnel plot showing the pseudo confidence interval, indicating the region within which we would expect 95% of studies to lie if the studies are all estimating the same underlying effect. The vertical line is the line of no effect. *Source*: Pérez-Piñar, et al. (2017). Reproduced with permission of Elsevier.

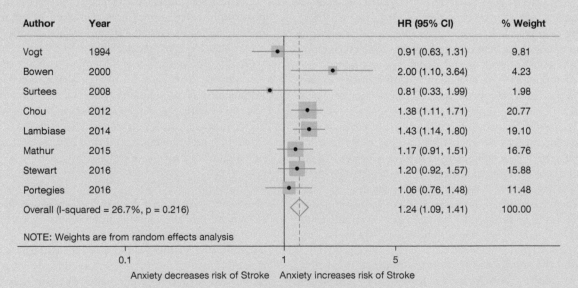

Author	Year		HR (95% CI)	% Weight
Vogt	1994		0.91 (0.63, 1.31)	9.81
Bowen	2000		2.00 (1.10, 3.64)	4.23
Surtees	2008		0.81 (0.33, 1.99)	1.98
Chou	2012		1.38 (1.11, 1.71)	20.77
Lambiase	2014		1.43 (1.14, 1.80)	19.10
Mathur	2015		1.17 (0.91, 1.51)	16.76
Stewart	2016		1.20 (0.92, 1.57)	15.88
Portegies	2016		1.06 (0.76, 1.48)	11.48
Overall (I-squared = 26.7%, p = 0.216)			1.24 (1.09, 1.41)	100.00

NOTE: Weights are from random effects analysis

0.1   1   5

Anxiety decreases risk of Stroke   Anxiety increases risk of Stroke

Figure 43.2 Forest plot of the hazard ratio (HR), with 95% confidence interval, of stroke in patients with anxiety disorders. *Source*: Pérez-Piñar et al. (2017). Reproduced with permission of Elsevier.

risk of stroke in those with anxiety disorders in two studies to increases in risk in the other studies, all confidence intervals overlap to some extent.

A more formal assessment of heterogeneity was provided by **Cochran's Chi-squared test for homogeneity**, which gave a non-significant result (test statistic $Q = 9.55$, degrees of freedom $= 8 - 1 = 7$, $P = 0.216$). However, $I^2 = 100 \times (Q - df)/Q = 100 \times 0.267 = 26.7\%$, suggesting moderate inconsistency across the studies and advocating a cautious approach to interpreting the combined estimate of HR for all trials. In view of this and the fact

that the Chi-squared test has low power to detect heterogeneity when the number of studies is small, the authors adopted the more conservative random effects approach to the analysis. The combined estimated HR was 1.24 (95% CI 1.09 to 1.41), indicating that there was evidence of an association between anxiety and stroke, with a pooled risk of stroke increased by 24% amongst patients suffering anxiety disorders. However, with the available evidence, it was not possible to differentiate between disparate anxiety disorders, and further research is required to determine the impact of specific anxiety disorders on different types of stroke.

Table 43.1 Characteristics of the eight observational studies included in the review.*

	Vogt 1994	Bowen 2000	Surtees 2008	Chou 2012	Lambiase 2014	Mathur 2015	Portegies 2016	Stewart 2016
Country	USA	Canada	UK	Taiwan	USA	UK	Netherlands	USA
Data source	E	MR	E	MR	E	MR	E	E
n	1529	2657	20627	390309	6019	524952	2625	2041
Age (years)	>15	>15	41-80	<20	25-74	>20	>45	>60
Female (%)	54	59	57	46	54	47	55	73
Follow-up (years)	15	12	12	10	22	10	20	9
Anxiety, n (%)	817 (53.4%)	866 (32.6%)	NR	1725 (0.4%)	1953 (31.9%)	22,128 (4.2%)	343 (13.1%)	849 (41.6%)
Stroke, n (%)	NR	44 (1.6%)	595 (2.9%)	19148 (4.9%)	419 (7.0%)	987 (0.2%)	332 (12.6%)	235 (11.5%)
Stroke assessment	ICD-7	ICD-9	ICD-9, ICD-10	ICD-9	ICD-9	MR	MR	ICD-9, ICD-10
Anxiety assessment	Bradburn worries index	ICD-9 DSM-III DSM-IIIR	Health and life experience (GAD)	ICD-9 DSM-IV TR (PD)	General wellbeing scale	Primary care scale	Hospital anxiety depression scale	Patient questionnaire
Adjustment for covariates	A, S, smoking, health status, SES, duration of health plan membership	A, S	A, S, CV risk factors, SES, PMH: MI, FH stroke, antidepressant use	A, S, comorbidities, regular medication	A, S, ethnicity, education, marital status	A, S, ethnicity	A, S	A, S, ethnicity, CV risk factors

*Only first author named in table.

A, age; CV risk factors: blood pressure, cholesterol, diabetes, smoking and obesity; E, epidemiological; FH, family history; GAD, generalized anxiety disorder; MI, myocardial infarction; MR, medical records; NR, not reported; PD, panic disorder; PMH, past medical history; S, sex; SES, socioeconomic status.

Source: Pérez-Piñar et al. (2017). Reproduced with permission of Elsevier.

44 Survival analysis

Survival data are concerned with the time it takes an individual to reach an endpoint of interest (often, but not always, death) and are characterized by the following two features.

- It is the **length of time** for the patient to reach the endpoint, rather than whether or not she or he reaches the endpoint, that is of primary importance. For example, we may be interested in length of survival in patients admitted with cirrhosis.
- Data may often be **censored** (see below).

Standard methods of analysis, such as logistic regression or a comparison of the mean time to reach the endpoint in patients with and without a new treatment, can give misleading results because of the censored data. Therefore, a number of statistical techniques, known as **survival methods**[1], have been developed to deal with these situations.

Censored data

Survival times are calculated from some baseline date that reflects a natural 'starting point' for the study (e.g. time of surgery or diagnosis of a condition) until the time that a patient reaches an endpoint of interest (e.g. death from the condition or a relapse). Often, however, we may not know when the patient reached the endpoint, only that she or he remained free of the endpoint while in the study. For example, patients in a trial of a new drug for the treatment of cancer, in which progression of cancer is the endpoint of interest, may be in cancer remission when they leave the study. This may either be because the trial ended while they were still in remission, because these individuals withdrew from the trial early before their cancer returned, or because they died of other non-cancer causes before the end of follow-up. Such data are described as **right-censored**. These patients were known *not* to have reached the endpoint when they were last under follow-up, and this information should be incorporated into the analysis.

Where follow-up does not begin until after the baseline date, survival times can also be **left-censored**.

Displaying survival data

A separate horizontal line can be drawn for each patient, its length indicating the survival time. Lines are drawn from left to right, and patients who reach the endpoint and those who are censored can be distinguished by the use of different symbols at the end of the line (Fig. 44.1). However, these plots do not summarize the data and it is difficult to get a feel for the survival experience overall.

A **survival curve**, usually calculated by the **Kaplan–Meier** method, displays the cumulative probability (the **survival probability**) of an individual remaining free of the endpoint at any time after baseline (Fig. 44.2). The survival probability will only change when an endpoint occurs, and thus the resulting 'curve' is drawn as a series of steps, starting at a survival probability of 1 (or 100%) at baseline (time 0) and dropping towards 0 as time increases. We may also display the **cumulative incidence** of the endpoint; this is calculated as (1 – survival probability) at each time point and the resulting curve is the inverse of the survival curve (i.e. it starts at a survival probability of 0 and moves up towards 1 as time increases). Although the information contained in both displays is the same, the cumulative incidence curve is generally preferred to the cumulative survival curve when the endpoint is rare (and so the survival probability remains high throughout the study) as this allows maximum detail to be shown without a break in the scale. An alternative method of calculating survival probabilities, using a **lifetable** approach, can be used when the time to reach the endpoint is only known to within a particular time interval (e.g. within a year). The survival probabilities using either the Kaplan–Meier or lifetable approaches may be obtained easily from most statistical packages.

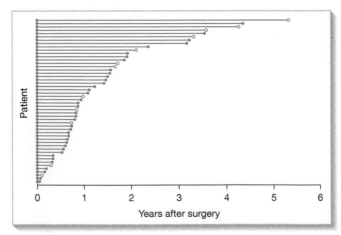

Figure 44.1 Survival experience of a random sample of 50 of 1358 patients with advanced pancreatic cancer who underwent either pancreaticoduodenectomy with portal vein resection, standard pancreaticoduodenectomy or surgical bypass. Filled orange circles indicate patients who died, open circles indicate those who remained alive at the end of follow-up.

Medical Statistics at a Glance, Fourth Edition. Aviva Petrie and Caroline Sabin. © 2020 Aviva Petrie and Caroline Sabin. Published 2020 by John Wiley & Sons Ltd.
Companion Website: www.medstatsaag.com

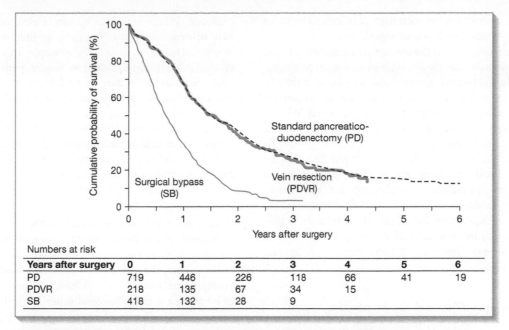

Figure 44.2 Kaplan–Meier curves showing the survival probability, expressed as a percentage, among patients with advanced pancreatic cancer undergoing pancreaticoduodenectomy with vein resection (PDVR), standard pancreaticoduodenectomy (PD) or surgical bypass (SB) – see Example.

Summarizing survival

We often summarize survival by quoting survival probabilities (with confidence intervals) at certain time points on the curve, for example the 5-year survival rates in patients after treatment for breast cancer. Alternatively, the median time to reach the endpoint (the time at which 50% of the individuals have *progressed*) can be quoted.

Comparing survival

We may wish to assess the impact of a number of factors of interest on survival, e.g. treatment or disease severity. Survival curves can be plotted separately for subgroups of patients; they provide a means of assessing visually whether different groups of patients reach the endpoint at different rates (Fig. 44.2). We can test formally whether there are any significant differences in progression rates between the different groups by, for example, using the log-rank test or regression models.

The log-rank test

This non-parametric test addresses the null hypothesis that there are no differences in survival times in the groups being studied, and compares events occurring at all time points on the survival curve. We cannot assess the independent roles of more than one factor on the time to the endpoint using the log-rank test.

Regression models

We can generate a regression model to quantify the relationships between one or more factors of interest and survival. At any point in time, t, an individual, i, has an instantaneous risk of reaching the endpoint, often known as the **hazard** or $\lambda_i(t)$, given that she or he has not reached it up to that point in time. For example, if death is the endpoint, the hazard is the risk of dying at time t. This instantaneous hazard is usually very small and is of limited interest. However, we may want to know whether there are any systematic differences between the hazards, over all time points, of individuals with different characteristics. For example,

is the hazard generally reduced in individuals treated with a new therapy compared with those treated with a placebo, when we take into account other factors, such as age or disease severity?

We can use the **Cox proportional hazards model** to test the independent effects of a number of explanatory variables (factors) on the hazard. It is of the form

$$\lambda_i(t) = \lambda_0(t) \exp\{\beta_1 x_1 + \beta_2 x_2 + \ldots + \beta_k x_k\}$$

where $\lambda_i(t)$ is the hazard for individual i at time t, $\lambda_0(t)$ is an arbitrary baseline hazard (in which we are not interested), $x_1, \ldots, x_k$ are explanatory variables in the model and $\beta_1, \ldots, \beta_k$ are the corresponding coefficients. We obtain estimates, $b_1, \ldots, b_k$, of these parameters using a form of maximum likelihood known as **partial likelihood**. The exponential of these values (i.e. $\exp\{b_1\} = e^{b_1}$) are the estimated **relative hazards** or **hazard ratios**. For a particular value of x_1, the hazard ratio is the estimated hazard of disease for $(x_1 + 1)$ relative to the estimated hazard of disease for x_1, while adjusting for all other x's in the equation. The relative hazard is interpreted in a similar manner to the odds ratio in logistic regression (Chapter 30) or the relative rate in Poisson regression (Chapter 31); therefore values above one indicate a raised hazard, values below one indicate a decreased hazard and values equal to one indicate that there is no increased or decreased hazard of the endpoint. A confidence interval can be calculated for the relative hazard and a significance test performed to assess its departure from one.

The relative hazard is assumed to be constant over time in this model (i.e. the hazards for the groups to be compared are assumed to be *proportional*). It is important to check this assumption[1]: we can, for example:

• use graphical methods – the simplest approach is to check that the two or more curves corresponding to the categories of a single covariate in a Kaplan–Meier survival plot move apart progressively over time. Alternatively, a plot of ln[−ln(survival probability)] versus ln(time) for each category of the covariate (sometimes referred to as a log log plot, and available in most statistical packages) should exhibit roughly parallel lines. In particular, lines that cross indicate a serious deviation from proportional hazards;

• incorporate an interaction between the covariate and ln(time) in the model and ensure that it is non-significant;

• perform a formal test, such as the global Chi-squared test based on Schoenfeld residuals, usually available in statistical packages.

If the proportional hazards assumption is violated, it may be possible to split the follow-up time into two or more intervals over which the hazards are known to be proportional. We can then perform a separate Cox regression analysis in each interval and report the results from each.

Other models can be used to describe survival data, e.g. the **Exponential**, **Weibull** or **Gompertz** models, each of which assumes a specific probability distribution for the hazard function. **Frailty models** are used when the observations on survival are not independent (i.e. there is correlation within clusters, such as within geographical areas because of shared environmental factors). However, all these models are beyond the scope of this book[1].

Problems encountered in survival analysis

Informative censoring

In any survival analysis we make the assumption that the probability that an individual's follow-up is censored is independent of (i.e. unrelated to) the probability that the individual will develop the outcome of interest (e.g. death). For example, an individual's follow-up may be censored because she or he moved from the area and was lost to follow-up; at the time of censoring, this person has the same chance of developing the outcome of interest as individuals who had been followed for the same period of time but whose follow-up was not censored. Where this assumption is violated, we say that we have **informative censoring** (and we must accommodate this in our statistical analysis). For example, in a study of the survival of patients with acute liver failure, patients who undergo liver transplantation may be withdrawn from the study early and their follow-up censored. As these individuals are likely to have a different prognosis to those who did not undergo transplantation, their follow-up will have been informatively censored. **Administrative censoring**, whereby patient follow-up is censored simply because the study ends on a particular date, is generally non-informative.

Competing risks

Occasionally, a study may have a number of different outcomes of interest. If the development of one or more of these outcomes precludes the development (or measurement) of any of the others, the outcomes are termed **competing risks**. For example, individuals with chronic kidney disease are known to be at higher risk of several other clinical events, including cardiovascular disease. If we are interested in assessing the risk factors for dying from end-stage renal disease after a diagnosis of chronic kidney disease, then an individual who dies from any cause other than end-stage renal disease after his/her diagnosis (e.g. if she or he experiences a fatal myocardial infarction) will no longer be at risk of death from end-stage renal disease. In this instance, the fatal myocardial infarction acts as a competing risk (as this event precludes the development of end-stage renal disease).

Reference

1 Collett, D. (2015) *Modelling Survival Data in Medical Research*. 3rd edition. London: Chapman and Hall/CRC.

Example

Pancreatic cancer is a common form of cancer in many resource-rich settings. However, survival after a diagnosis of pancreatic cancer remains poor. Over the last 15 years, improvements in surgical technique have enabled more aggressive surgical methods that may offer a better survival prognosis. In particular, there have been reports that pancreaticoduodenectomy with portal vein resection (PDVR) may offer survival advantages over standard pancreaticoduodenectomy (PD) or standard surgical bypass (SB). Ravikumar *et al.* undertook a retrospective data analysis to assess the post-surgical outcomes of 1588 patients with advanced pancreatic cancer. Of the 1358 patients with mortality information available, 218 had undergone PDVR, 719 had undergone PD and 418 had undergone SB. The patients were followed for a median of 1.1 (interquartile range 0.5, 1.9) years after surgery. The experience of a random sample of 50 of these patients is illustrated in Fig. 44.1. Over the follow-up period (the patients were followed for a maximum of 11 years), 1058 patients died. **Kaplan–Meier curves** showing the cumulative survival percentage at any time point after baseline are displayed separately for individuals in the three surgical groups (Fig. 44.2).

The computer output for the **log-rank test** contained the following information:

Test	Chi-square	df	P-value
Log-rank	222.5875	2	<0.0001

Thus there is a significant difference ($P < 0.0001$) between survival times in the three groups. By 1 year after surgery, 67.3% of those undergoing PDVR and 67.1% of those undergoing PD remained alive, compared to only 34.0% of those undergoing SB (Fig. 44.2).

A **Cox proportional hazards regression model** was used to investigate whether these differences in survival could be explained by differences in the sex of the patient (there may be differences in mortality outcomes between men and women), his/her age at the time of surgery (older people are likely to have a poorer prognosis) or the date on which the surgery was performed (outcomes are known to have improved over time). Graphical methods suggested that the proportional hazards assumption was reasonable for these variables. The results of this model are shown in Table 44.1.

The results in Table 44.1 indicate that individuals who have undergone pancreaticoduodenectomy have a lower hazard of mortality after surgery than those undergoing a standard surgical bypass, regardless of whether the surgery involved portal vein resection, even after adjusting for other factors known to be associated with a poorer outcome. In particular, individuals undergoing PDVR had a mortality hazard that was 0.41 (= exp{−0.89}) times that of individuals undergoing a SB (i.e. the mortality hazard was reduced by 59%, $P < 0.0001$) after adjusting for other factors, and individuals undergoing PD had a mortality hazard that was 0.40 (= exp{−0.92}) times that of individuals undergoing a SB (i.e. the mortality hazard was reduced by 60%, $P < 0.0001$) after adjustment. In addition, older age (hazard increases by 4% per additional 5 years of age) and surgery in 2003 or earlier (hazard increases by 31%) were both associated with a higher mortality hazard after surgery.

Table 44.1 Results of Cox proportional hazards regression analysis.

Variable*	Coding	df	Parameter estimate	Standard error	P-value	Estimated relative hazard	95% confidence interval for relative hazard
Type of surgery	SB		reference		-		
	PDVR	1	−0.89	0.10	<0.0001	0.41	(0.34–0.50)
	PD	1	−0.92	0.07	<0.0001	0.40	(0.35–0.46)
Sex of patient	Male (0)		reference				
	Female (1)	1	0.02	0.06	0.76	1.02	(0.90–1.15)
Age of patient at time of surgery	(/5 years older)	1	0.04	0.02	0.02	1.04	(1.01–1.08)
Year of surgery	2003 or earlier	1	0.27	0.09	0.004	1.31	(1.09–1.58)
	2004–2005	1	0.08	0.10	0.40	1.08	(0.90–1.31)
	2006–2007		reference				
	2008–2009	1	−0.06	0.09	0.52	0.94	(0.79–1.13)
	2010 and later	1	0.01	0.11	0.93	1.01	(0.81–1.26)

*Codes for the binary variable, sex of patient, are shown in parentheses. Type of surgery and year of surgery were included by incorporating dummy variables to reflect the two types of surgery (PDVR and PD) and the four calendar periods (before 2004, 2004–2005, 2008–2009, 2010 and later) which were compared to the reference categories of SB and 2006–2007, respectively.

Data kindly provided by Miss R. Ravikumar, Royal Free Hospital, London, UK, and adapted from: Ravikumar, R., Sabin, C., Hilal, M.A., *et al.* (2014) Portal vein resection in borderline resectable pancreatic cancer: a United Kingdom Multicenter study. *Journal of the American College of Surgeons*, **218**, 401-411.

45 Bayesian methods

The frequentist approach

The hypothesis tests described in this book are based on the **frequentist** approach to probability (Chapter 7) and inference that considers the number of times an event would occur if we were to repeat the experiment a large number of times. This approach is sometimes criticized for the following reasons.

- It uses only information obtained from the current study, and does not incorporate into the inferential process any other information we might have about the effect of interest, e.g. a clinician's views about the relative effectiveness of two therapies before a clinical trial is undertaken.

- It does not directly address the issues of greatest interest. In a drug comparison, we are usually really interested in knowing whether one drug is *more effective* than the other. However, the frequentist approach tests the hypothesis that the two drugs are *equally effective*. Although we conclude that one drug is superior to the other if the *P*-value is small, this probability (i.e. the *P*-value) describes the chance of getting the observed results if the drugs are equally effective, rather than the chance that one drug is more effective than the other (our real interest).

- It tends to over-emphasize the role of hypothesis testing and whether or not a result is significant, rather than the implications of the results.

The Bayesian approach

An alternative, **Bayesian**[1], approach to inference reflects an individual's personal degree of belief in a hypothesis, possibly based on information already available. Individuals usually differ in their degrees of belief in a hypothesis; in addition, these beliefs may change as new information becomes available. The Bayesian approach calculates the probability that a hypothesis is *true* (our focus of interest) by updating *prior* opinions about the hypothesis as new data become available.

Conditional probability

A particular type of probability, known as **conditional probability**, is fundamental to Bayesian analyses. This is the probability of an event, given that another event has already occurred. As an illustration, consider an example. The incidence of haemophilia A in the general population is approximately 1 in 10,000 male births. However, if we know that a woman is a carrier for haemophilia, this incidence increases to around 1 in 2 male births. Therefore, the probability that a male child has haemophilia, given that his mother is a carrier, is very different to the unconditional probability that he has haemophilia if his mother's carrier status is unknown.

Bayes theorem

Suppose we are investigating a hypothesis (e.g. that a treatment effect equals some value). Bayes theorem converts a **prior probability**, describing an individual's belief in the hypothesis *before* the study is carried out, into a **posterior probability**, describing his/her belief *afterwards*. The posterior probability is, in fact, the conditional probability of the hypothesis, given the results from the study. **Bayes theorem** states that the **posterior probability** is proportional to the **prior probability** multiplied by a value, the **likelihood** of the observed results which describes the plausibility of the observed results if the hypothesis is true (Chapter 32).

Diagnostic tests in a Bayesian framework

Almost all clinicians intuitively use a Bayesian approach in their reasoning when making a diagnosis. They build a picture of the patient based on clinical history and/or the presence of symptoms and signs. From this, they decide on the *most likely* diagnosis, having eliminated other diagnoses on the presumption that they are unlikely to be true, given what they know about the patient. They may subsequently confirm or amend this diagnosis in the light of new evidence, e.g. if the patient responds to treatment or a new symptom develops.

When an individual attends a clinic, the clinician usually has some idea of the probability that the individual has the disease – the **prior** or **pre-test probability**. If nothing else is known about the patient, this is simply the **prevalence** (Chapters 12 and 38) of the disease in the population. We can use Bayes theorem to change the prior probability into a posterior probability. This is most easily achieved if we incorporate the **likelihood ratio** (Chapter 32), based on information obtained from the most recent investigation (e.g. a diagnostic test result), into Bayes theorem. The likelihood ratio of a positive test result is the chance of a positive test result if the patient has disease, divided by that if he or she is disease-free. We discussed the likelihood ratio in this context in Chapter 38 and showed that it could be used to indicate the usefulness of a diagnostic test. We now use it to express Bayes theorem in terms of odds (Chapter 16)

$$\textbf{Posterior odds of disease} = \textbf{prior odds} \times \textbf{likelihood ratio}$$
$$\textbf{of a positive test result}$$

where

$$\text{Prior odds} = \frac{\text{prior probability}}{(1 - \text{prior probability})}$$

Medical Statistics at a Glance, Fourth Edition. Aviva Petrie and Caroline Sabin. © 2020 Aviva Petrie and Caroline Sabin. Published 2020 by John Wiley & Sons Ltd.
Companion Website: www.medstatsaag.com

The posterior odds is simple to calculate but, for easier interpretation, we convert the odds back into a probability using the relationship

$$\text{Posterior probability} = \frac{\text{posterior odds}}{(1 + \text{posterior odds})}$$

This **posterior** or **post-test probability** is the probability that the patient has the disease, given a positive test result. It is similar to the positive predictive value (PPV, Chapter 38) but the clinician will not be able to determine the PPV unless he or she has access to the test results from a sample of patients, each of whom has a definitive diagnosis from a gold standard test (Table 38.1). Furthermore, the main factor that affects the PPV is the prevalence, and there may be reasons why an individual's underlying risk of disease is known to be higher or lower than the overall population prevalence. Thus, in this situation, even if the clinician could calculate the PPV, it may not give a reasonable indication of his or her belief, after the test result is known, that the patient has the disease. Therefore, it is preferable to calculate the post-test probability in this situation.

A simpler way to calculate the post-test probability is to use **Fagan's nomogram** (Fig. 45.1); by connecting the pre-test probability (expressed as a percentage) to the likelihood ratio and extending the line, we can evaluate the post-test probability.

Disadvantages of Bayesian methods

As part of any Bayesian analysis, it is necessary to specify the prior probability of the hypothesis (e.g. the pre-test probability that a patient has disease). Because of the subjective nature of these priors, individual researchers and clinicians may choose different values for them. For this reason, Bayesian methods are often criticized as being arbitrary. Where the most recent evidence from the study (i.e. the likelihood) is very strong, however, the influence of the prior information is minimized (at its extreme, the results will be completely uninfluenced by the prior information).

The calculations involved in many Bayesian analyses are complex, usually requiring sophisticated statistical packages that are highly computer intensive. Therefore, despite being intuitively appealing, Bayesian methods have not been used widely. However, the availability of powerful personal computers means that their use is becoming more common.

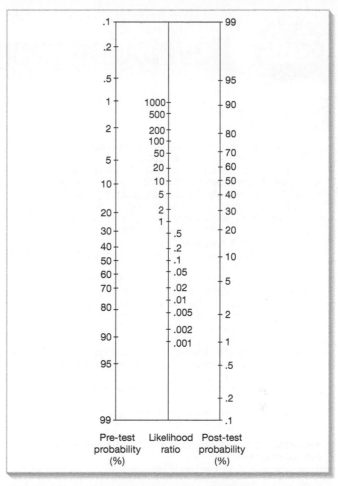

Figure 45.1 Fagan's nomogram for interpreting a diagnostic test result. *Source*: Sackett et al. (1997). Reproduced with permission of Elsevier.

Reference

1 Freedman, L. (1996) Bayesian statistical methods. A natural way to assess clinical evidence. *British Medical Journal*, 313, 569–570.

Example

In the example in Chapter 38 we showed that, in patients with hepatitis aged under 20 years, a ceruloplasmin concentration <16.6 mg/dL had a sensitivity of 91.2% and specificity of 94.9% to predict Wilson's disease (WD). The likelihood ratio for a positive test for this cut-off was 17.9.

If we believe that the prevalence of WD in those patients with hepatitis under 20 years of age is 6.4% (as observed in the Korean sample), the prior probability of periodontitis in such patients equals 0.064.

$$\text{Prior odds} = \frac{0.064}{0.936} = 0.068$$

$$\text{Posterior odds} = 0.068 \times \text{likelihood ratio}$$

$$= 0.068 \times 17.9$$

$$= 1.22$$

$$\text{Posterior probability} = \frac{1.22}{(1 + 1.22)} = 0.550$$

Therefore, if the patient has a ceruloplasmin concentration <16.6 mg/dL, and we assume a pre-test probability of 0.064, then we believe that the patient has a 55% chance of having WD. This can also be estimated directly from Fagan's nomogram (Fig 45.1) by connecting the pre-test probability of 6.4% to a likelihood ratio of 17.9 and extending the line to cut the post-test probability axis. In contrast, if we believe the probability that a patient has WD is as low as 2% then the post-test probability will equal 27%.

In both cases, the post-test probability is substantially higher than the pre-test probability, indicating the usefulness of using ceruloplasmin concentration <16.6 mg/dL as an indicator of WD in young children and young adults with hepatitis.

46 Developing prognostic scores

Why do we do it?

Given a large number of demographic or clinical features of an individual, we may want to *predict* whether that individual is likely to experience an event of interest. This event may either reflect a positive outcome for the individual (e.g. a good response to treatment, a cure) or a negative outcome (e.g. disease, death). We generate a **prognostic score** (often referred to as a **prognostic index** or, when predicting a negative outcome, a **risk score**) for each individual that provides a graded measure of the likelihood that the individual will experience the event.

- At its simplest, if considering an event with well-established risk factors (e.g. cardiovascular disease), a score can be generated by counting the number of risk factors possessed by each individual (e.g. male sex, older age, current smoker, family history of cardiovascular disease, diabetes mellitus, dyslipidaemia, hypertension) – this score should provide a crude indication of an individual's risk of the event (with a higher number indicating a higher risk of cardiovascular disease). However, this approach assumes that each factor contributes equally to the chance of experiencing the event.
- A preferred alternative is to use a formal statistical analysis (often a logistic regression (Chapter 30) or a similar method known as discriminant analysis) which identifies factors that are significantly associated with the event and provides an assessment of the relative importance of each of these factors in determining the chance of experiencing the event. The prognostic score can then be calculated for an individual, using the coefficients from the model to provide a weighted sum of its components (i.e. z in Chapter 30). Although the range of values of this score depends on how the score is

derived, a higher score generally indicates a greater chance of experiencing the event.

Sometimes patients are categorized by their scores, e.g. into those at low, moderate or high risk of experiencing the event. Alternatively, if a logistic regression has been performed, we can use the generated score for an individual to obtain a direct estimate of his or her predicted probability of the event (Chapter 30); as this is a probability, it takes a value from 0 to 1.

However, when using a regression model to generate a prognostic score, a model that explains a large proportion of the variability in the data may not necessarily be good at predicting which patients will develop the event. Furthermore, any score, even if based on known risk factors for the event, may provide misleading information on an individual's prognosis. Therefore, once we have derived a predictive score based on a model, we should assess the validity of that score.

Assessing the performance of a prognostic score

In order to demonstrate that our score will be useful, we should assess its performance by investigating whether it is accurate, able to discriminate between those who do and do not experience the event, correctly calibrated and transportable to other populations; we describe each of these qualities in the sections that follow (where we assume that a higher score indicates a greater chance of experiencing the event). In addition to good performance, a score should also demonstrate clinical value, i.e. it should lead to an improvement in the clinical management of patients. In other words, the score should provide prognostic information and demonstrate better performance than existing risk scores or the raw data. For example, a score based on a patient's age, sex and blood pressure must demonstrate that it leads to clinical decisions that are different to (and more effective than) those that would have been made based on knowledge of these factors on their own.

1 How accurate is the score?

We wish to describe the extent to which the score is able to predict the event correctly.

- We produce a **classification table** (Chapter 30 and Appendix C) showing the number of individuals in whom we correctly and incorrectly predict the event (similar to the table in Chapter 38) and calculate relevant measures such as:
  - the sensitivity and specificity;
  - the total accuracy of the score. This is equal to the number of individuals correctly predicted to experience or not experience the event, divided by the total number of individuals – the closer the value is to one, the better the accuracy (a perfect score would correctly predict 100% of individuals).
- When we have used logistic regression to generate the score, we can calculate the **mean Brier score** for all n individuals in the sample. The Brier score for the ith individual is the squared difference between the predicted probability of that individual

experiencing the event (P_i) and his or her observed outcome ($X_i = 1$ or 0 if he or she did or did not experience the event, respectively); the mean Brier score is $\Sigma(P_i - X_i)^2/n$. It gives an indication of model accuracy, taking a value from 0 (able to predict the event perfectly) to 0.25 (of no value). The mean Brier score is closely related to the model R^2 (Chapter 27).

2 How well can the score discriminate between those who do and do not experience the event?

We wish to assess the ability of the score to rank individuals according to their chance of experiencing the event.

- We categorize individuals according to their scores (e.g. into 5–10 equally sized groups determined by the relevant percentiles) and consider the event rates in each category (see Example). We should observe a trend towards increased event rates in those with higher scores.
- We draw a **receiver operating characteristic (ROC) curve**, which is a plot of the sensitivity of the score against (1 – specificity). The curve for a score that has good discriminative ability lies in the upper left-hand quadrant of the plot and that for a score that is no better than chance at discriminating will lie along the 45° diagonal (Fig. 38.1, see also Chapters 30 and 38). The area under the ROC curve (sometimes referred to as **AUROC**) gives an indication of the ability of the score to discriminate between those who do and do not experience the event. If we randomly select two individuals from our sample, one of whom experiences the event and one of whom does not, AUROC gives the probability that the individual with the event has a higher score than the individual without the event; AUROC will equal 1 for a score that discriminates perfectly, but will equal 0.5 for a score that performs no better than chance.
- We calculate **Harrell's c statistic**, which is a measure of discrimination that is equivalent to AUROC. We select *all* 'pairs' of individuals in the sample with discordant events (i.e. we match every individual who experiences the event to every individual who does not experience the event) – the number of such pairs is our denominator – and calculate the percentage of these pairs in whom the predicted score is higher in the individuals with the event. Where the predicted score in the two individuals is equal, the numerator is increased by 0.5. The c statistic depends on the distribution of the score and/or predicted probabilities – if the sample is relatively homogeneous (i.e. the scores or predicted probabilities are all fairly similar to each other), then c will be close to 0.5. The **D statistic** is an alternative measure of discrimination that can be used for survival data when censoring is present. When comparing two or more prognostic scores, the score with the higher D statistic has greater discriminative ability.

3 Is the score correctly calibrated?

Where we have used logistic regression to generate the predicted probabilities of the event, we may wish to know whether there is good agreement between these predicted probabilities and the observed probabilities (either 0 or 1) of the event occurring. It is possible for a prognostic score to discriminate well between individuals who do and do not experience the event (i.e. scores may be higher in those who experience the event) while still providing a poor estimate of the risk of the event occurring. This may occur when a prognostic score is applied in a different population to the one from which it was originally derived (e.g. when applying a cardiovascular risk score derived from a population in northern Europe to a population in southern Europe where the underlying risk of cardiovascular disease is much lower). This is of importance if clinical decisions are based on the predicted probability of the event, as poor calibration may result in patients receiving inappropriate care.

To determine model calibration we calculate the **Hosmer–Lemeshow goodness of fit** statistic which assesses the agreement between the observed event probabilities and those predicted by the score. Individuals in the sample are stratified into g groups (we usually take $g = 10$ and base the groups on the deciles of the distribution of predicted probabilities from the score; other classifications, e.g. using eight groups, may result in different conclusions being drawn). The expected frequency of the event in each group is the sum of the predicted probabilities of the event for the individuals in that group. This is compared with the observed frequency of those with the event in the corresponding group by calculating a test statistic that follows a Chi-squared distribution with ($g - 2$) degrees of freedom (Chapter 8). A P-value < 0.05 suggests that the model is not well calibrated.

4 Is the score transportable or generalizable?

We wish to know whether the score will work well in populations that are different from the one from which it was derived. Any prognostic score will always perform well on the data set that was used to derive the score and estimates of model performance (i.e. measures of accuracy, discrimination and calibration) from this data set (**internal validation**) will be overly optimistic. Thus, we generally require validation on at least one independent data set (**external validation**) to give a true assessment of the performance of the score; good performance on this independent data set provides evidence that the score is transportable or generalizable.

Where external validation is impractical, a number of alternative methods of internal validation may be used.

- We separate the data into two subsamples – the **training sample**, used to derive the score, and the **validation sample**, used to validate the score. Generally, the training sample, chosen randomly, is larger than the validation sample (e.g. the training sample may contain 70% of the individuals in the original sample).
- We perform **cross-validation** where we partition the data set into subsets; we derive the risk score on a single subset initially and then validate it on the remaining subsets. When performing **k-fold cross-validation**, we split the data set into k subsets; we derive the score using one of the subsets and validate it on the remaining ($k - 1$) subsets. After repeating this process for each of the k subsets, we average the resulting risk score estimates and measures of model performance (e.g. AUROC) over all the subsets. **Leave-one-out cross-validation** (analogous to jackknifing – Chapter 11) is similar, but we remove each individual from the data set one at a time, and develop and validate the score on the remaining ($n - 1$) individuals in the sample. Again, we then average the estimates from the subsets.
- We can use **bootstrapping** (Chapter 11) to estimate the prognostic score and assess its performance.
- When the score is derived from a multicentre study (Chapter 12), we can perform an **internal–external cross-validation** that excludes a different centre from the data set for each analysis. Although the participating studies in a multicentre study generally follow the same study protocol, this approach will provide some evidence of model transportability as the centres are often in different settings.

Developing prognostic indices and risk scores for other types of data

While many of the methods that we have described are most suitable for a binary outcome, using logistic regression or discriminant analysis to estimate the model and produce a risk score, it is possible to generate prognostic scores based on other types of data (e.g. survival data with censoring (Chapter 44), Poisson regression models (Chapter 31)). Many of the tests have been modified to deal with these other types of data although some tests (e.g. the Hosmer–Lemeshow test) are inappropriate when using different models.

Reporting guidelines

TRIPOD, another component of the EQUATOR network (Appendix D and Chapter 37), provides a checklist for improving the quality of prediction model development and validation (www.equator-network.org/reporting-guidelines/tripod-statement/).

Example

Given the short supply of donor organs for liver transplantation, there is a need to allocate organs to individuals on the transplant waiting list in a fair and transparent manner that optimizes the outcomes of those who receive a transplant. One way to achieve this is through the development of a validated score that indicates an individual's short-term (i.e. 3-month) risk of mortality following transplant based on donor and recipient characteristics. This score can then be used to identify the most suitable recipient on the waiting list when a donor organ becomes available. In order to generate such a score, information on both donor and recipient characteristics at the time of transplant was obtained for 31,094 individuals who had received a first liver transplantation in one of 23 European countries from 1988 to 2003.

A group of 21,605 individuals from the data set were selected at random for inclusion into the training set, of whom 2540 (12%) had died by 3 months. A logistic regression model was used to identify factors associated with 3-month mortality and the coefficients from this model were used to generate a prognostic score for each individual, which could then be used to estimate an individual's probability of dying in the first 3 months after transplant (Chapter 30).

The final model used to generate the score comprised nine covariates: year of transplant (1988–1991, 1992–1995, 1996–1999 or 2000–2003); cause of liver failure (acute liver failure, hepatocellular carcinoma, alcoholic cirrhosis, hepatitis C virus cirrhosis, primary biliary cirrhosis or other); age of donor (categorized as ≤40, 41–60 or >60 years); donor–recipient blood group status (identical, compatible or incompatible); hepatitis B surface antigen positivity of recipient; whether the patient had received a split or reduced organ graft; the patient's health status (classified using the United Network of Organ Sharing (UNOS) score with values ranging from 1 (patient in intensive care) to 4 (patient at home with normal function)) at the time of surgery; the total ischaemia time (categorized as ≤13 or >13 hours); and the experience of the centre where the surgery was performed, based on the number of transplants performed at that centre in the year of the transplant (categorized as ≤36, 37–69 or ≥70 transplants).

We show measures of accuracy, discrimination and calibration of the score for the training sample in Table 46.1. Overall, the score ranged from −4.13 (corresponding to a 3-month mortality probability of 1.6%) to 1.34 (79.3%). Using a ROC curve (Fig. 46.1), a cut-off of −2.1 was identified as an optimal threshold for the score, with individuals who had scores that were higher than this being predicted to die within 3 months of transplant. Using this cut-off, the model correctly predicted the outcomes of 64.4% of patients in the training sample;

Table 46.1 Estimates of model accuracy, discrimination and calibration from the training and validation samples.

	Training sample	Validation sample
Sample size	21605	9489
Number of deaths observed	2540	1138
Score range	−4.13 to 1.34	−4.06 to 0.87
3-month predicted mortality probability; range	1.6% to 79.3%	1.7% to 70.5%
Model accuracy (using a cut-off of −2.1)		
Total model accuracy	64.4%	64.5%
Sensitivity	62.5%	60.0%
Specificity	64.7%	65.1%
Mean Brier score	0.1	0.1
Harrell's c statistic	0.691	0.688
Hosmer–Lemeshow P-value	0.95	0.83

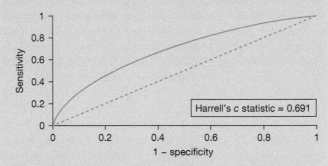

Figure 46.1 ROC curve for the predicted score (based on the training sample) with the 45° line (dashed line) indicating a score that would be no better than chance.

the sensitivity and specificity of the score were 62.5% and 64.7%, respectively. The mean Brier score of the model was 0.1, indicating reasonable model accuracy. Harrell's c statistic and the P-value from the Hosmer–Lemeshow test suggested a reasonable ability of the score to discriminate between those who died and those who remained alive at 3 months and good calibration (i.e. no evidence of lack of fit).

Burroughs, A.K., Sabin, C.A., Rolles, K., *et al.* (2006) 3-month and 12-month mortality after first liver transplant in adults in Europe: predictive models for outcome. *Lancet*, **367**, 225–232. Reproduced with permission of Elsevier.

Appendices

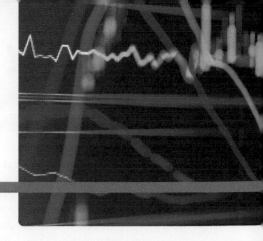

Appendices

Appendix A: Statistical tables

This appendix contains statistical tables discussed in the text. We have provided only limited P-values because data are usually analysed using a computer, and P-values are included in its output. Other texts, such as that by Fisher and Yates[1], contain more comprehensive tables. You can also obtain the P-value directly from some computer packages, given a value of the test statistic. Empty cells in a table are an indication that values do not exist.

Table A1 contains the probability in the two tails of the distribution of a variable, z, which follows the Standard Normal distribution. The P-values in Table A1 relate to the absolute values of z, so if z is negative, we ignore its sign. For example, if a test statistic that follows the Standard Normal distribution has the value 1.1, $P = 0.271$.

Table A2 and **Table A3** contain the probability in the two tails of a distribution of a variable that follows the t-distribution (Table A2) or the Chi-squared distribution (Table A3) with given degrees of freedom (df). To use Table A2 or Table A3, if the absolute value of the test statistic (with given df) lies between the tabulated values in two columns, then the two-tailed P-value lies between the P-values specified at the top of these columns. If the test statistic is to the right of the final column, then $P < 0.001$; if it is to the left of the second column, then $P > 0.10$. For example, (i) Table A2: if the test statistic is 2.62 with $df = 17$, then $0.01 < P < 0.05$; (ii) Table A3: if the test statistic is 2.62 with $df = 17$, then $P < 0.001$.

Table A4 contains often used P-values and their corresponding values for z, a variable with a Standard Normal distribution. This table may be used to obtain multipliers for the calculation of confidence intervals (CI) for Normally distributed variables. For example, for a 95% confidence interval, the multiplier is 1.96.

Table A5 contains P-values for a variable that follows the F-distribution with specified degrees of freedom in the numerator and denominator. When comparing variances (Chapter 35), we usually use a two-tailed P-value. For the analysis of variance (Chapter 22), we use a one-tailed P-value. For given degrees of freedom in the numerator and denominator, the test is significant at the level of P quoted in the table if the test statistic is greater than the tabulated value. For example, if the test statistic is 2.99 with $df = 5$ in the numerator and $df = 15$ in the denominator, then $P < 0.05$ for a one-tailed test.

Table A6 contains two-tailed P-values of the sign test of r responses of a particular type out of a total of n' responses. For a one-sample test, r equals the number of values above (or below) the median (Chapter 19). For a paired test, r equals the number of positive (or negative) differences (Chapter 20) or the number of preferences for a particular treatment (Chapter 23). n' equals the number of values not equal to the median, non-zero differences or actual preferences, as relevant. For example, if we observed three positive differences out of eight non-zero differences, then $P = 0.726$.

Table A7 contains the ranks of the values that determine the upper and lower limits of the approximate 90%, 95% and 99% confidence intervals (CI) for the median. For example, if the sample size is 23, then the limits of the 95% confidence interval are defined by the 7th and 17th ordered values.

For sample sizes greater than 50, find the observations that correspond to the ranks (to the nearest integer) equal to: (i) $n/2 - z\sqrt{n}/2$; and (ii) $1 + n/2 - z\sqrt{n}/2$; where n is the sample size and $z = 1.64$ for a 90% CI, $z = 1.96$ for a 95% CI, and $z = 2.58$ for a 99% CI (the values of z being obtained from the Standard Normal distribution, Table A4). These observations define (i) the lower, and (ii) the upper confidence limits for the median.

Table A8 contains the range of values for the sum of the ranks (T_+ or T_-) that determines significance in the Wilcoxon signed ranks test (Chapter 20). If the sum of the ranks of the positive (T_+) or negative (T_-) differences, out of n' non-zero differences, is equal to or outside the tabulated limits, the test is significant at the P-value quoted. For example, if there are 16 non-zero differences and $T_+ = 21$, then $0.01 < P < 0.05$.

Table A9 contains the range of values for the sum of the ranks (T) that determines significance for the Wilcoxon rank sum test (Chapter 21) at (a) the 5% level, and (b) the 1% level. Suppose we have two samples of sizes n_S and n_L, where $n_S \le n_L$. If the sum of the ranks of the group with the smaller sample size, n_S, is equal to or outside the tabulated limits, the test is significant at (a) the 5% level, or (b) the 1% level. For example, if $n_S = 6$ and $n_L = 8$, and the sum of the ranks in the group of six observations equals 39, then $P > 0.05$.

Table A10 and **Table A11** contain two-tailed P-values for Pearson's (Table A10) and Spearman's (Table A11) correlation coefficients when testing the null hypothesis that the relevant correlation coefficient is zero (Chapter 26). Significance is achieved, for a given sample size, at the stated P-value if the absolute value (i.e. ignoring its sign) of the sample value of the correlation coefficient exceeds the tabulated value. For example, if the sample size equals 24 and Pearson's $r = 0.58$, then $0.001 < P < 0.01$. If the sample size equals 7 and Spearman's $r_s = -0.63$, then $P > 0.05$.

Table A12 contains the digits 0–9 arranged in random order.

Reference

1 Fisher, R.A. and Yates, F. (1963) *Statistical Tables for Biological, Agricultural and Medical Research*. 6th edition. Edinburgh: Oliver and Boyd.

Medical Statistics at a Glance, Fourth Edition. Aviva Petrie and Caroline Sabin. © 2020 Aviva Petrie and Caroline Sabin. Published 2020 by John Wiley & Sons Ltd.
Companion Website: www.medstatsaag.com

Table A1 Standard Normal distribution.	
z	2-tailed P-value
0.0	1.000
0.1	0.920
0.2	0.841
0.3	0.764
0.4	0.689
0.5	0.617
0.6	0.549
0.7	0.484
0.8	0.424
0.9	0.368
1.0	0.317
1.1	0.271
1.2	0.230
1.3	0.194
1.4	0.162
1.5	0.134
1.6	0.110
1.7	0.089
1.8	0.072
1.9	0.057
2.0	0.046
2.1	0.036
2.2	0.028
2.3	0.021
2.4	0.016
2.5	0.012
2.6	0.009
2.7	0.007
2.8	0.005
2.9	0.004
3.0	0.003
3.1	0.002
3.2	0.001
3.3	0.001
3.4	0.001
3.5	0.000

Derived using Microsoft Excel Version 5.0.

Table A2 t-distribution.

	Two-tailed P-value			
df	0.10	0.05	0.01	0.001
1	6.314	12.706	63.656	636.58
2	2.920	4.303	9.925	31.600
3	2.353	3.182	5.841	12.924
4	2.132	2.776	4.604	8.610
5	2.015	2.571	4.032	6.869
6	1.943	2.447	3.707	5.959
7	1.895	2.365	3.499	5.408
8	1.860	2.306	3.355	5.041
9	1.833	2.262	3.250	4.781
10	1.812	2.228	3.169	4.587
11	1.796	2.201	3.106	4.437
12	1.782	2.179	3.055	4.318
13	1.771	2.160	3.012	4.221
14	1.761	2.145	2.977	4.140
15	1.753	2.131	2.947	4.073
16	1.746	2.120	2.921	4.015
17	1.740	2.110	2.898	3.965
18	1.734	2.101	2.878	3.922
19	1.729	2.093	2.861	3.883
20	1.725	2.086	2.845	3.850
21	1.721	2.080	2.831	3.819
22	1.717	2.074	2.819	3.792
23	1.714	2.069	2.807	3.768
24	1.711	2.064	2.797	3.745
25	1.708	2.060	2.787	3.725
26	1.706	2.056	2.779	3.707
27	1.703	2.052	2.771	3.689
28	1.701	2.048	2.763	3.674
29	1.699	2.045	2.756	3.660
30	1.697	2.042	2.750	3.646
40	1.684	2.021	2.704	3.551
50	1.676	2.009	2.678	3.496
100	1.660	1.984	2.626	3.390
200	1.653	1.972	2.601	3.340
5000	1.645	1.960	2.577	3.293

Derived using Microsoft Excel Version 5.0.

Table A3 Chi-squared distribution.

	Two-tailed P-value			
df	0.10	0.05	0.01	0.001
1	2.706	3.841	6.635	10.827
2	4.605	5.991	9.210	13.815
3	6.251	7.815	11.345	16.266
4	7.779	9.488	13.277	18.466
5	9.236	11.070	15.086	20.515
6	10.645	12.592	16.812	22.457
7	12.017	14.067	18.475	24.321
8	13.362	15.507	20.090	26.124
9	14.684	16.919	21.666	27.877
10	15.987	18.307	23.209	29.588
11	17.275	19.675	24.725	31.264
12	18.549	21.026	26.217	32.909
13	19.812	22.362	27.688	34.527
14	21.064	23.685	29.141	36.124
15	22.307	24.996	30.578	37.698
16	23.542	26.296	32.000	39.252
17	24.769	27.587	33.409	40.791
18	25.989	28.869	34.805	42.312
19	27.204	30.144	36.191	43.819
20	28.412	31.410	37.566	45.314
21	29.615	32.671	38.932	46.796
22	30.813	33.924	40.289	48.268
23	32.007	35.172	41.638	49.728
24	33.196	36.415	42.980	51.179
25	34.382	37.652	44.314	52.619
26	35.563	38.885	45.642	54.051
27	36.741	40.113	46.963	55.475
28	37.916	41.337	48.278	56.892
29	39.087	42.557	49.588	58.301
30	40.256	43.773	50.892	59.702
40	51.805	55.758	63.691	73.403
50	63.167	67.505	76.154	86.660
60	74.397	79.082	88.379	99.608
70	85.527	90.531	100.43	112.32
80	96.578	101.88	112.33	124.84
90	107.57	113.15	124.12	137.21
100	118.50	124.34	135.81	149.45

Derived using Microsoft Excel Version 5.0.

Table A4 Standard Normal distribution.

	Two-tailed *P*-value				
	0.50	**0.10**	**0.05**	**0.01**	**0.001**
Relevant CI	50%	90%	95%	99%	99.9%
z (i.e. CI multiplier)	0.67	1.64	1.96	2.58	3.29

Derived using Microsoft Excel Version 5.0.

Table A6 Two-tailed *P*-values for the sign test.

	r = number of 'positive differences' (see explanation)					
n'	**0**	**1**	**2**	**3**	**4**	**5**
4	0.125	0.624	1.000			
5	0.062	0.376	1.000			
6	0.032	0.218	0.688	1.000		
7	0.016	0.124	0.454	1.000		
8	0.008	0.070	0.290	0.726	1.000	
9	0.004	0.040	0.180	0.508	1.000	
10	0.001	0.022	0.110	0.344	0.754	1.000

Derived using Microsoft Excel Version 5.0.

Table A5 The *F*-distribution.

df of denominator	2-tailed *P*-value	1-tailed *P*-value	Degrees of freedom (*df*) of the numerator												
			1	**2**	**3**	**4**	**5**	**6**	**7**	**8**	**9**	**10**	**15**	**25**	**500**
1	**0.05**	**0.025**	**647.8**	**799.5**	**864.2**	**899.6**	**921.8**	**937.1**	**948.2**	**956.6**	**963.3**	**968.6**	**984.9**	**998.1**	**1017.0**
1	0.10	0.05	161.4	199.5	215.7	224.6	230.2	234.0	236.8	238.9	240.5	241.9	245.9	249.3	254.1
2	**0.05**	**0.025**	**38.51**	**39.00**	**39.17**	**39.25**	**39.30**	**39.33**	**39.36**	**39.37**	**39.39**	**39.40**	**39.43**	**39.46**	**39.50**
2	0.10	0.05	18.51	19.00	19.16	19.25	19.30	19.33	19.35	19.37	19.38	19.40	19.43	19.46	19.49
3	**0.05**	**0.025**	**17.44**	**16.04**	**15.44**	**15.10**	**14.88**	**14.73**	**14.62**	**14.54**	**14.47**	**14.42**	**14.25**	**14.12**	**13.91**
3	0.10	0.05	10.13	9.55	9.28	9.12	9.01	8.94	8.89	8.85	8.81	8.79	8.70	8.63	8.53
4	**0.05**	**0.025**	**12.22**	**10.65**	**9.98**	**9.60**	**9.36**	**9.20**	**9.07**	**8.98**	**8.90**	**8.84**	**8.66**	**8.50**	**8.27**
4	0.10	0.05	7.71	6.94	6.59	6.39	6.26	6.16	6.09	6.04	6.00	5.96	5.86	5.77	5.64
5	**0.05**	**0.025**	**10.01**	**8.43**	**7.76**	**7.39**	**7.15**	**6.98**	**6.85**	**6.76**	**6.68**	**6.62**	**6.43**	**6.27**	**6.03**
5	0.10	0.05	6.61	5.79	5.41	5.19	5.05	4.95	4.88	4.82	4.77	4.74	4.62	4.52	4.37
6	**0.05**	**0.025**	**8.81**	**7.26**	**6.60**	**6.23**	**5.99**	**5.82**	**5.70**	**5.60**	**5.52**	**5.46**	**5.27**	**5.11**	**4.86**
6	0.10	0.05	5.99	5.14	4.76	4.53	4.39	4.28	4.21	4.15	4.10	4.06	3.94	3.83	3.68
7	**0.05**	**0.025**	**8.07**	**6.54**	**5.89**	**5.52**	**5.29**	**5.12**	**4.99**	**4.90**	**4.82**	**4.76**	**4.57**	**4.40**	**4.16**
7	0.10	0.05	5.59	4.74	4.35	4.12	3.97	3.87	3.79	3.73	3.68	3.64	3.51	3.40	3.24
8	**0.05**	**0.025**	**7.57**	**6.06**	**5.42**	**5.05**	**4.82**	**4.65**	**4.53**	**4.43**	**4.36**	**4.30**	**4.10**	**3.94**	**3.68**
8	0.10	0.05	5.32	4.46	4.07	3.84	3.69	3.58	3.50	3.44	3.39	3.35	3.22	3.11	2.94
9	**0.05**	**0.025**	**7.21**	**5.71**	**5.08**	**4.72**	**4.48**	**4.32**	**4.20**	**4.10**	**4.03**	**3.96**	**3.77**	**3.60**	**3.35**
9	0.10	0.05	5.12	4.26	3.86	3.63	3.48	3.37	3.29	3.23	3.18	3.14	3.01	2.89	2.72
10	**0.05**	**0.025**	**6.94**	**5.46**	**4.83**	**4.47**	**4.24**	**4.07**	**3.95**	**3.85**	**3.78**	**3.72**	**3.52**	**3.35**	**3.09**
10	0.10	0.05	4.96	4.10	3.71	3.48	3.33	3.22	3.14	3.07	3.02	2.98	2.85	2.73	2.55
15	**0.05**	**0.025**	**6.20**	**4.77**	**4.15**	**3.80**	**3.58**	**3.41**	**3.29**	**3.20**	**3.12**	**3.06**	**2.86**	**2.69**	**2.41**
15	0.10	0.05	4.54	3.68	3.29	3.06	2.90	2.79	2.71	2.64	2.59	2.54	2.40	2.28	2.08
20	**0.05**	**0.025**	**5.87**	**4.46**	**3.86**	**3.51**	**3.29**	**3.13**	**3.01**	**2.91**	**2.84**	**2.77**	**2.57**	**2.40**	**2.10**
20	0.10	0.05	4.35	3.49	3.10	2.87	2.71	2.60	2.51	2.45	2.39	2.35	2.20	2.07	1.86
30	**0.05**	**0.025**	**5.57**	**4.18**	**3.59**	**3.25**	**3.03**	**2.87**	**2.75**	**2.65**	**2.57**	**2.51**	**2.31**	**2.12**	**1.81**
30	0.10	0.05	4.17	3.32	2.92	2.69	2.53	2.42	2.33	2.27	2.21	2.16	2.01	1.88	1.64
50	**0.05**	**0.025**	**5.34**	**3.97**	**3.39**	**3.05**	**2.83**	**2.67**	**2.55**	**2.46**	**2.38**	**2.32**	**2.11**	**1.92**	**1.57**
50	0.10	0.05	4.03	3.18	2.79	2.56	2.40	2.29	2.20	2.13	2.07	2.03	1.87	1.73	1.46
100	**0.05**	**0.025**	**5.18**	**3.83**	**3.25**	**2.92**	**2.70**	**2.54**	**2.42**	**2.32**	**2.24**	**2.18**	**1.97**	**1.77**	**1.38**
100	0.10	0.05	3.94	3.09	2.70	2.46	2.31	2.19	2.10	2.03	1.97	1.93	1.77	1.62	1.31
1000	**0.05**	**0.025**	**5.04**	**3.70**	**3.13**	**2.80**	**2.58**	**2.42**	**2.30**	**2.20**	**2.13**	**2.06**	**1.85**	**1.64**	**1.16**
1000	0.10	0.05	3.85	3.00	2.61	2.38	2.22	2.11	2.02	1.95	1.89	1.84	1.68	1.52	1.13

Derived using Microsoft Excel Version 5.0.

	Table A7 Ranks for confidence intervals for the median.				**Table A8** Critical ranges for the Wilcoxon signed ranks test.		

Table A7 Ranks for confidence intervals for the median.

Sample size	Approximate		
	90% CI	95% CI	99% CI
6	1,6	1,6	—
7	1,7	1,7	—
8	2,7	1,8	—
9	2,8	2,8	1,9
10	2,9	2,9	1,10
11	3,9	2,10	1,11
12	3,10	3,10	2,11
13	4,10	3,11	2,12
14	4,11	3,12	2,13
15	4,12	4,12	3,13
16	5,12	4,13	3,14
17	5,13	4,14	3,15
18	6,13	5,14	4,15
19	6,14	5,15	4,16
20	6,15	6,15	4,17
21	7,15	6,16	5,17
22	7,16	6,17	5,18
23	8,16	7,17	5,19
24	8,17	7,18	6,19
25	8,18	8,18	6,20
26	9,18	8,19	6,21
27	9,19	8,20	7,21
28	10,19	9,20	7,22
29	10,20	9,21	8,22
30	11,20	10,21	8,23
31	11,21	10,22	8,24
32	11,22	10,23	9,24
33	12,22	11,23	9,25
34	12,23	11,24	9,26
35	13,23	12,24	10,26
36	13,24	12,25	10,27
37	14,24	13,25	11,27
38	14,25	13,26	11,28
39	14,26	13,27	11,29
40	15,26	14,27	12,29
41	15,27	14,28	12,30
42	16,27	15,28	13,30
43	16,28	15,29	13,31
44	17,28	15,30	13,32
45	17,29	16,30	14,32
46	17,30	16,31	14,33
47	18,30	17,31	15,33
48	18,31	17,32	15,34
49	19,31	18,32	15,35
50	19,32	18,33	16,35

Derived using Microsoft Excel Version 5.0.

Table A8 Critical ranges for the Wilcoxon signed ranks test.

n'	Two-tailed P-value		
	0.05	0.01	0.001
6	0–21	—	—
7	2–26	—	—
8	3–33	0–36	—
9	5–40	1–44	—
10	8–47	3–52	—
11	10–56	5–61	0–66
12	13–65	7–71	1–77
13	17–74	9–82	2–89
14	21–84	12–93	4–101
15	25–95	15–105	6–114
16	29–107	19–117	9–127
17	34–119	23–130	11–142
18	40–131	27–144	14–157
19	46–144	32–158	18–172
20	52–158	37–173	21–189
21	58–173	42–189	26–205
22	66–187	48–205	30–223
23	73–203	54–222	35–241
24	81–219	61–239	40–260
25	89–236	68–257	45–280

Adapted from Altman, D.G. (1991) *Practical Statistics for Medical Research.* Copyright CRC Press, Boca Raton.

Table A9(a) Critical ranges for the Wilcoxon rank sum test for a two-tailed $P = 0.05$.

n_L	n_S (the number of observations in the smaller sample)											
	4	**5**	**6**	**7**	**8**	**9**	**10**	**11**	**12**	**13**	**14**	**15**
4	10–26	16–34	23–43	31–53	40–64	49–77	60–90	72–104	85–119	99–135	114–152	130–170
5	11–29	17–38	24–48	33–58	42–70	52–83	63–97	75–112	89–127	103–144	118–162	134–181
6	12–32	18–42	26–52	34–64	44–76	55–89	66–104	79–119	92–136	107–153	122–172	139–191
7	13–35	20–45	27–57	36–69	46–82	57–96	69–111	82–127	96–144	111–162	127–181	144–201
8	14–38	21–49	29–61	38–74	49–87	60–102	72–118	85–135	100–152	115–171	131–191	149–211
9	14–42	22–53	31–65	40–79	51–93	62–109	75–125	89–142	104–160	119–180	136–200	154–221
10	15–45	23–57	32–70	42–84	53–99	65–115	78–132	92–150	107–169	124–188	141–209	159–231
11	16–48	24–61	34–74	44–89	55–105	68–121	81–139	96–157	111–177	128–197	145–219	164–241
12	17–51	26–64	35–79	46–94	58–110	71–127	84–146	99–165	115–185	132–206	150–228	169–251
13	18–54	27–68	37–83	48–99	60–116	73–134	88–152	103–172	119–193	136–215	155–237	174–261
14	19–57	28–72	38–88	50–104	62–122	76–140	91–159	106–180	123–201	141–223	160–246	179–271
15	20–60	29–76	40–92	52–109	65–127	79–146	94–166	110–187	127–209	145–232	164–256	184–281

Table A9(b) Critical ranges for the Wilcoxon rank sum test for a two-tailed $P = 0.01$.

n_L	n_S (the number of observations in the smaller sample)											
	4	**5**	**6**	**7**	**8**	**9**	**10**	**11**	**12**	**13**	**14**	**15**
4	—	—	21–45	28–56	37–67	46–80	57–93	68–108	81–123	94–140	109–157	125–175
5	—	15–40	22–50	29–62	38–74	48–87	59–101	71–116	84–132	98–149	112–168	128–187
6	10–34	16–44	23–55	31–67	40–80	50–94	61–109	73–125	87–141	101–159	116–178	132–198
7	10–38	16–49	24–60	32–73	42–86	52–101	64–116	76–133	90–150	104–169	120–188	136–209
8	11–48	17–53	25–65	34–78	43–93	54–108	66–124	79–141	93–159	108–178	123–199	140–220
9	11–45	18–57	26–70	35–84	45–99	56–115	68–132	82–149	96–168	111–188	127–209	144–231
10	12–48	19–61	27–75	37–89	47–105	58–122	71–139	84–158	99–177	115–197	131–219	149–241
11	12–52	20–65	28–80	38–95	49–111	61–128	73–147	87–166	102–186	118–207	135–229	153–252
12	13–55	21–69	30–84	40–100	51–117	63–135	76–154	90–174	105–195	122–216	139–239	157–263
13	13–59	22–73	31–89	41–106	53–123	65–142	79–161	93–182	109–203	125–226	143–249	162–273
14	14–62	22–78	32–94	43–111	54–130	67–149	81–169	96–190	112–212	129–235	147–259	166–284
15	15–65	23–82	33–99	44–117	56–136	69–156	84–176	99–198	115–221	133–244	151–269	171–294

Source: Diem (1970). Reproduced with permission of John Wiley & Sons.

Table A10 Pearson's correlation coefficient.

Sample size	Two-tailed P-value		
	0.05	0.01	0.001
5	0.878	0.959	0.991
6	0.811	0.917	0.974
7	0.755	0.875	0.951
8	0.707	0.834	0.925
9	0.666	0.798	0.898
10	0.632	0.765	0.872
11	0.602	0.735	0.847
12	0.576	0.708	0.823
13	0.553	0.684	0.801
14	0.532	0.661	0.780
15	0.514	0.641	0.760
16	0.497	0.623	0.742
17	0.482	0.606	0.725
18	0.468	0.590	0.708
19	0.456	0.575	0.693
20	0.444	0.561	0.679
21	0.433	0.549	0.665
22	0.423	0.537	0.652
23	0.413	0.526	0.640
24	0.404	0.515	0.629
25	0.396	0.505	0.618
26	0.388	0.496	0.607
27	0.381	0.487	0.597
28	0.374	0.479	0.588
29	0.367	0.471	0.579
30	0.361	0.463	0.570
35	0.334	0.430	0.532
40	0.312	0.403	0.501
45	0.294	0.380	0.474
50	0.279	0.361	0.451
55	0.266	0.345	0.432
60	0.254	0.330	0.414
70	0.235	0.306	0.385
80	0.220	0.286	0.361
90	0.207	0.270	0.341
100	0.197	0.257	0.324
150	0.160	0.210	0.266

Source: Diem (1970). Reproduced with permission of John Wiley & Sons.

Table A11 Spearman's correlation coefficient.

Sample size	Two tailed P-value		
	0.05	0.01	0.001
5	1.000		
6	0.886	1.000	
7	0.786	0.929	1.000
8	0.738	0.881	0.976
9	0.700	0.833	0.933
10	0.648	0.794	0.903

Adapted from Siegel, S. & Castellan, N.J. (1988) *Nonparametric Statistics for the Behavioural Sciences*. 2nd edition. New York: McGraw-Hill.

Table A12 Random numbers.

34814	68020	28998	51687	40088	35458	24708	01815	53776
99106	50899	07394	91071	22411	61643	64435	62552	64316
47185	31782	48894	68790	51852	36918	05737	90653	61123
81354	57296	39329	52263	43194	51624	42429	61367	41207
83467	85622	95778	05347	00445	51334	29445	99176	30091
27924	34167	57060	57535	32278	16949	04960	04116	91467
58319	88164	94130	07743	16917	15681	93572	99753	49117
49732	66702	72425	99117	49298	87265	14195	83391	19794
69594	26749	68743	39139	44495	11944	12970	56523	62411
30074	97517	97450	54251	51777	21073	03909	26519	39578
81147	57508	93479	87826	28965	74474	97468	80149	17834
74689	28933	59819	93052	61325	83145	44684	72958	91824
14802	25982	48024	15461	37570	44685	47386	09504	77831
68501	34194	85355	38411	46559	41694	99678	88268	86674
48734	92671	85252	85985	34228	91289	56331	14683	36493
84102	81699	97352	54509	93196	51204	43351	11818	41179
28432	32873	83834	09862	12720	64569	42218	26726	80866
91458	82524	75523	01276	19591	47473	90251	99103	72947
45435	30389	69732	81962	30243	96199	33546	39672	83760
23557	78437	44957	98728	65674	34701	83398	54102	65845
30395	91850	52004	04844	28848	19728	96571	13317	70859
69991	12755	97916	57639	43445	90463	85556	35469	19749
32980	43608	20592	72527	63583	46443	53929	87219	55198
59776	37035	53765	55196	68659	71429	25225	91942	51132
73714	79868	23880	92254	72984	07792	81306	24277	82366
61547	16575	68520	59869	67299	73565	77316	96682	18031
87737	01058	76012	76247	75616	51335	70364	78942	40564
98669	08334	40520	78389	56498	74336	02434	48599	67579
81535	46690	92814	44456	29227	48122	30522	13852	48436
05975	47110	32733	46929	98261	52193	83215	53192	83109

Derived using Microsoft Excel Version 5.0.

Appendix B: Altman's nomogram for sample size calculations (Chapter 36)

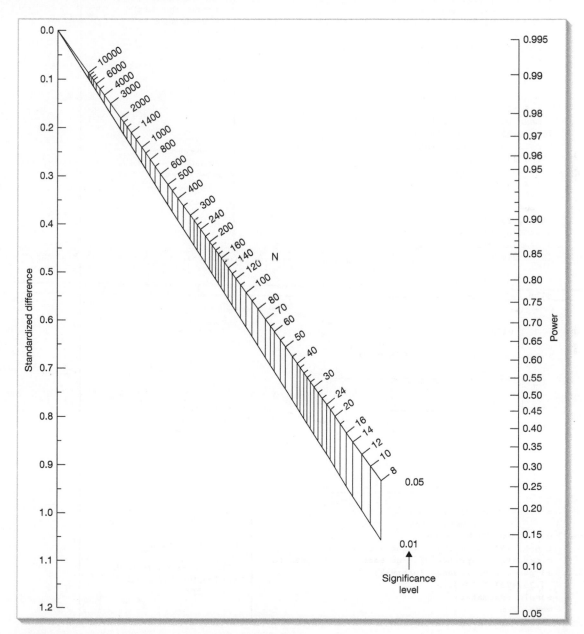

Source: Altman (1982). Reproduced with permission from John Wiley & Sons.

Medical Statistics at a Glance, Fourth Edition. Aviva Petrie and Caroline Sabin. © 2020 Aviva Petrie and Caroline Sabin. Published 2020 by John Wiley & Sons Ltd.
Companion Website: www.medstatsaag.com

Appendix C: Typical computer output

Analysis of plasma leptin data described in Chapter 20, generated by R

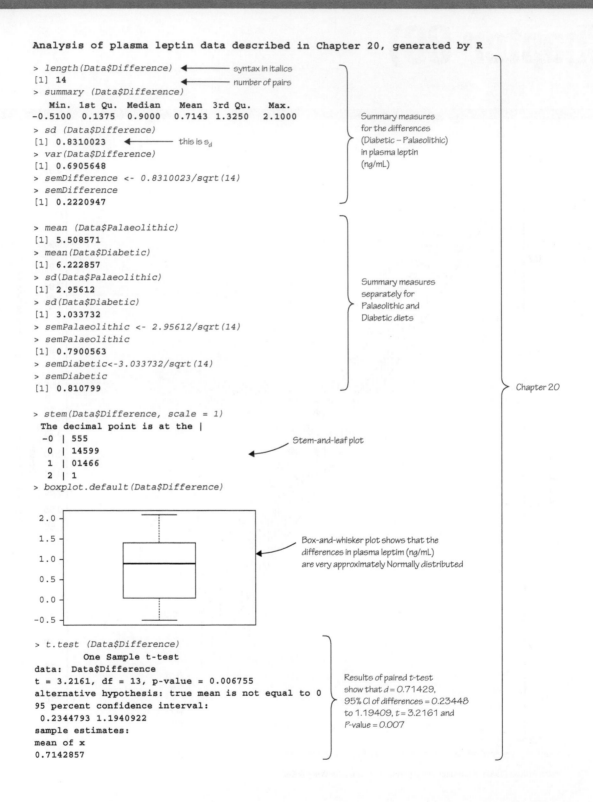

```
> length(Data$Difference)        ◄—— syntax in italics
[1] 14                           ◄—— number of pairs
> summary (Data$Difference)
    Min. 1st Qu. Median   Mean 3rd Qu.   Max.
 -0.5100  0.1375  0.9000 0.7143  1.3250 2.1000
> sd (Data$Difference)
[1] 0.8310023                    ◄—— this is s_d
> var(Data$Difference)
[1] 0.6905648
> semDifference <- 0.8310023/sqrt(14)
> semDifference
[1] 0.2220947
```

Summary measures for the differences (Diabetic – Palaeolithic) in plasma leptin (ng/mL)

```
> mean (Data$Palaeolithic)
[1] 5.508571
> mean(Data$Diabetic)
[1] 6.222857
> sd(Data$Palaeolithic)
[1] 2.95612
> sd(Data$Diabetic)
[1] 3.033732
> semPalaeolithic <- 2.95612/sqrt(14)
> semPalaeolithic
[1] 0.7900563
> semDiabetic<-3.033732/sqrt(14)
> semDiabetic
[1] 0.810799
```

Summary measures separately for Palaeolithic and Diabetic diets

Chapter 20

```
> stem(Data$Difference, scale = 1)
  The decimal point is at the |
  -0 | 555
   0 | 14599
   1 | 01466
   2 | 1
> boxplot.default(Data$Difference)
```

Stem-and-leaf plot

Box-and-whisker plot shows that the differences in plasma leptim (ng/mL) are very approximately Normally distributed

```
> t.test (Data$Difference)
        One Sample t-test
data: Data$Difference
t = 3.2161, df = 13, p-value = 0.006755
alternative hypothesis: true mean is not equal to 0
95 percent confidence interval:
 0.2344793 1.1940922
sample estimates:
mean of x
0.7142857
```

Results of paired *t*-test show that $d = 0.71429$, 95% CI of differences = 0.23448 to 1.19409, $t = 3.2161$ and P-value = 0.007

Medical Statistics at a Glance, Fourth Edition. Aviva Petrie and Caroline Sabin. © 2020 Aviva Petrie and Caroline Sabin. Published 2020 by John Wiley & Sons Ltd.
Companion Website: www.medstatsaag.com

Analysis of platelet data described in Chapter 22, generated by SPSS

```
EXAMINE VARIABLES=Platelet BY Group
  /PLOT=BOXPLOT
  /STATISTICS=NONE
  /NOTOTAL.
```
← Syntax

Explore Group

Case Processing Summary

Table with information on the number of patients in each group

		Cases					
		Valid		Missing		Total	
	Group	N	Percent	N	Percent	N	Percent
Platelet count (x10^9/L)	Caucasian	90	100.0%	0	0.0%	90	100.0%
	Afro-Caribbean	21	100.0%	0	0.0%	21	100.0%
	Mediterranean	19	100.0%	0	0.0%	19	100.0%
	Other	20	100.0%	0	0.0%	20	100.0%

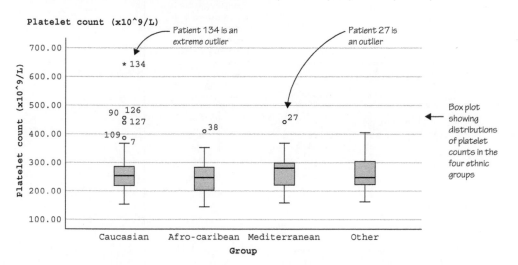

Box plot showing distributions of platelet counts in the four ethnic groups

```
ONEWAY Platelet BY Group
  /STATISTICS DESCRIPTIVES HOMOGENEITY
  /MISSING ANALYSIS.
```

Oneway

Descriptives

Summary measures for each of the four groups

Platelet count (x10^9/L)

	N	Mean	Std. Deviation	Std. Error	95% Confidence Interval for Mean		Minimum	Maximum
					Lower Bound	Upper Bound		
Caucasian	90	268.10	77.078	8.125	251.96	284.24	156.00	651.00
Afro-Caribbean	21	254.29	67.500	14.730	223.56	285.01	148.00	414.00
Mediterranean	19	281.05	71.093	16.310	246.79	315.32	165.00	449.00
Other	20	273.30	63.424	14.182	243.62	302.98	170.00	414.00
Total	150	268.50	73.045	5.964	256.71	280.29	148.00	651.00

Test of Homogeneity of Variances

'Sig' is the P-value in SPSS. All approaches give $P = 0.99$, indicating that there is no evidence that the variances are different in the four groups

		Levene Statistic	df1	df2	Sig.
Platelet count (x10^9/L)	Based on Mean	.041	3	146	.989
	Based on Median	.025	3	146	.995
	Based on Median and with adjusted df	.025	3	136.4	.995
	Based on trimmed mean	.027	3	146	.994

ANOVA — This is the ANOVA table

Platelet count (x10^9/L)

	Sum of Squares	df	Mean Square	F	Sig.
Between Groups	7711.967	3	2570.656	.477	.699
Within Groups	787289.533	146	5392.394		
Total	795001.500	149			

← P-value

Chapter 22

Analysis of FEV1 data described in Chapter 21 (Example 1), generated by SAS

```
                    The SAS System
         OBS        GRP           FEV
          1        Placebo       1.28571
          2        Placebo       1.31250
          3        Placebo       1.60000
          4        Placebo       1.41250
          5        Placebo       1.60000
         49        Treated       1.60000
         50        Treated       1.80000
         51        Treated       1.94286
         52        Treated       1.84286
         53        Treated       1.90000
```

Print out of first five observations in each group

```
...............Treatment Group=Placebo...............
                  Univariate Procedure
    Variable=FEV
                       Moments
         N              48      Sum Wgts           48
         Mean       1.536759    Sum            73.76441
         Std Dev    0.245819    Variance       0.060427
         Skewness   0.272608    Kurtosis       0.500457
         USS        116.1981    CSS            2.840059
         CV         15.99592    Std Mean       0.035481
         T:Mean=0   43.31232    Pr> |T|          0.0001
         Num ^=0        48      Num > 0            48
         M (Sign)       24      Pr>=|M|          0.0001
         Sgn Rank      588      Pr>=|S|          0.0001

                     Quantiles (Def=5)
         100% Max     2.1875        99%      2.1875
          75% Q3        1.7         95%     1.91429
          50% Med    1.551785       90%     1.85714
          25% Q1     1.36905        10%     1.28571
           0% Min        1           5%     1.12857
                                     1%         1
         Range        1.1875
         Q3-Q1        0.33095
         Mode         1.3875

                        Extremes
       Lowest      Obs       Highest       Obs
            1(     21)      1.85714(      47)
         1.04(     33)          1.9(      26)
      1.12857(     45)      1.91429(      46)
      1.18571(     12)       2.1125(      27)
      1.28571(      1)       2.1875(      20)
```

Median

Univariate summary statistics showing that the mean and median are fairly similar in the placebo group. Thus we believe that the values are approximately Normally distributed

Chapter 21

Continued

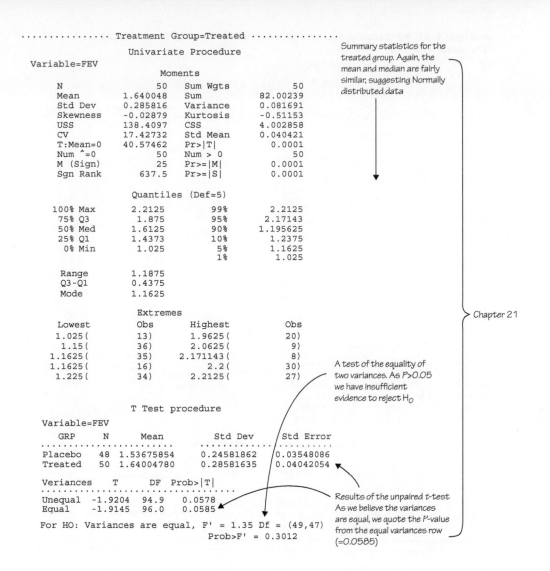

```
............... Treatment Group=Treated ...............
                    Univariate Procedure
Variable=FEV
                          Moments
    N                  50    Sum Wgts            50
    Mean         1.640048    Sum          82.00239
    Std Dev      0.285816    Variance     0.081691
    Skewness     -0.02879    Kurtosis     -0.51153
    USS          138.4097    CSS          4.002858
    CV           17.42732    Std Mean     0.040421
    T:Mean=0     40.57462    Pr>|T|         0.0001
    Num ^=0            50    Num > 0             50
    M (Sign)           25    Pr>=|M|        0.0001
    Sgn Rank        637.5    Pr>=|S|        0.0001

                    Quantiles (Def=5)

    100% Max       2.2125    99%            2.2125
     75% Q3         1.875    95%           2.17143
     50% Med       1.6125    90%          1.195625
     25% Q1        1.4373    10%            1.2375
      0% Min        1.025    5%             1.1625
                             1%              1.025

    Range          1.1875
    Q3-Q1          0.4375
    Mode           1.1625

                      Extremes
    Lowest       Obs      Highest       Obs
    1.025(      13)       1.9625(       20)
     1.15(      36)       2.0625(        9)
    1.1625(     35)      2.171143(       8)
    1.1625(     16)          2.2(       30)
    1.225(      34)       2.2125(       27)


                    T Test procedure
Variable=FEV
    GRP     N       Mean          Std Dev      Std Error
    ....................     ..............  ..............
    Placebo  48  1.53675854    0.24581862     0.03548086
    Treated  50  1.64004780    0.28581635     0.04042054

    Veriances    T      DF   Prob>|T|
    ....................     ..............
    Unequal  -1.9204   94.9   0.0578
    Equal    -1.9145   96.0   0.0585

    For HO: Variances are equal, F' = 1.35 Df = (49,47)
                                    Prob>F' = 0.3012
```

Summary statistics for the treated group. Again, the mean and median are fairly similar, suggesting Normally distributed data

Chapter 21

A test of the equality of two variances. As $P>0.05$ we have insufficient evidence to reject H_O

Results of the unpaired t-test As we believe the variances are equal, we quote the P-value from the equal variances row (=0.0585)

Analysis of anthropometric data described in Chapters 26, 28 and 29, generated by SAS

OBS	SBP	Height	Weight	Sex
1	91.00	119.7	20.0	0
2	122.50	124.6	42.5	0
3	109.50	111.3	19.8	0
4	100.50	110.3	18.9	0
5	99.00	112.5	19.0	0
6	103.50	115.1	19.3	0
7	101.00	116.3	19.6	0
8	103.00	111.1	17.1	1
9	106.50	117.2	20.7	1
10	102.50	113.2	22.1	1

Print out of data from first 10 children

Correlation Analysis

4 'VAR' Variables: SBP   Height   Weight   Age

Simple Statistics

Variable	N	Mean	Std Dev	Sum
SBP	100	104.414700	9.430933	10441
Height	100	120.054000	6.439986	12005
Weight	100	22.826000	4.223303	2282.600000
Age	100	6.696900	0.731717	669.690000

Simple Statistics

Variable	Minimum	Maximum
SBP	81.500000	128.850000
Height	107.1000000	136.800000
Weight	15.900000	42.500000
Age	5.130000	8.840000

Summary statistics for each variable

Pearson Correlation Coefficients/Prob>|R| under Ho:Rho=0
/N=100

	SBP	Height	Weight	Age
SBP	1.00000	0.33066	0.51774	0.16373
	0.0	0.0008	0.0001	0.1036
Height	0.33066	1.00000	0.69151	0.64486
	0.0008	0.0	0.0001	0.0001
Weight	0.51774	0.69151	1.00000	0.38935
	0.0001	0.0001	0.0	0.0001
Age	0.16373	0.64486	0.38935	1.00000
	0.1036	0.0001	0.0001	0.0

Pearson's correlation coefficient between SBP and age

Associated P-value

Spearman Correlation Coefficients/Prob>|R| under Ho:Rho=0
/N=100

	SBP	Height	Weight	Age
SBP	1.00000	0.31519	0.45453	0.14778
	0.0	0.0014	0.0001	0.1423
Height	0.31519	1.00000	0.82298	0.61491
	0.0014	0.0	0.0001	0.0001
Weight	0.45453	0.82298	1.00000	0.51260
	0.0001	0.0001	0.0	0.0001
Age	0.14778	0.61491	0.51260	1.00000
	0.1423	0.0001	0.0001	0.0

Spearman's correlation coefficient between height and age

P-value

Chapter 26

```
Model:MODEL1
Dependent Variable:SBP
                    Analysis of Variance

Source        DF      Sum of        Mean      F Value    Prob>F
                      Squares       Square

Model          1     962.71441    962.71441    12.030    0.0008          ANOVA table
Error         98    7842.59208     80.02645
C Total       99    8805.30649

       Root MSE         8.94575    R-square     0.1093
       Dep Mean       104.41470    Adj R-sq     0.1002
            C.V.         8.56752
```

Results from simple linear regression of SBP (systolic blood pressure) on height Chapter 28

```
                    Parameter Estimates

   Intercept, a
                   Parameter      Standard     T for HO:
Variable    DF     Estimate       Error      Parameter=0

Intercep     1     46.281684    16.78450788     2.757
Height       1      0.484224     0.13960927     3.468

Variable DF      Prob>|T|              Slope, b

Intercep     1     0.0070
Height       1     0.0008
```

```
Model:MODEL1
Dependent Variable:SBP
                    Analysis of Variance

Source        DF      Sum of        Mean      F Value    Prob>F
                      Squares       Square

Model          3    2804.04514    934.68171    14.952    0.0001
Error         96    6001.26135     62.51314
C Total       99    8805.30649

     Root MSE           7.90653    R-square     0.3184
     Dep Mean         104.41470    Adj R-sq     0.2972
     C.V.               7.57223
```

Results from multiple linear regression of SBP on height weight and gender Chapter 29

```
                    Parameter Estimates

Variable    DF   Parameter      Standard     T for HO:
                 Estimate       Error      Parameter=0

Intercep     1    79.439541    17.11822110     4.641
Height       1    -0.031023     0.17170250    -0.181
Weight       1     1.179495     0.26139400     4.512
Sex          1     4.229540     1.61054848     2.626

Variable    DF   Prob>|T|            Estimated partial
                                     regression
Intercep     1    0.0001             coefficients
Height       1    0.8570
weight       1    0.0001
Sex          1    0.0101
```

Analysis of HHV-8 data described in Chapters 23, 24 and 30, generated by Stata

```
. list   hhv8 gonorrho syphilis hsv2 hiv age in 1/10
```

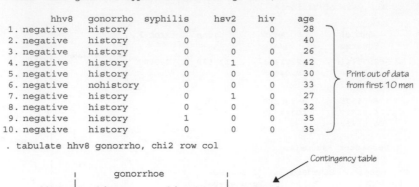

```
            hhv8     gonorrho   syphilis     hsv2      hiv      age
 1. negative   history        0          0        0       28
 2. negative   history        0          0        0       40
 3. negative   history        0          0        0       26
 4. negative   history        0          1        0       42
 5. negative   history        0          0        0       30
 6. negative   nohistory      0          0        0       33
 7. negative   history        0          1        0       27
 8. negative   history        0          0        0       32
 9. negative   history        1          0        0       35
10. negative   history        0          0        0       35
```

Print out of data from first 10 men

```
. tabulate hhv8 gonorrho, chi2 row col
```

Contingency table

```
                         gonorrhoe
        hhv8 | no histor      history   |     Total
-------------+----------------------------+----------
    negative |    192           29       |      221      ← Row marginal total
             |   86.88        13.12      |    100.00
             |   84.21        67.44      |     81.55
-------------+----------------------------+----------
    positive |     36           14       |       50      Observed frequency
             |   72.00        28.00      |    100.00
             |   15.79        32.56      |     18.45
-------------+----------------------------+----------
       Total |    228           43       |      271      Column marginal total
             |   84.13        15.87      |    100.00
             |  100.00       100.00      |    100.00      Overall total

        Pearson chi2(1) =  6.7609     Pr = 0.009
```

Row % → ; *Column %* →

Chi-squared test results

Chapter 24

Start of logistic regression output →
```
. logit   hhv8 gonorrho syphilis hsv2 hiv age, or tab

Iteration 0:  Log Likelihood =-122.86506
Iteration 1:  Log Likelihood =-111.87072
Iteration 2:  Log Likelihood =-110.58712
Iteration 3:  Log Likelihood =-110.56596
Iteration 4:  Log Likelihood =-110.56595
```

Number of men with complete information on all variables

```
Logit Estimates                     Number of obs =     260
                                    chi2(5)       =   24.60
                                    Prob > chi2   = 0.0002
     Log Likelihood = -110.56595    Pseudo R2     = 0.1001
```

Wald test statistic

Chi-square for covariates and its P-value

Deviance = −2 log likelihood = 221.13

```
------------------------------------------------------------------------------
        hhv8 |     Coef.    Std. Err.      z       P>|z|    [95% Conf. Interval]
-------------+----------------------------------------------------------------
    gonorrho |   .5093263    .4363219    1.167    0.243    -.345849    1.364502
    syphilis |   1.192442    .7110707    1.677    0.094    -.201231    2.586115
        hsv2 |   .7910041    .3871114    2.043    0.041    .0322798    1.549728
         hiv |   1.635669    .6028147    2.713    0.007    .4541736    2.817164
         age |   .0061609    .0204152    0.302    0.763    -.0338521    .046174
    constant |  -2.224164    .6511603   -3.416    0.001   -3.500415   -.9479135
------------------------------------------------------------------------------
```

$$\frac{Deviance}{df} = \frac{221.13}{260-6} = 0.87$$

No evidence of extra-Binomial variation

Results from multivariable logistic regression Chapter 30

P-value

```
------------------------------------------------------------------------------
        hhv8 | Odds Ratio  Std. Err.      z       P>|z|    [95% Conf. Interval]
-------------+----------------------------------------------------------------
    gonorrho |   1.66417    .7261137    1.167    0.243    .7076193    3.913772
    syphilis |   3.295118   2.343062    1.677    0.094    .8177235    13.27808
        hsv2 |   2.20561    .8538167    2.043    0.041    1.032806    4.710191
         hiv |   5.132889   3.094181    2.713    0.007    1.574871    16.72934
         age |   1.00618    .0205413    0.302    0.763    .9667145    1.047257
------------------------------------------------------------------------------
```

CI's exclude 1

Significant findings, P < 0.05

```
. lroc

Logistic model for hhv8

number of observations =     260
area under ROC curve   =   0.6868
```

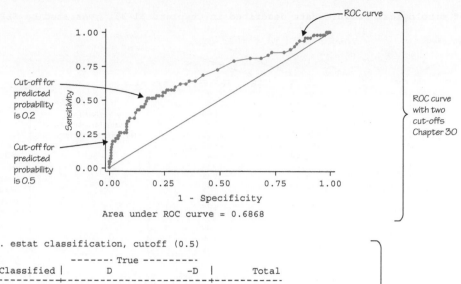

Cut-off for predicted probability is 0.2

Cut-off for predicted probability is 0.5

ROC curve

ROC curve with two cut-offs Chapter 30

Area under ROC curve = 0.6868

```
. estat classification, cutoff (0.5)
                 ------- True ---------
Classified |      D           -D    |     Total
-----------+------------------------+----------
     +     |      9            5     |      14
     -     |     38          208     |     246
-----------+------------------------+----------
   Total   |     47          215     |     260

Classified + if predicted Pr(D) >= .5
-----------------------------------------------
Sensitivity                  Pr( +| D)   19.15%
Specificity                  Pr( -|-D)   97.65%
Positive predictive value    Pr( D| +)   64.29%
Negative predictive value    Pr(-D| -)   84.55%
-----------------------------------------------
False + rate for true -D     Pr( +|-D)    2.35%
False - rate for true D      Pr( -| D)   80.85%
False + rate for classified +  Pr(-D| +) 35.71%
False - rate for classified -  Pr( D| -) 15.45%
-----------------------------------------------
Correctly classified                     83.46%
```

Poor sensitivity
Good specificity

Assessing predictive efficiency, cut-off 0.5 Chapter 30

```
. estat classification, cutoff (0.2)
                 ------- True ---------
Classified|       D           -D    |     Total
----------+-------------------------+----------
     +    |      24           43     |      67
     -    |      23          170     |     193
----------+-------------------------+----------
   Total  |      47          213     |     260

Classified + if predicted pr(D) >= .2
-----------------------------------------------
Sensitivity                  Pr( +| D)   51.06%
Specificity                  Pr( -|-D)   79.81%
Positive predictive value    Pr( D| +)   35.82%
Negative predictive value    Pr(-D| -)   88.08%
-----------------------------------------------
False + rate for true -D     Pr( +|-D)   20.19%
False - rate for true D      Pr( -| D)   48.94%
False + rate for classified +  Pr(-D| +) 64.18%
False - rate for classified -  Pr( D| -) 11.92%
-----------------------------------------------
Correctly classified                     74.62%
-----------------------------------------------
```

Lower cut-off

Sensitivity increased
Specificity decreased

Total correctly classified decreased

Assessing predictive efficiency, cut-off 0.2 Chapter 30

Analysis of virological failure data described in Chapters 31-33, generated by SAS

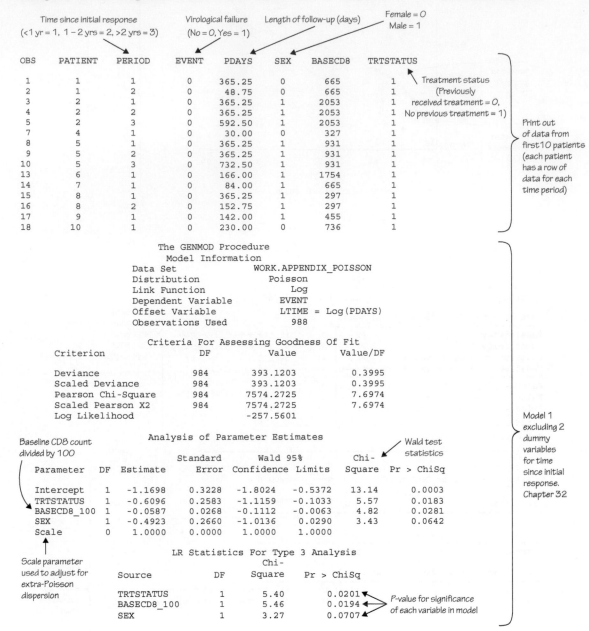

Time since initial response
(<1 yr = 1, 1 – 2 yrs = 2, >2 yrs = 3)

Virological failure
(No = 0, Yes = 1)

Length of follow-up (days)

Female = 0
Male = 1

OBS	PATIENT	PERIOD	EVENT	PDAYS	SEX	BASECD8	TRTSTATUS
1	1	1	0	365.25	0	665	1
2	1	2	0	48.75	0	665	1
3	2	1	0	365.25	1	2053	1
4	2	2	0	365.25	1	2053	1
5	2	3	0	592.50	1	2053	1
7	4	1	0	30.00	0	327	1
8	5	1	0	365.25	1	931	1
9	5	1	0	365.25	1	931	1
10	5	3	0	732.50	1	931	1
13	6	1	0	166.00	1	1754	1
14	7	1	0	84.00	1	665	1
15	8	1	0	365.25	1	297	1
16	8	2	0	152.75	1	297	1
17	9	1	0	142.00	1	455	1
18	10	1	0	230.00	0	736	1

Treatment status
(Previously
received treatment = 0,
No previous treatment = 1)

Print out
of data from
first 10 patients
(each patient
has a row of
data for each
time period)

The GENMOD Procedure
Model Information

Data Set	WORK.APPENDIX_POISSON
Distribution	Poisson
Link Function	Log
Dependent Variable	EVENT
Offset Variable	LTIME = Log(PDAYS)
Observations Used	988

Criteria For Assessing Goodness Of Fit

Criterion	DF	Value	Value/DF
Deviance	984	393.1203	0.3995
Scaled Deviance	984	393.1203	0.3995
Pearson Chi-Square	984	7574.2725	7.6974
Scaled Pearson X2	984	7574.2725	7.6974
Log Likelihood		-257.5601	

Analysis of Parameter Estimates

Baseline CD8 count
divided by 100

Wald test
statistics

Parameter	DF	Estimate	Standard Error	Wald 95% Confidence Limits		Chi-Square	Pr > ChiSq
Intercept	1	-1.1698	0.3228	-1.8024	-0.5372	13.14	0.0003
TRTSTATUS	1	-0.6096	0.2583	-1.1159	-0.1033	5.57	0.0183
BASECD8_100	1	-0.0587	0.0268	-0.1112	-0.0063	4.82	0.0281
SEX	1	-0.4923	0.2660	-1.0136	0.0290	3.43	0.0642
Scale	0	1.0000	0.0000	1.0000	1.0000		

Scale parameter
used to adjust for
extra-Poisson
dispersion

LR Statistics For Type 3 Analysis

Source	DF	Chi-Square	Pr > ChiSq
TRTSTATUS	1	5.40	0.0201
BASECD8_100	1	5.46	0.0194
SEX	1	3.27	0.0707

P-value for significance
of each variable in model

Model 1
excluding 2
dummy
variables
for time
since initial
response.
Chapter 32

```
                           Model Information
                   Data Set            WORK.APPENDIX_POISSON
                   Distribution              Poisson
                   Link Function                Log
                   Dependent Variable         EVENT
                   Offset Variable            LTIME
                   Observations Used            988

                        Class Level Information

                   Class      Levels    Values
                   PERIOD3       3       1 2 3

                 Criteria For Assessing Goodness Of Fit
        Criterion                 DF        Value      Value/DF

        Deviance                 982      387.5904      0.3947
        Scaled Deviance          982      387.5904      0.3947
        Pearson Chi-Square       982     5890.6342      5.9986
        Scaled Pearson X2        982     5890.6342      5.9986
        Log Likelihood                   -254.7952

                 Analysis Of Parameter Estimates

                             Standard      Wald 95%        Chi-
Parameter        DF  Estimate   Error  Confidence Limits  Square  Pr > ChiSq

Intercept         1   -1.2855  0.3400  -1.9518  -0.6192   14.30    0.0002
TRTSTATUS         1   -0.5871  0.2587  -1.0942  -0.0800    5.15    0.0233
BASECD8_100       1   -0.0558  0.0267  -0.1083  -0.0034    4.36    0.0369
SEX               1   -0.4868  0.2664  -1.0089   0.0353    3.34    0.0676
PERIOD      1     0    0.0000  0.0000   0.0000   0.0000     .        .
PERIOD      2     1    0.4256  0.2702  -0.1039   0.9552    2.48    0.1152
PERIOD      3     1   -0.5835  0.4825  -1.5292   0.3622    1.46    0.2265
Scale             0    1.0000  0.0000   1.0000   1.0000

                 LR Statistics For Type 3 Analysis
                                   Chi-
            Source         DF     Square    Pr > ChiSq

            TRTSTATUS       1      5.00       0.0253
            BASECD8_100     1      4.91       0.0267
            SEX             1      3.19       0.0742
            PERIOD          2      5.53       0.0630
```

LRS or deviance gives *P* > 0.99 for evaluating goodness of fit

Degrees of freedom

This is substantially <1, indicating underdispersion

Estimates of model parameters shown in Table 31.1.—Relative rates obtained by antilogging estimates

CI for model coefficients

Zeros in this row indicate that Period 1 is reference category

Test statistic = difference in deviances of 2 models = 393.1203 − 387.5904

P-value for test of difference in deviancies from models with and without dummy variables for time since initial response

Degrees of freedom = difference in number of parameters in Models 1 and 2

Model 2 including 2 dummy variables for time since initial response and CD8 count as a numerical variable. Chapters 31 and 32

```
                           Model Information
                   Data Set            WORK.APPENDIX_POISSON
                   Distribution              Poisson
                   Link Function                Log
                   Dependent Variable         EVENT
                   Offset Variable            LTIME
                   Observations Used            988


                        Class Level Information
                   Class      Levels    Values
                   PERIOD        3       1 2 3

                 Criteria For Assessing Goodness Of Fit

        Criterion                 DF        Value      Value/DF

        Deviance                 983      392.5001      0.3993
        Scaled Deviance          983      392.5001      0.3993
        Pearson Chi-Square       983     5580.2152      5.6767
        Scaled Pearson X2        983     5580.2152      5.6767
        Log Likelihood                   -257.2501

                 Analysis Of Parameter Estimates

                             Standard      Wald 95%        Chi-
Parameter        DF  Estimate   Error  Confidence Limits  Square  Pr > ChiSq

Intercept         1   -1.7549  0.2713  -2.2866  -1.2232   41.85   <.0001
TRTSTATUS         1   -0.6290  0.2577  -1.1340  -0.1240    5.96    0.0146
SEX               1   -0.5444  0.2649  -1.0637  -0.0252    4.22    0.0399
PERIOD      1     0    0.0000  0.0000   0.0000   0.0000     .        .
PERIOD      2     1    0.4191  0.2701  -0.1103   0.9485    2.41    0.1207
PERIOD      3     1   -0.6481  0.4814  -1.5918   0.2955    1.81    0.1782
Scale             0    1.0000  0.0000   1.0000   1.0000

                 LR Statistics For Type 3 Analysis
                                   Chi-
            Source         DF     Square    Pr > ChiSq

            TRTSTATUS       1      5.77       0.0163
            SEX             1      4.00       0.0455
            PERIOD          2      6.08       0.0478
```

Model excluding baseline CD8 count. Chapter 33

```
                    Model Information
        Data Set              WORK.APPENDIX_POISSON
        Distribution          Poisson
        Link Function         Log
        Dependent Variable    EVENT
        Offset Variable       LTIME
        Observations Used     988

              Class Level Information
        Class       Levels    Values

        PERIOD         3       1  2  3
        CD8GRP         5       1  2  3  4  5

              Criteria For Assessing Goodness Of Fit
        Criterion             DF        Value       Value/DF

        Deviance             979      387.1458       0.3955
        Scaled Deviance      979      387.1458       0.3955
        Pearson Chi-Square   979     5852.1596       5.9777
        Scaled Pearson X2    979     5852.1596       5.9777
        Log Likelihood               -254.5729

              Analysis Of Parameter Estimates

                              Standard      Wald 95%          Chi-
Parameter        DF  Estimate   Error   Confidence Limits   Square   Pr > ChiSq

Intercept         1   -1.2451   0.6116   -2.4439   -0.0463    4.14     0.0418
TRTSTATUS         1   -0.5580   0.2600   -1.0677   -0.0483    4.60     0.0319
SEX               1   -0.4971   0.2675   -1.0214    0.0272    3.45     0.0631
PERIOD      1     0    0.0000   0.0000    0.0000    0.0000     .         .
PERIOD      2     1    0.4550   0.2715   -0.0771    0.9871    2.81     0.0937
PERIOD      3     1   -0.5386   0.4849   -1.4890    0.4119    1.23     0.2667
CD8GRP      1     1   -0.2150   0.6221   -1.4343    1.0044    0.12     0.7297
CD8GRP      2     1   -0.3646   0.7648   -1.8636    1.1345    0.23     0.6336
CD8GRP      3     0    0.0000   0.0000    0.0000    0.0000     .         .
CD8GRP      4     1   -0.3270   1.1595   -2.5996    1.9455    0.08     0.7779
CD8GRP      5     1   -0.8264   0.6057   -2.0136    0.3608    1.86     0.1725
Scale             0    1.0000   0.0000    1.0000    1.0000

              LR Statistics For Type 3 Analysis
                                   Chi-
        Source           DF       Square    Pr > ChiSq

        TRTSTATUS         1        4.48       0.0342
        SEX               1        3.30       0.0695
        PERIOD            2        5.54       0.0628
        CD8GRP            4        5.35       0.2528
```

Model including baseline CD8 count as a series of dummy variables. Chapter 33

Parameter estimates for dummy variables for baseline CD8 count where category 3 (≥825, <1100) is reference category

Number of additional variables in larger model

Test statistic = 392.5001 − 387.1458

P-value for test of significance of baseline CD8 count when incorporated as a categorical variable

Analysis of periodontal data used in Chapter 42, generated by Stata

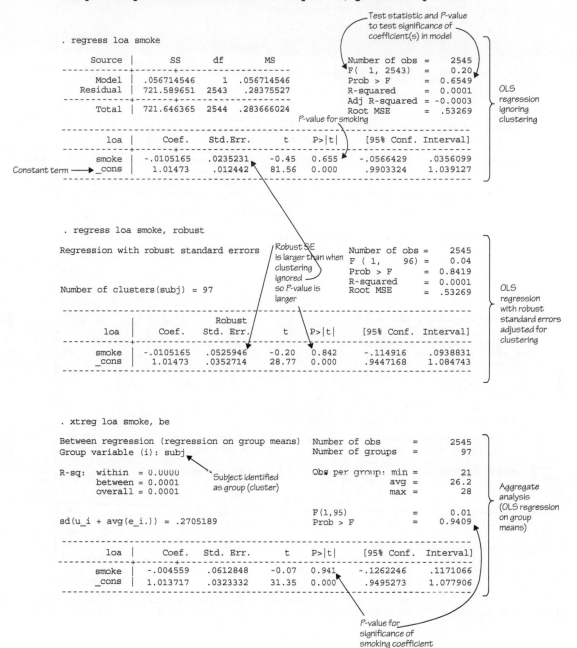

Test statistic and *P*-value to test significance of coefficient(s) in model

. regress loa smoke

Source	SS	df	MS
Model	.056714546	1	.056714546
Residual	721.589651	2543	.28375527
Total	721.646365	2544	.283666024

Number of obs = 2545
F(1, 2543) = 0.20
Prob > F = 0.6549
R-squared = 0.0001
Adj R-squared = -0.0003
Root MSE = .53269

P-value for smoking

OLS regression ignoring clustering

loa	Coef.	Std.Err.	t	P>|t|	[95% Conf. Interval]
smoke	-.0105165	.0235231	-0.45	0.655	-.0566429 .0356099
_cons	1.01473	.012442	81.56	0.000	.9903324 1.039127

Constant term →

. regress loa smoke, robust

Regression with robust standard errors

Robust SE is larger than when clustering ignored so *P*-value is larger

Number of obs = 2545
F (1, 96) = 0.04
Prob > F = 0.8419
R-squared = 0.0001
Root MSE = .53269

Number of clusters(subj) = 97

OLS regression with robust standard errors adjusted for clustering

loa	Coef.	Robust Std. Err.	t	P>|t|	[95% Conf. Interval]
smoke	-.0105165	.0525946	-0.20	0.842	-.114916 .0938831
_cons	1.01473	.0352714	28.77	0.000	.9447168 1.084743

. xtreg loa smoke, be

Between regression (regression on group means)
Group variable (i): subj

Number of obs = 2545
Number of groups = 97

Subject identified as group (cluster)

R-sq: within = 0.0000
between = 0.0001
overall = 0.0001

Obs per group: min = 21
avg = 26.2
max = 28

Aggregate analysis (OLS regression on group means)

sd(u_i + avg(e_i.)) = .2705189

F(1,95) = 0.01
Prob > F = 0.9409

loa	Coef.	Std. Err.	t	P>|t|	[95% Conf. Interval]
smoke	-.004559	.0612848	-0.07	0.941	-.1262246 .1171066
_cons	1.013717	.0323332	31.35	0.000	.9495273 1.077906

P-value for significance of smoking coefficient

```
. iis subj
. xtreg loa smoke, pa robust corr(exchangeable)

Iteration 1: tolerance = .00516018
Iteration 2: tolerance = 2.204e-07
```

Correlation structure
identified as
exchangeable

Model Chi-square to test
significance of coefficient
in model

P-value
for model
Chi-square

```
GEE population-averaged model            Number of obs      =      2545
Group variable:                  subj    Number of groups   =        97
Link:                        identity    Obs per group: min =        21
Family:                      Gaussian                   avg =      26.2
Correlation:             exchangeable                   max =        28
                                         Wald chi2(1)       =      0.01
Scale parameter:              .2835381    Prob > chi2        =    0.9198
```

GEE with
robust
standard
errors and
exchangeable
correlation
structure

```
                    (standard errors adjusted for clustering on subj)
------------------------------------------------------------------------------
             |               Semi-robust
         loa |      Coef.   Std. Err.      z    P>|z|     [95% Conf. Interval]
-------------+----------------------------------------------------------------
       smoke |  -.0053018   .0526501    -0.10   0.920    -.1084941    .0978905
       _cons |   1.013841   .0347063    29.21   0.000     .9458185    1.081865
------------------------------------------------------------------------------
```

Wald test statistic

```
. xtreg loa smoke, mle

Fitting constant-only model:
Iteration 0:    log likelihood = -1785.7026
Iteration 1:    log likelihood = -1785.7004
```

difference = −0.0038 so
− 2 log likelihood ratio
= 2 × 0.0038
= 0.0076
≃ 0.01

```
Fitting full model:
Iteration 0:    log likelihood = -1785.7027
Iteration 1:    log likelihood = -1785.6966
Iteration 2:    log likelihood = -1785.6966
```

final
iteration
provides
stable
estimates

```
Random-effects ML regression            Number of obs      =      2545
Group variable (i): subj                Number of groups   =        97

Random effects u_i - Gaussian           Obs per group:  min =        21
                                                        avg =      26.2
                                                        max =        28
```

Degrees of
freedom

Random
effects
model

LRS = −2 log likelihood ratio

```
                                         LR chi2(1)         =      0.01
Log likelihood  = -1785.6966             Prob > chi2        =    0.9302
```

P-value

```
------------------------------------------------------------------------------
         loa |      Coef.   Std. Err.      z    P>|z|     [95% Conf. Interval]
-------------+----------------------------------------------------------------
       smoke |  -.0053168   .0607203    -0.09   0.930    -.1243265    .1136928
       _cons |   1.013844    .032046    31.64   0.000     .951035    1.076653
-------------+----------------------------------------------------------------
     /sigma_u |   .2519226   .0204583    12.31   0.000     .2118251    .2920201
     /sigma_e |   .4684954   .0066952    69.98   0.000     .4553731    .4816176
-------------+----------------------------------------------------------------
         rho |   .2242953   .0288039                       .1719879    .2846119
------------------------------------------------------------------------------
Likelihood-ratio test of sigma_u=0: chibar2(01)=  443.21 Prob>=chibar2 = 0.000
```

σ_c ⟶ /sigma_u
σ ⟶ /sigma_e

Intracluster
correlation
coefficient

$$= \frac{0.2519226^2}{0.2519226^2 + 0.4684954^2}$$

Appendix D: Checklists and trial profile from the EQUATOR network and critical appraisal templates

In 2008, the **EQUATOR** (Enhancing the **QUA**lity and Transparency **O**f Health **R**esearch) Network was initiated with the objectives of providing resources and training for the reporting of health research, as well as assistance in the development, dissemination and implementation of reporting guidelines. The international collaboration is led by experts in the area of research methodology, reporting and editorial work. Its website (www.equator-network.org) provides links to a substantial number of guidelines which are often updated in the light of new evidence. In view of this evolving process, we present the guidelines (correct at the time of printing) only for randomized controlled trials (the CONSORT checklist (Table D1) and flow chart (Fig. D1)) and observational studies (the STROBE checklist (Table D2)), two common study designs. Guidelines for the presentation of study results are now available for many other types of study[1]. We provide website addresses (the guidelines may also be accessed from the EQUATOR website) in the following table for some of these designs, all relevant to the content of this book, so that you can find them online in the most up to date versions.

Name	Derivation	Use	Website or reference	Chapter
CONSORT	**CON**solidated Standards **O**f Reporting Trials	Randomized controlled trials	www.consort-statement.org	14
SPIRIT	**S**tandard **P**rotocol **I**tems: **R**ecommendations for **I**nterventional **T**rials	Clinical trial protocols	www.spirit-statement.org	14
STROBE	**ST**rengthening the **R**eporting of **OB**servational studies in **E**pidemiology	Observational studies	www.strobe-statement.org	15, 16
SAMPL	**S**tatistical **A**nalyses and **M**ethods in the **P**ublished **L**iterature	Basic statistical methods and results	www.equator-network.org/reporting-guidelines/sampl/	37
STARD	**STA**ndards for **R**eporting **D**iagnostic accuracy studies	Diagnostic accuracy	www.stard-statement.org	38
GRRAS	**G**uidelines for **R**eporting **R**eliability and **A**greement **S**tudies	Reliability and agreement	www.equator-network.org/reporting-guidelines/guidelines-for-reporting-reliability-and-agreement-studies-grras-were-proposed/	39
PRISMA	**P**referred **R**eporting **I**tems for **S**ystematic reviews and **M**eta-**A**nalyses	Systematic reviews and meta-analysis of healthcare interventions	www. prisma-statement.org	43
MOOSE	**M**eta-analysis **O**f **O**bservational **S**tudies in **E**pidemiology	Meta-analysis of observational studies	Stroup, D.F., Berlin, J.A., Morton, S.C., *et al.* (2000) Meta-analysis of observational studies in epidemiology: a proposal for reporting. Meta-analysis Of Observational Studies in Epidemiology (MOOSE) group. *JAMA*, **283**, 2008–2012.	43
TRIPOD	**T**ransparent **R**eporting of a multivariable prediction model for **I**ndividual **P**rognosis **O**r **D**iagnosis	Model development and validation	www.tripod-statement.org	46

Reference

1 Moher, D., Altman, D.G., Schulz, K., Simera, I and Wager, E. (eds) (2014) *Guidelines for Reporting Health Research: A User's Manual*. Oxford: Wiley-Blackwell.

Equator Network Statements

Table D1 CONSORT (Consolidation of Standards for Reporting Trials) 2010 Statement* – checklist of information to include when reporting a randomized trial.

Section/topic	Item no	Checklist item	Reported on page no.
Title and abstract			
	1a	Identification as a randomised trial in the title	_____
	1b	Structured summary of trial design, methods, results, and conclusions (for specific guidance see CONSORT for abstracts)	_____
Introduction			
Background and objectives	2a	Scientific background and explanation of rationale	_____
	2b	Specific objectives or hypotheses	_____
Methods			
Trial design	3a	Description of trial design (such as parallel, factorial) including allocation ratio	_____
	3b	Important changes to methods after trial commencement (such as eligibility criteria), with reasons	_____
Participants	4a	Eligibility criteria for participants	_____
	4b	Settings and locations where the data were collected	_____
Interventions	5	The interventions for each group with sufficient details to allow replication, including how and when they were actually administered	_____
Outcomes	6a	Completely defined pre-specified primary and secondary outcome measures, including how and when they were assessed	_____
	6b	Any changes to trial outcomes after the trial commenced, with reasons	_____
Sample size	7a	How sample size was determined	_____
	7b	When applicable, explanation of any interim analyses and stopping guidelines	_____
Randomisation:			_____
Sequence generation	8a	Method used to generate the random allocation sequence	_____
	8b	Type of randomisation; details of any restriction (such as blocking and block size)	_____
Allocation concealment mechanism	9	Mechanism used to implement the random allocation sequence (such as sequentially numbered containers), describing any steps taken to conceal the sequence until interventions were assigned	_____
Implementation	10	Who generated the random allocation sequence, who enrolled participants, and who assigned participants to interventions	_____
Blinding	11a	If done, who was blinded after assignment to interventions (for example, participants, care providers, those assessing outcomes) and how	_____
	11b	If relevant, description of the similarity of interventions	_____
Statistical methods	12a	Statistical methods used to compare groups for primary and secondary outcomes	_____
	12b	Methods for additional analyses, such as subgroup analyses and adjusted analyses	_____
Results			
Participant flow (a diagram is strongly recommended)	13a	For each group, the numbers of participants who were randomly assigned, received intended treatment, and were analysed for the primary outcome	_____
	13b	For each group, losses and exclusions after randomisation, together with reasons	_____
Recruitment	14a	Dates defining the periods of recruitment and follow-up	_____
	14b	Why the trial ended or was stopped	_____
Baseline data	15	A table showing baseline demographic and clinical characteristics for each group	_____
Numbers analysed	16	For each group, number of participants (denominator) included in each analysis and whether the analysis was by original assigned groups	_____

continued

Section/topic	Item no	Checklist item	Reported on page no.
Outcomes and estimation	17a	For each primary and secondary outcome, results for each group, and the estimated effect size and its precision (such as 95% confidence interval)	_____
	17b	For binary outcomes, presentation of both absolute and relative effect sizes is recommended	_____
Ancillary analyses	18	Results of any other analyses performed, including subgroup analyses and adjusted analyses, distinguishing pre-specified from exploratory	_____
Harms	19	All important harms or unintended effects in each group (for specific guidance see CONSORT for harms)	_____
Discussion			
Limitations	20	Trial limitations, addressing sources of potential bias, imprecision, and, if relevant, multiplicity of analyses	_____
Generalisability	21	Generalisability (external validity, applicability) of the trial findings	_____
Interpretation	22	Interpretation consistent with results, balancing benefits and harms, and considering other relevant evidence	_____
Other information			
Registration	23	Registration number and name of trial registry	_____
Protocol	24	Where the full trial protocol can be accessed, if available	_____
Funding	25	Sources of funding and other support (such as supply of drugs), role of funders	_____

*It is strongly recommend that this statement is read in conjunction with the *CONSORT 2010 Explanation and Elaboration* for important clarifications on all the items. If relevant, it is also recommended that the CONSORT extensions for cluster randomised trials, non-inferiority and equivalence trials, non-pharmacological treatments, herbal interventions, and pragmatic trials are also read. For up to date references relevant to this checklist, see www.consort-statement.org.

Source: Schulz (2010). Reproduced with permission of BMJ Publishing Group Ltd.

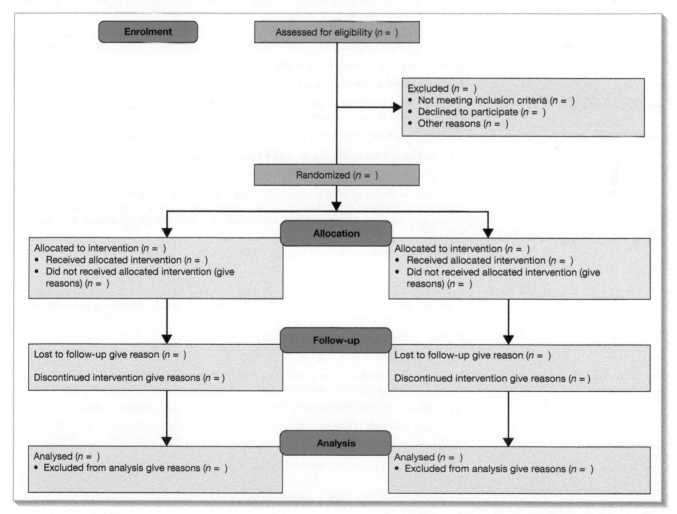

Figure D1 The CONSORT Statement's 2010 trial profile of a randomized controlled trial's progress. *Source:* Schulz (2010). Reproduced with permission of BMJ Publishing Group Ltd.

Table D.2 STROBE Statement – checklist of items that should be included in reports of observational studies.

	Item no.	Recommendation
Title and abstract	1	(a) Indicate the study's design with a commonly used term in the title or the abstract
		(b) Provide in the abstract an informative and balanced summary of what was done and what was found
Introduction		
Background/rationale	2	Explain the scientific background and rationale for the investigation being reported
Objectives	3	State specific objectives, including any prespecified hypotheses
Methods		
Study design	4	Present key elements of study design early in the paper
Setting	5	Describe the setting, locations, and relevant dates, including periods of recruitment, exposure, follow-up, and data collection
Participants	6	(a) *Cohort study*—Give the eligibility criteria, and the sources and methods of selection of participants. Describe methods of follow-up *Case-control study*—Give the eligibility criteria, and the sources and methods of case ascertainment and control selection. Give the rationale for the choice of cases and controls *Cross-sectional study*—Give the eligibility criteria, and the sources and methods of selection of participants
		(b) *Cohort study*—For matched studies, give matching criteria and number of exposed and unexposed *Case-control study*—For matched studies, give matching criteria and the number of controls per case
Variables	7	Clearly define all outcomes, exposures, predictors, potential confounders, and effect modifiers. Give diagnostic criteria, if applicable
Data sources/measurement	8*	For each variable of interest, give sources of data and details of methods of assessment (measurement). Describe comparability of assessment methods if there is more than one group
Bias	9	Describe any efforts to address potential sources of bias
Study size	10	Explain how the study size was arrived at
Quantitative variables	11	Explain how quantitative variables were handled in the analyses. If applicable, describe which groupings were chosen and why
Statistical methods	12	(a) Describe all statistical methods, including those used to control for confounding
		(b) Describe any methods used to examine subgroups and interactions
		(c) Explain how missing data were addressed
		(d) *Cohort study*—If applicable, explain how loss to follow-up was addressed *Case-control study*—If applicable, explain how matching of cases and controls was addressed *Cross-sectional study*—If applicable, describe analytical methods taking account of sampling strategy
		(e) Describe any sensitivity analyses
Results		
Participants	13*	(a) Report numbers of individuals at each stage of study—eg numbers potentially eligible, examined for eligibility, confirmed eligible, included in the study, completing follow-up, and analysed
		(b) Give reasons for non-participation at each stage
		(c) Consider use of a flow diagram
Descriptive data	14*	(a) Give characteristics of study participants (eg demographic, clinical, social) and information on exposures and potential confounders
		(b) Indicate number of participants with missing data for each variable of interest
		(c) *Cohort study*—Summarise follow-up time (eg, average and total amount)
Outcome data	15*	*Cohort study*—Report numbers of outcome events or summary measures over time
		Case-control study—Report numbers in each exposure category, or summary measures of exposure
		Cross-sectional study—Report numbers of outcome events or summary measures

continued

	Item no.	Recommendation
Main results	16	(*a*) Give unadjusted estimates and, if applicable, confounder-adjusted estimates and their precision (eg, 95% confidence interval). Make clear which confounders were adjusted for and why they were included
		(*b*) Report category boundaries when continuous variables were categorized
		(*c*) If relevant, consider translating estimates of relative risk into absolute risk for a meaningful time period
Other analyses	17	Report other analyses done—eg analyses of subgroups and interactions, and sensitivity analyses
Discussion		
Key results	18	Summarise key results with reference to study objectives
Limitations	19	Discuss limitations of the study, taking into account sources of potential bias or imprecision. Discuss both direction and magnitude of any potential bias
Interpretation	20	Give a cautious overall interpretation of results considering objectives, limitations, multiplicity of analyses, results from similar studies, and other relevant evidence
Generalisability	21	Discuss the generalisability (external validity) of the study results
Other information		
Funding	22	Give the source of funding and the role of the funders for the present study and, if applicable, for the original study on which the present article is based

*Give information separately for cases and controls in case-control studies and, if applicable, for exposed and unexposed groups in cohort and cross-sectional studies.

Note: An *Explanation and Elaboration* article discusses each checklist item and gives methodological background and published examples of transparent reporting. The STROBE checklist is best used in conjunction with this article (freely available on the websites of *PLoS Medicine* at http://www.plosmedicine.org/, *Annals of Internal Medicine* at http://www.annals.org/, and *Epidemiology* at http://www.epidem.com/). Information on the STROBE Initiative is available at www.strobe-statement.org.

Source: von Elm (2007). Reproduced with permission of Elsevier.

Critical Appraisal Templates

Template D1 Critical appraisal and evaluating the evidence in published papers reporting randomized controlled trials (RCTs)

1. Title and abstract

a. Is the trial identified as a RCT in the title?

b. Does the abstract summarize the trial primary objective, design, methods, results and conclusions?

2. Introduction

a. Is a proper description provided of the scientific background and is the rationale for the trial explained sufficiently? Has all the relevant information from previous studies and other available evidence been included?

b. Is the primary aim of the trial indicated, preferably in relation to a relevant hypothesis based on the outcome of interest, and are secondary objectives described?

3. Methods

a. Trial design

Is the trial design described adequately? Are any aspects of the design utilized to avoid bias fully described? For example:

i. Randomization Are full details of the randomization process provided, including the method used to generate the random allocation sequence, the type of randomization, steps taken to conceal the allocation sequence and details of the implementation of the randomization (e.g. who enrolled the participants and who assigned the participants to the interventions)?

ii. Blinding To what extent was the study blind? If relevant, is a description provided of the similarity of the interventions?

iii. Allocation concealment Was the allocation sequence concealed from the staff recruiting patients for the trial?

b. Participants

i. Is there a complete description of the eligibility (inclusion and exclusion) criteria for the participants?

ii. Was the study conducted using an appropriate spectrum of patients?

c. Interventions

i. Is the intervention (treatment and/or placebo if appropriate) for each group described in sufficient detail?

ii. Were the groups treated in similar fashion, aside from the fact that they received different interventions?

d. Outcomes

i. Is consideration given to all the important outcomes?

ii. Are the primary and secondary outcomes defined precisely?

iii. Were there any changes to the outcomes after the trial started?

e. Sample size

i. Is there a power statement to justify the overall sample size? Does this power statement indicate the form of the statistical analysis on which it is based and does it include a specification of the values of all the factors that affect sample size for this calculation?

ii. If relevant, is there a full explanation of any interim analysis, including the steps taken to reduce the Type I error rate?

iii. If subgroup analyses have been performed, is there a justification for the subgroup sample sizes, based on power calculations, and a description of the steps taken to reduce the Type I error rate? Alternatively, are these subgroup analyses specified as being *exploratory* in nature, with an indication that they may be underpowered?

f. Statistical methods

i. Are all the statistical methods used to compare groups for primary and secondary outcomes identified?

ii. Are the statistical methods appropriate (e.g. have underlying assumptions been verified; have dependencies in the data (e.g. pairing) been taken into account in the analysis?)?

iii. Is there a description of additional analyses, such as subgroup analyses? Were any additional analyses undertaken specified *a priori* or were they *post hoc* analyses?

4. Results

a. Participant numbers and dates

i. Is there a full explanation (preferably in a participant flow chart), for each treatment group, of the numbers of participants who were randomly assigned, received the intended treatment and were analysed for the primary outcome?

ii. If relevant, are numbers of and reasons for losses to follow-up and exclusions after randomization documented?

iii. Are dates provided which define the periods of recruitment and follow-up?

continued

b. Baseline data

    i. Is there a table which shows the baseline demographic and clinical characteristics for each group?

    ii. Are the groups comparable?

c. Numbers analysed

    i. Is there a specification of whether an 'intention-to-treat' (ITT) analysis was performed? Is a justification given for the choice of analysis (ITT or other) and is this appropriate?

    ii. If there were protocol deviations, was a sensitivity analysis performed (e.g. a per protocol analysis or an analysis with imputed data for missing observations)?

d. Outcomes of interest

    i. Main outcome of interest Is an appropriate summary measure given for the main outcome variable (i.e. that which relates to the primary aim of the study) for each comparison group? For example, the rate/risk/odds of occurrence of the outcome (e.g. death) if the outcome variable is *binary*, stating results in absolute numbers when feasible; or the mean (median) if the outcome variable is *numerical*?

    ii. Magnitude of the effect of interest Is there an indication of the magnitude of the effect of interest? For example, a ratio such as the relative rate/risk/odds or a difference such as the absolute difference in risk if the outcome variable is *binary*; or a difference in means (medians) if the main outcome variable is *numerical*?

    iii. Precision of the effect of interest Is there an indication of the precision of the effect of interest (e.g. a 95% confidence interval or standard error)?

e. Additional analyses If additional (e.g. subgroup) analyses were performed, are their results provided, and are any exploratory analyses distinguished from those that were pre-specified?

f. Harms Are all important harms in each group documented?

5. Discussion

a. Deciding whether the results are important

    i. Are the key findings summarized with reference to the trial objectives?

    ii. Do the results make **biological sense**?

    iii. If a **confidence interval** for the effect of interest (e.g. the difference in treatment means) has been provided:

        – Would you regard the observed effect clinically important (irrespective of whether or not the result of the relevant hypothesis test is statistically significant) if the lower limit of the confidence interval represented the true value of the effect?

        – Would you regard the observed effect clinically important if the upper limit of the confidence interval represented the true value of the effect?

        – Are your answers to the above two points sufficiently similar to declare the results of the study unambiguous and important?

    iv. Is there an evaluation of the **number of patients needed to treat** (NNT) with the experimental treatment rather than the control treatment in order to prevent one of them developing the 'bad' outcome?

b. Limitations Is there a discussion of all the trial limitations, including sources of potential bias and imprecision?

c. Generalizability Is there a discussion of the generalizability (external validity) of the trial findings (i.e. the extent to which the participants are representative of the wider population)?

d. Interpretation Taking the benefits and harms into consideration, as well as the limitations of the trial, any multiple testing and subgroup analyses, is the interpretation of the trial findings consistent with the results?

6. Other information

a. Registration Are the trial registration number and the name of the trial registry provided?

b. Protocol Is there information about where the protocol can be accessed?

c. Funding Are sources of funding documented and is there a conflict of interest statement for each of the investigators?

1. Title and abstract

a. Is the study design (i.e. cohort, case–control or cross-sectional study) clearly identified in the title?

b. Does the abstract provide a balanced summary of the study design, methods, results, conclusions and any major limitations?

2. Introduction

a. Is there a proper description of the scientific background and rationale for the current investigation? Has all the relevant information from any previous studies and other available evidence been included?

b. Is the primary objective of the current investigation indicated and are secondary objectives described? Were all the objectives pre-specified? If a cohort study, were there any modifications to the original study protocol, including the formulation of additional objectives, following the publication of new evidence after the cohort study was initiated?

3. Methods

a. Study design Is the study design described adequately? In particular, is the type of study identified and a description provided of the study setting, location and any relevant dates (including periods of recruitment, exposure, follow-up and data collection)?

b. Participants

   i. Are eligibility criteria (inclusion and exclusion) provided for the study participants? Are the source and methods of selection of participants described?

   ii. If a case–control study, is the rationale for the choice of cases and controls explained?

   iii. If a cohort study, is the method of follow-up described?

   iv. Was the study conducted using an appropriate spectrum of participants?

   v. If the study was matched, is information provided on the matching criteria and number of exposed/unexposed participants (cohort study) or controls per case (case–control study)?

c. Variables

   i. Is there a clear description of outcomes, exposures, predictors, potential confounders, and effect modifiers (with details of methods of assessment and diagnostic criteria, if applicable)?

   ii. Are details provided on the comparability of assessment methods if there is more than one group?

d. Bias Have any efforts been made to address potential sources of bias? Are these fully described?

e. Sample size Is there a full explanation of how the study size was determined?

f. Statistical methods

   i. Is there a description of how quantitative variables were handled in the analysis, including any choice of groupings?

   ii. Are all the statistical methods used, including those adopted to control for confounding, fully described?

   iii. If relevant, are the methods used to examine subgroups and interactions described?

   iv. Is there a description of how missing data have been dealt with in all relevant analyses?

   v. Is there a description of how losses to follow-up (cohort studies), matching (case–control studies) or sampling strategy (cross-sectional studies) have been dealt with?

   vi. Are all sensitivity analyses fully described?

4. Results

a. Participant numbers and dates

   i. Is there a report of the number of individuals included at each stage of the study (e.g. the numbers potentially eligible, examined for eligibility, confirmed eligible, included in study, completed follow-up, included in the analysis), preferably through the use of a flow chart?

   ii. If relevant, are reasons for non-participation at any stage documented?

continued

b. Descriptive data

    i. Are the characteristics of study participants (demographic, clinical and social) and information on exposures and potential confounders provided?

    ii. Is there an indication of the number of participants with missing data for each variable of interest?

    iii. If a cohort study, is the follow-up time summarized (e.g. average and total amount)?

c. Main results

    i. Main outcome measures Is there full information on outcomes, e.g. the number of outcome events or summary measures over time (cohort studies), numbers in each exposure category or summary measures of exposure (case–control studies) or number of outcome events or summary measures (cross-sectional studies)?

    ii. Magnitude of effects of interest Are unadjusted estimates and, if applicable, confounder-adjusted estimates provided?

    iii. Precision of effects of interest Is there an indication of the precision (e.g. 95% confidence intervals) of the estimates?

    iv. If applicable, is there a clear indication of which **confounders** were adjusted for in the analysis and why they were selected?

d. Other analyses Are the results reported of all other analyses performed, including analyses of subgroups and interactions and any sensitivity analyses?

5. Discussion

a. Summary of key results

    i. Is there a summary of the key findings with reference to the study objectives?

    ii. Do the results make **biological sense**?

    iii. Consider the **confidence interval** for the any effect of interest:

       – Would you regard the observed effect clinically important (irrespective of whether or not the result of the relevant hypothesis test is statistically significant) if the lower limit of the confidence interval represented the true value of the effect?

       – Would you regard the observed effect clinically important if the upper limit of the confidence interval represented the true value of the effect?

       – Are your answers to the above two points sufficiently similar to declare the results of the study unambiguous and important?

    iv. If feasible, have any estimates of relative 'risk' (e.g. relative risk, odds ratio) been translated into absolute 'risks' for a meaningful time period?

b. Limitations Is there a discussion of all the study limitations, including the sources of imprecision and the sources and effect (i.e. direction and magnitude) of any potential bias?

c. Generalizability Is there a discussion of the generalizability (external validity) of the study findings (i.e. the extent to which the participants are representative of the wider population)?

d. Interpretation Are the study findings interpreted in a cautious way, taking full consideration of the study objectives, the limitations of the study, any multiple testing, the results from other similar studies and any other relevant evidence?

6. Other information

a. Funding sources Are the sources of funding documented, both for the original study on which the article is based, if relevant, and for the present study, and is the role of the funders described?

b. Conflict of interest Is there a clear and transparent conflict of interest statement for each of the investigators?

2 × 2 table: A contingency table of frequencies with two rows and two columns

−2log likelihood: See likelihood ratio statistic

Accuracy: Refers to the way in which an observed value of a quantity agrees with the true value

Adjusted odds ratio: The odds ratio for a factor (explanatory variable) in a multivariable logistic regression model which is controlled for the effects of other covariates

Administrative censoring: Follow-up is censored because of administrative reasons (e.g. the study ends on a particular date) and is generally non-informative

All subsets model selection: See automatic model selection

Allocation bias: A systematic distortion of the data resulting from the way in which individuals are assigned to treatment groups. Sometimes called channelling bias

Alternative hypothesis: The hypothesis about the effect of interest that disagrees with the null hypothesis and is true if the null hypothesis is false

Altman's nomogram: A diagram that relates the sample size of a statistical test to the power, significance level and standardized difference

AMSTAR 2. A critical appraisal tool for systematic reviews that include randomized and non-randomized studies

Analysis of covariance (ANCOVA): A special form of analysis of variance that compares mean values of a dependent variable between groups of individuals after adjusting for the effect of one or more explanatory variables

Analysis of variance (ANOVA): A general term for analyses that compare the population means of groups of observations by splitting the total variance of a variable into its component parts, each attributed to a particular factor

ANCOVA: See analysis of covariance

ANOVA: See analysis of variance

Arithmetic mean: A measure of location obtained by dividing the sum of the observations by the number of observations. Often called the mean

Ascertainment bias: May occur when the sample included in a study is not randomly selected from the population and differs in some important respects from that population

ASCII or text file format: A data file in plain text format that can be read/imported by most software packages. The data values in each row are typically delimited by spaces or commas

Assessment bias: See observer bias

Attrition bias: When those who are lost to follow-up in a longitudinal study differ in a systematic way from those who are not lost to follow-up

AUROC: Area under a ROC curve

Automatic model selection: A method of selecting explanatory variables to be included in a mathematical model, e.g. forward, backward, stepwise, all subsets

Average: A general term for a measure of location

Backward selection: See automatic model selection

Bar or column chart: A diagram that illustrates the distribution of a categorical or discrete variable by showing a separate horizontal or vertical bar for each 'category', its length being proportional to the (relative) frequency in that 'category'

Bartlett's test: Used to compare variances

Bayes theorem: The posterior probability of an event/hypothesis is proportional to the product of its prior probability and the likelihood

Bayesian approach to inference: Uses not only current information (e.g. from a trial) but also an individual's previous belief (often subjective) about a hypothesis to evaluate the posterior belief in the hypothesis

Bias: A systematic difference between the results obtained from a study and the true state of affairs

Bimodal distribution: Data whose distribution has two 'peaks'

Binary variable: A categorical variable with two categories. Also called a dichotomous variable

Binomial distribution: A discrete probability distribution of a binary random variable; useful for inferences about proportions

Bioequivalence trial: A type of trial in which we are interested in showing that the rate and extent of absorption of a new formulation of a drug is the same as that of an old formulation, when the drugs are given at the same dose

Blinding: When the patients, clinicians and the assessors of response to treatment in a clinical trial are unaware of the treatment allocation (double-blind), or when the patient is aware of the treatment received but the assessor of response is not (single-blind). Also called masking

Block: A homogeneous group of experimental units that share similar characteristics. Sometimes called a stratum

Bonferroni correction (adjustment): A *post hoc* adjustment to the P-value to take account of the number of tests performed in multiple hypothesis testing

Bootstrapping: A simulation process that can be used to derive a confidence interval for a parameter. It involves estimating the parameter from each of many random samples of size *n* obtained by sampling with replacement from the original sample of size *n*; the confidence interval is derived by considering the variability of the distribution of these estimates

Box (box-and-whisker) plot: A diagram illustrating the distribution of a variable; it indicates the median, upper and lower quartiles, and, often, the maximum and minimum values

Brier score: Measures the squared difference between an individual's predicted probability of an event and his/her observed outcome. The mean Brier score is used to assess the accuracy of a prognostic score

British Standards Institution repeatability coefficient: The maximum difference that is likely to occur between two repeated measurements

c statistic: Measures the area under a ROC curve and may be used to assess the ability of a prognostic score or diagnostic test to discriminate between those with and without a particular condition; can be used to compare two or more such scores or tests. $c = 1$ when the discriminatory ability is perfect and $c = 0.5$ when the procedure performs no better than chance. See also Harrell's *c* statistic

Carry-over effect: The residual effect of the previous treatment in a cross-over trial

Case: An individual with the outcome of interest (e.g. disease) in an investigation

Case–control study: Groups of individuals with the disease (the cases) and without the disease (the controls) are identified, and exposures to risk factors in these groups are compared

Medical Statistics at a Glance, Fourth Edition. Aviva Petrie and Caroline Sabin. © 2020 Aviva Petrie and Caroline Sabin. Published 2020 by John Wiley & Sons Ltd.
Companion Website: www.medstatsaag.com

Categorical (qualitative) variable: Each individual belongs to one of a number of distinct categories of the variable

Causal modelling: Statistical methods that describe and test the underlying causal relationships between an exposure of interest and an outcome

Causal pathway: The chain of events or factors leading in sequence to an outcome, when the effect of any step in the sequence is dependent on the event in the previous step(s)

Cell of a contingency table: The designation of a particular row and a particular column of the table

Censored data: Occur in survival analysis because there is incomplete information on outcome. See also left- and right-censored data

Census: A cross-sectional study that collects information from every individual in a population

Central tendency bias: Responders tend to move towards the midpoint of the scale of measurement

Centring: A process used to improve the interpretation of a parameter in a regression model; achieved by subtracting a constant (often the sample mean of the explanatory variable) from the value of the explanatory variable for each individual

Channelling bias: See allocation bias

Chi-squared (χ^2) distribution: A right-skewed continuous distribution characterized by its degrees of freedom; useful for analysing categorical data

Chi-squared test: Used on frequency data, it tests the null hypothesis that there is no association between the factors that define a contingency table. Also used to test differences in proportions

CI: See confidence interval for a parameter

Clinical cohort: A group of patients with the same clinical condition whose outcomes are observed over time

Clinical heterogeneity: Exists when the trials included in a meta-analysis have differences in the patient population, definition of variables, etc., which create problems of non-compatibility

Clinical trial: Any form of planned experiment on humans that is used to evaluate a new 'treatment' on a clinical outcome

Cluster randomization: Groups of individuals, rather than separate individuals, are randomly (by chance) allocated to treatments

Cluster randomized trial: Each group or cluster of individuals, rather than each individual, is randomly (using a method based on chance) allocated to a treatment

Cochrane Collaboration: An international network of clinicians, methodologists and consumers who continually update systematic reviews and make them available to others

Coefficient of variation: The standard deviation divided by the mean (often expressed as a percentage)

Cohen's kappa (κ): A measure of agreement between two sets of categorical measurements on the same individuals. If $\kappa = 1$, then there is perfect agreement; if $\kappa = 0$, then there is no better than chance agreement

Cohort study: A group of individuals, all without the outcome of interest (e.g. disease), is followed (usually prospectively) to study the effect on future outcomes of exposure to a risk factor

Collinearity: Pairs of explanatory variables in a regression analysis are very highly correlated, i.e. with correlation coefficients very close to ± 1

Competing risks: The development of one or more of the outcomes of interest precludes the development (or measurement) of any of the others

Complete randomized design: Experimental units assigned randomly to treatment groups

Composite endpoint: An outcome that is considered to have occurred if any of several different events is observed

Conditional logistic regression: A form of logistic regression used when individuals in a study are matched

Conditional probability: The probability of an event, given that another event has occurred

Confidence interval (CI) for a parameter: Broadly interpreted as the range of values within which we are (usually) 95% confident that the true population parameter lies. Strictly, after repeated sampling, 95% of confidence limits so determined will contain the parameter

Confidence limits: The upper and lower values of a confidence interval

Confounding: When one or more explanatory variables are related to the outcome and each other so that it is difficult to assess the independent effect of each one on the outcome variable

CONSORT Statement: Facilitates critical appraisal and interpretation of RCTs by providing guidance, in the form of a checklist and flowchart, to authors about how to report their trials

Contingency table: A (usually) two-way table in which the entries are frequencies

Continuity correction: A correction applied to a test statistic to adjust for the approximation of a discrete distribution by a continuous distribution

Continuous probability distribution: The random variable defining the distribution is continuous

Continuous variable: A numerical variable in which there is no limitation on the values that the variable can take other than that restricted by the degree of accuracy of the measuring technique

Control: An individual without the disease under investigation in a case–control study, or not receiving the new treatment in a clinical trial

Control group: A term used in comparative studies, e.g. clinical trials, to denote a comparison group. See also negative and positive controls

Convenience sample: A group of individuals believed to be representative of the population from which it is selected, but chosen because it is close at hand rather than being randomly selected

Correlation coefficient (Pearson's): A quantitative measure, ranging from −1 to +1, of the extent to which points in a scatter diagram conform to a straight line. See also Spearman's rank correlation coefficient

Covariate: See explanatory variable

Covariate pattern: A particular set of values for the explanatory variables in a regression model held by one or more individuals in the study

Cox proportional hazards regression model: See proportional hazards regression model

Cross-over design: Each individual receives more than one treatment under investigation, one after the other in random order

Cross-sectional study: Carried out at a single point in time

Cross-sectional time series model: See panel model

Cross-validation: We partition the data set into subsets, derive the measure of interest or model on a single subset initially and then validate it on the remaining subsets

Cumulative frequency: The number of individuals who have values below and including the specified value of a variable

Cumulative meta-analysis: The studies are added one by one in a specified order (usually according to date of publication) and a separate meta-analysis is performed on the accumulated studies after each addition

Data: Observations on one or more variables

Data dredging: The results of a study are analysed in many different ways, with a view to obtaining a significant finding, without prior specification of the hypothesis of interest

Deciles: Those values that divide the ordered observations into 10 equal parts

Degrees of freedom (df) of a statistic: The sample size minus the number of parameters that have to be estimated to calculate the statistic; they indicate the extent to which the observations are 'free' to vary

Dependent variable: A variable (usually denoted by y) that is predicted by the explanatory variable in regression analysis. Also called the response or outcome variable

Deviance: See likelihood ratio statistic

df: See degrees of freedom of a statistic

Diagnostic test: Used to aid or make a diagnosis of a particular condition

Dichotomous variable: See binary variable

Discrete probability distribution: The random variable defining the distribution takes discrete values

Discrete variable: A numerical variable that can only take integer values

Discriminant analysis: A method, similar to logistic regression, which can be used to identify factors that are significantly associated with a binary response

Disease register: See clinical cohort

Distribution-free tests: See non-parametric tests

Dot plot: A diagram in which each observation on a variable is represented by one dot on a horizontal (or vertical) line

Double-blind: See blinding

Dummy variables: The $k - 1$ binary variables that are created from a nominal or ordinal categorical variable with $k > 2$ categories, affording a comparison of each of the $k - 1$ categories with a reference category in a regression analysis. Also called indicator variables

Ecological fallacy: We believe mistakenly that an association that we observe between variables at the group or aggregate level (e.g. region) reflects the corresponding association at an individual level (the individuals in the regions) in the same population

Ecological study: A particular type of epidemiological study in which the unit of observation is a community or group of individuals rather than the individual

Effect modifier: See interaction

Effect of interest: The value of the response variable that reflects the comparison of interest, e.g. the difference in means

Empirical distribution: The observed distribution of a variable

Endpoint: A clearly defined outcome for an individual; it must be specified before the data are collected

Epidemiological studies: Concerned with the distribution and determinants of disease in specified populations

EQUATOR Network: Initiated to provide resources and training for the reporting of health research and assistance in the development, dissemination and implementation of reporting guidelines

Equivalence trial: Used to show that two treatments are clinically equivalent

Error: The difference between the observed and true value. Measurement error has random (due to chance) and possibly systematic (non-random) components; sampling error arises because only a sample of the population is investigated

Error variation: See residual variation

Estimate: A quantity obtained from a sample that is used to represent a population parameter

Evidence-based medicine (EBM): The use of current best evidence in making decisions about the care of individual patients

Exchangeable model: Assumes the estimation procedure is not affected if two observations within a cluster are interchanged

Expected frequency: The frequency that is expected under the null hypothesis

Experimental study: The investigator intervenes in some way to affect the outcome

Experimental unit: The smallest group of individuals who can be regarded as independent for analysis purposes

Explanatory variable: A variable (usually denoted by x) that is used to predict the dependent variable in a regression analysis. Also called the independent, exposure or predictor variable or a covariate

Exposure variable: See explanatory variable

External validation: A substantiation of the findings (e.g. a prognostic index) obtained from one data set using at least one other independent data set

Extra-Binomial variation: The variation in the data, after adjusting for covariates, is greater (overdispersion) or less (underdispersion) than that expected in a Binomial model

Extra-Poisson variation: Occurs when the residual variance is greater (overdispersion) or less (underdispersion) than that expected in a Poisson model

F-distribution: A right-skewed continuous distribution characterized by the degrees of freedom of the numerator and denominator of the ratio that defines it; useful for comparing two variances, and more than two means using the analysis of variance

F-test: See variance ratio test

Factorial experiment: Allows the simultaneous analysis of a number of factors of interest

Fagan's nomogram: A diagram relating the pre-test probability of a diagnostic test result to the likelihood and the post-test probability. It is usually used to convert the former into the latter

False negative: An individual who has the disease but is diagnosed as disease-free

False positive: An individual who is free of the disease but is diagnosed as having the disease

Fisher–Freeman–Halton test: A test evaluating exact probabilities in a contingency table that has more than two rows and/or columns

Fisher's exact test: A test that evaluates exact probabilities (i.e. does not rely on approximations to the Chi-squared distribution) in a contingency table (often a 2×2 table); recommended when the expected frequencies are small

Fitted value: The predicted value of the response variable in a regression analysis corresponding to the particular value(s) of the explanatory variable(s)

Fixed effect: One where the levels of the factor make up the entire population of interest (e.g. the factor 'treatment' whose levels are drug, surgery and radiotherapy). It contrasts with a random effect where the levels represent a sample from the population (e.g. the factor 'patient' whose levels are the 20 patients in a RCT)

Fixed effect model: Contains only fixed effects; used in a meta-analysis when there is no evidence of statistical heterogeneity

Follow-up: The time that an individual is in a study, from entry until she or he experiences the outcome (e.g. develops the disease) or leaves the study or until the conclusion of the study

Forest plot: A diagram used in a meta-analysis showing the estimated effect in each trial and their average (with confidence intervals)

Forward selection: See automatic model selection

Frailty model: Used in survival analysis when there are random effects (clustered data)

Free-format data: Each variable in the computer file is separated from the next by some delimiter, often a space or comma

Frequency: The number of times an event occurs

Frequency distribution: Shows the frequency of occurrence of each possible observation, class of observations or category, as appropriate

Frequency matching: The individuals in two or more comparative groups are matched on a *group* basis so that the average value of each of the relevant potential risk factors of each group is similar to that in every other group. Also called group matching

Frequentist probability: Proportion of times an event would occur if we were to repeat the experiment a large number of times

Funding bias: A tendency to report findings in the direction favoured by the funding body

Funnel plot: A scatter diagram, used in a meta-analysis, with some measure of study size (usually) on the vertical axis and the treatment effect (usually) on the horizontal axis. The plot will be asymmetrical with a gap towards the bottom left-hand corner if publication bias is present

G-estimation: A form of causal modelling that is used to adjust for time-varying confounding

Gaussian distribution: See Normal distribution

GEE: See generalized estimating equation

Generalizability: See transportability

Generalized estimating equation (GEE): Used in a two-level hierarchical structure to estimate parameters and their standard errors to take into account the clustering of the data without referring to a parametric model for the random effects; sometimes referred to as population-averaged or marginal models

Generalized linear model (GLM): A regression model that is expressed in a general form via a link function which relates the mean value of the dependent variable (with a known probability distribution such as Normal, Binomial or Poisson) to a linear function of covariates

Geometric mean: A measure of location for data whose distribution is skewed to the right; it is the antilog of the arithmetic mean of the log data

GLM: See generalized linear model

Gold standard test: Provides a definitive diagnosis of a particular condition

Goodness of fit: A measure of the extent to which the values obtained from a model agree with the observed data

Group matching: See frequency matching

GRRAS guidelines: For reporting reliability and agreement studies

Harrell's c statistic: A measure of discrimination equivalent to the area under the ROC curve

Hazard: The instantaneous risk of reaching the endpoint in survival analysis

Hazard ratio: See relative hazard

Healthy entrant effect: By choosing disease-free individuals to participate in a study, the response of interest (typically mortality) is lower in the first period of the study than would be expected in the general population

Heterogeneity of variance: Unequal variances

Hierarchical model: See multilevel model

Hierarchical repeated measures ANOVA: An extension of repeated measures analysis of variance; individuals are nested within groups and each individual has repeated measures (e.g. over time). Also called nested repeated measures ANOVA

Histogram: A diagram that illustrates the (relative) frequency distribution of a continuous variable by using connected bars. The bar's area is proportional to the (relative) frequency in the range specified by the boundaries of the bar

Historical controls: Individuals who are not assigned to a treatment group at the start of the study but who received treatment some time in the past and are used as a comparison group

Homoscedasticity: Equal variances; also described as homogeneity of variance

Hosmer–Lemeshow goodness of fit statistic: Assesses the agreement between the observed event probabilities and those predicted by a logistic model or prognostic score

Hypothesis test: The process of using a sample to assess how much evidence there is against a null hypothesis about the population. Also called a significance test

I^2: An index that can be used to quantify the impact of statistical heterogeneity between the studies in a meta-analysis

ICC: See intraclass correlation coefficient

Imputation: The process of replacing missing data with substituted values

Incidence: The number of new cases of a disease in a defined period

Incidence rate: The number of new cases of a disease in a defined period divided by the person-years of follow-up of individuals susceptible at the start of the period

Incidence rate ratio (IRR): A relative rate defined as the ratio of two incidence rates

Incident cases: Patients who have just been diagnosed

Independent samples: Every unit in each sample is unrelated to the units in the other samples

Independent variable: See explanatory variable

Indicator variables: See dummy variables

Inference: The process of drawing conclusions about the population using sample data

Influence plot: In meta-analysis it is used to assess the influence of each of k studies: every one of the k studies is deleted in turn, a meta-analysis is used to estimate the effect of interest from the remaining $k - 1$ studies, and these estimates, with confidence intervals, are drawn in a diagram similar to a forest plot

Influential point: An observation which, if omitted from a regression analysis, will lead to a change in one or more of the parameter estimates of the model

Information bias: Occurs during data collection when measurements on exposure and/or disease outcome are incorrectly recorded in a systematic manner

Informative censoring: The probability that an individual will develop the outcome of interest if he or she has survived to a particular time is different in an individual whose follow-up is censored at that time (e.g. if he or she is withdrawn from the study because of a deterioration in his or her condition) from an individual who remains under follow-up

Intention-to-treat (ITT) analysis: All patients in the clinical trial are analysed in the groups to which they were originally assigned

Interaction: Occurs between two explanatory variables in a regression analysis when the effect of one of the variables on the dependent variable varies according to the level of the other. In the context of ANOVA, an interaction exists between two factors when the difference between the levels of one factor is different for two or more levels of the second factor. Also called effect modification

Intercept: The value of the dependent variable in a regression equation when the value(s) of the explanatory variable(s) is (are) zero

Interdecile range: The difference between the 10th and 90th percentiles; it contains the central 80% of the ordered observations

Interim analyses: Pre-planned analyses at intermediate stages of a study

Intermediate variable: A variable that lies on the causal pathway between the explanatory variable and the outcome of interest

Internal–external cross-validation: Used in a multicentre study where we exclude a different centre from the data set for each analysis, and develop and validate the measure of interest on the remaining centres

Internal pilot study: A small-scale preliminary investigation whose data are included in the main study results; usually used to evaluate the variability of observations which then enables the initial overall sample size estimate to be revised

Internal validation: A substantiation of the findings (e.g. the value of a prognostic index) using the data set from which they were derived

Interpolate: Estimate the required value that lies between two known values

Interquartile range: The difference between the 25th and 75th percentiles; it contains the central 50% of the ordered observations

Interval estimate: A range of values within which we believe the population parameter lies

Intraclass correlation coefficient (ICC): In a two-level structure, it expresses the variation between clusters as a proportion of the total variation; it represents the correlation between any two randomly chosen level 1 units in one randomly chosen cluster

IRR: See incidence rate ratio

ITT: See intention-to-treat analysis

Jackknifing: A method of estimating parameters and confidence intervals; each of n individuals is successively removed from the sample, the parameters are estimated from the remaining $n - 1$ individuals, and finally the estimates of each parameter are averaged

k-fold cross-validation: We split the data set into k subsets, derive the measure of interest or model on one of the subsets, and validate it on the remaining $k - 1$ subsets, repeating the procedure for each subset

Kaplan–Meier plot: A survival curve in which the survival probability (or 1 – survival probability) is plotted against the time from baseline. It is used when exact times to reach the endpoint are known

Kolmogorov–Smirnov test: Determines whether data are Normally distributed

Kruskal–Wallis test: A non-parametric alternative to the one-way ANOVA; used to compare the distributions of more than two independent groups of observations

Lead-time bias: Occurs particularly in studies assessing changes in survival over time where the development of more accurate diagnostic procedures may mean that patients entered later into the study are diagnosed at an earlier stage in their disease, resulting in an apparent increase in survival from the time of diagnosis

Leave-one-out cross-validation: We remove each individual from the data set one at a time, and develop and validate the measure of interest on the remaining $n - 1$ individuals in the sample

Left-censored data: Come from patients in whom follow-up did not begin until after the baseline date

Lehr's formulae: Can be used to calculate the optimal sample sizes required for some hypothesis tests when the power is specified as 80% or 90% and the significance level as 0.05

Level: A particular category of a categorical variable or factor

Level 1 unit: The 'individual' at the lowest level of a hierarchical structure; individual level 1 units (e.g. patients) are nested within a level 2 unit (e.g. ward)

Level 2 unit: The 'individual' at the second lowest level in a hierarchical structure; each level 2 unit (e.g. ward) comprises a cluster of level 1 units (e.g. patients)

Level of evidence: A measure of the strength of findings from any particular study design; studies are often ranked in terms of the levels of evidence they provide, starting with the strongest and leading to the weakest evidence

Levene's test: Tests the null hypothesis that two or more variances are equal

Leverage: A measure of the extent to which the value of the explanatory variable(s) for an individual differs from the mean of the explanatory variable(s) in a regression analysis

Lifetable approach to survival analysis: A way of determining survival probabilities when the time to reach the endpoint is only known to within a particular time interval

Likelihood: The probability of the data, given the model. In the context of a diagnostic test, it describes the plausibility of the observed test result if the disease is present (or absent)

Likelihood ratio (LR): A ratio of two likelihoods; for diagnostic tests, the LR is the ratio of the chances of getting a particular test result in those having and not having the disease

Likelihood ratio statistic (LRS): Equal to -2 times the ratio of the log likelihood of a saturated model to that of the model of interest. It is used to assess adequacy of fit and may be called the deviance or, commonly, $-2\log$ likelihood. The difference in the LRS in two nested models can be used to compare the models

Likelihood ratio test: Uses the likelihood ratio statistic to compare the fit of two regression models or to test the significance of one or a set of parameters in a regression model

Likert scale: A scale with a small number of graded responses, such as very poor, poor, no opinion, good and excellent

Limits of agreement: In an assessment of repeatability, it is the range of values between which we expect 95% of the differences between repeated measurements in the population to lie

Linear regression line: The straight line that is defined by an algebraic expression linking two variables

Linear relationship: Implies a straight-line relationship between two variables

Link function: In a generalized linear model, it is a transformation of the mean value of the dependent variable which is modelled as a linear combination of the covariates

Lin's concordance correlation coefficient: A measure of agreement between pairs of observations measured on the same scale. It modifies the Pearson correlation coefficient that assesses the tightness of the data about the line of best fit (precision) when one member of the pair of observations is plotted against the other using the same scale. It includes a bias correction factor that measures how far the line of best fit is from the 45° line through the origin (accuracy)

Log-rank test: A non-parametric approach to comparing two survival curves

Logistic regression: A form of generalized linear model used to relate one or more explanatory variables to the logit of the expected proportion of individuals with a particular outcome when the response is binary

Logistic regression coefficient: The partial regression coefficient in a logistic regression equation

Logit (logistic) transformation: A transformation applied to a proportion or probability, p, such that $\text{logit}(p) = \ln[p/(1-p)] = \ln(\text{odds})$

Lognormal distribution: A right-skewed probability distribution of a random variable whose logarithm follows the Normal distribution

Longitudinal study: Follows individuals over a period of time

LRS: See likelihood ratio statistic

Main outcome variable: That which relates to the major objective of the study

Mann–Whitney U test: See Wilcoxon rank sum (two-sample) test

MAR: See missing at random

Marginal model: See generalized estimating equation

Marginal structural model: A form of causal modelling designed to adjust for time-dependent confounding in observational studies

Marginal total in a contingency table: The sum of the frequencies in a given row (or column) of the table

Masking: See blinding

Matching: A process of creating (usually) pairs of individuals who are similar with respect to variables that may influence the response of interest

Maximum likelihood estimation (MLE): An iterative process of estimation of a parameter that maximizes the likelihood

MCAR: See missing completely at random

McNemar–Bowker test: A test of symmetry in a $k \times k$ contingency table; it is an extension of the McNemar test for two related groups (e.g. two raters both assessing each of a number of individuals) when the outcome has $k > 2$ categories

McNemar's test: Compares proportions in two related groups using a Chi-squared test statistic

Mean: See arithmetic mean

Measurement bias: A systematic error is introduced by an inaccurate measurement tool

Median: A measure of location that is the middle value of the ordered observations

Meta-analysis (overview): A quantitative systematic review that combines the results of relevant studies to produce, and investigate, an estimate of the overall effect of interest

Meta-regression: An extension of meta-analysis that can be used to investigate heterogeneity of effects across studies. The estimated effect of interest (e.g. the relative risk) at the study level is regressed on one or more study-level characteristics (the explanatory variables)

Method of least squares: A method of estimating the parameters in a regression analysis, based on minimizing the sum of the squared residuals. Also called ordinary least squares (OLS)

Misclassification bias: Occurs when we incorrectly classify a categorical exposure and/or outcome variable

Missing at random (MAR): Missing values of a variable can be completely explained by non-missing values of one or more of the other variables

Missing completely at random (MCAR): Missing values are truly randomly distributed in the data set and the fact that they are missing is unrelated to any study variable

Missing not at random (MNAR): The chance that data on a particular variable are missing is strongly related to that variable

Mixed model: A model in which some of the variables have random effects and others have fixed effects. See also multilevel model and random effects model

MLE: See maximum likelihood estimation

MNAR: See missing not at random

Mode: The value of a single variable that occurs most frequently in a data set

Model: Describes, in algebraic terms, the relationship between two or more variables

Model Chi-squared test: Usually refers to a hypothesis test in a regression analysis that tests the null hypothesis that all the parameters associated with the covariates are zero; it is based on the difference in two likelihood ratio statistics

Model sensitivity: The extent to which estimates in a regression model are affected by one or more individuals in the data set or misspecification of the model

Mortality rate: The death rate

Multicentre study: A study conducted concurrently in more than one centre (e.g. hospital), each following the same protocol

Multilevel model: Used for the analysis of hierarchical data in which level 1 units (e.g. patients) are nested within level 2 units

Multinomial logistic regression: A form of logistic regression used when the nominal outcome variable has more than two categories. Also called polychotomous logistic regression

Multiple imputation: A number (generally up to 5) of imputed data sets are created from the original data set, with missing values replaced by imputed values. Standard statistical procedures are used on each complete imputed data set and, finally, the results from these analyses are combined

Multiple linear regression: A linear regression model in which there is a single numerical dependent variable and two or more explanatory variables. Also called multivariable linear regression

Multivariable regression model: Any regression model that has a single outcome variable and two or more explanatory variables

Multivariate analysis: Two or more outcomes of interest (response variables) are investigated simultaneously, e.g. multivariate ANOVA, cluster analysis, factor analysis

Multivariate regression model: Has two or more outcome variables and two or more explanatory variables

Mutually exclusive categories: Each individual can belong to only one category

Negative controls: Those patients in a comparative study (usually a RCT) who do not receive active treatment

Negative predictive value: The proportion of individuals with a negative test result who do not have the disease

Nested models: Two regression models, the larger of which includes the covariates in the smaller model, plus additional covariate(s)

Nested repeated measures ANOVA: See hierarchical repeated measures ANOVA

NNT: See number of patients needed to treat

Nominal significance level: The significance level chosen for each of a number of repeated hypothesis tests so that the overall significance level is kept at some specified value, typically 0.05

Nominal variable: A categorical variable whose categories have no natural ordering

Non-inferiority trial: Used to demonstrate that a given treatment is clinically not inferior to another

Non-parametric tests: Hypothesis tests that do not make assumptions about the distribution of the data. Sometimes called distribution-free tests or rank methods

Normal (Gaussian) distribution: A continuous probability distribution that is bell-shaped and symmetrical; its parameters are the mean and variance

Normal plot: A diagram for assessing, visually, the Normality of data; an appropriate straight line on the Normal plot implies Normality

Normal range: See reference interval

Null hypothesis, H_0: The statement that assumes no effect in the population

Number of patients needed to treat (NNT): The number of patients we need to treat with the experimental rather than the control treatment to prevent one of them developing the 'bad' outcome

Numerical (quantitative) variable: A variable that takes either discrete or continuous values

Observational study: The investigator does nothing to affect the outcome

Observer bias: One observer tends to under-report (or over-report) a particular variable. Also called assessment bias

Odds: The ratio of the probabilities of two complementary events, typically the probability of having a disease divided by the probability of not having the disease

Odds ratio: The ratio of two odds (e.g. the odds of disease in individuals exposed and unexposed to a factor). Sometimes taken as an estimate of the relative risk in a case–control study

Offset: An explanatory variable whose regression coefficient is fixed at unity in a generalized linear model. It is the log of the total person-years (or months/days, etc.) of follow-up in a Poisson model when the dependent variable is defined as the number of events occurring instead of a rate

OLS: Ordinary least squares. See method of least squares

On-treatment analysis: Patients in a clinical trial are only included in the analysis if they complete a full course of the treatment to which they were (randomly) assigned. Also called per protocol analysis

One-sample t-test: Investigates whether the population mean of a variable differs from some hypothesized value

One-tailed test: The alternative hypothesis specifies the direction of the effect of interest

One-way analysis of variance: A particular form of ANOVA used to compare the means of more than two independent groups of observations

Ordinal logistic regression: A form of logistic regression used when the ordinal outcome variable has more than two ordered categories

Ordinal variable: A categorical variable whose categories are ordered in some way

Ordinary least squares (OLS): See method of least squares

Outlier: An observation that is distinct from the main body of the data and is incompatible with the rest of the data

Overdispersion: Occurs when the residual variance is greater than that expected by the defined regression model (e.g. Binomial, Poisson)

Over-fitted model: A model containing too many variables, e.g. more than 1/10th of the number of individuals in a multiple linear regression model

Overview: See meta-analysis

P-value: The probability of obtaining our results, or something more extreme, if the null hypothesis is true

Paired observations: Relate to responses from matched individuals or the same individual in two different circumstances

Paired t-test: Tests the null hypothesis that the mean of a set of differences of paired observations in a population is equal to zero

Pairwise matching: The individuals in two or more comparative groups are matched on an *individual* basis, e.g. in a case–control study, each case is matched individually to a control who has similar potential risk factors

Panel model: Regression model used when each individual has repeated measurements over time. Also called cross-sectional time series model

Parallel trial: Each patient receives only one treatment when two or more treatments are being compared

Parameter: A summary measure (e.g. the mean, proportion) that characterizes a probability distribution. Its value relates to the population

Parametric test: Hypothesis test that makes certain distributional assumptions about the data

Partial regression coefficients: The parameters, other than the intercept, that describe a multivariable regression model

Pearson's correlation coefficient: See correlation coefficient

Per protocol analysis: See on-treatment analysis

Percentage point: The percentile of a distribution; it indicates the proportion of the distribution that lies to its right (i.e. in the right-hand tail), to its left (i.e. in the left-hand tail) or in both right- and left-hand tails

Percentiles: Those values that divide the ordered observations into 100 equal parts

Person-years of follow-up: The sum, over all individuals, of the number of years that each individual is followed-up in a study.

Pie chart: A diagram showing the frequency distribution of a categorical or discrete variable. A circular 'pie' is split into sectors, one for each 'category'; the area of each sector is proportional to the frequency in that category

Pilot study: Small-scale preliminary investigation

Placebo: An inert 'treatment', identical in appearance to the active treatment, that is compared with the active treatment in a negatively controlled clinical trial to assess the therapeutic effect of the active treatment by separating from it the effect of receiving treatment; also used to accommodate blinding

Point estimate: A single value, obtained from a sample, that estimates a population parameter

Point prevalence: The number of individuals with a disease (or percentage of those susceptible) at a particular point in time

Poisson distribution: A discrete probability distribution of a random variable representing the number of events occurring randomly and independently at a fixed average rate

Poisson regression model: A form of generalized linear model used to relate one or more explanatory variables to the log of the expected rate of an event (e.g. of disease) when the follow-up of the individuals varies but the rate is assumed constant over the study period

Polynomial regression: A non-linear (e.g. quadratic, cubic, quartic) relationship between a dependent variable and one or more explanatory variables

Population: The entire group of individuals in whom we are interested

Population-averaged model: See genereralized estimating equation

Positive controls: Those patients in a comparative study (usually a RCT) who receive some form of active treatment as a basis of comparison wi the novel treatment

Positive predictive value: The proportion of individuals with a positive diagnostic test result who have the disease

Post hoc **comparison adjustments:** Made to adjust the *P*-values when multiple comparisons are performed, e.g. Bonferroni

Posterior probability: An individual's belief, based on prior belief and new information (e.g. a test result), that an event will occur

Post-test probability: The posterior probability, determined from previous information and the diagnostic test result, that an individual has a disease

Power: The probability of rejecting the null hypothesis when it is false

Precision: A measure of sampling error. Refers to how well repeated observations agree with one another

Predictor variable: See explanatory variable

Pre-test probability: The prior probability, evaluated before a diagnostic test result is available, that an individual has a disease

Prevalence: The number (proportion) of individuals with a disease at a given point in time (point prevalence) or within a defined interval (period prevalence)

Prevalent cases: Patients who have the disease at a given point in time or within a defined interval but who were diagnosed at a previous time

Primary endpoint: The outcome that most accurately reflects the benefit of a new therapy in a clinical trial

Prior probability: An individual's belief, based on subjective views and/or retrospective observations, that an event will occur

PRISMA Statement: An evidence-based minimum set of items for reporting systematic reviews and meta-analyses

Probability: Measures the chance of an event occurring; it ranges from 0 to 1. See also conditional, posterior and prior probability

Probability density function: The equation that defines a probability distribution

Probability distribution: A theoretical distribution that is described by a mathematical model. It shows the probabilities of all possible values of a random variable

Prognostic index: See prognostic score

Prognostic score: A graded measure of the likelihood that an individual will experience an event. Also called a risk score or prognostic index

Propensity score methods: Used to remove the effects of confounding in an observational study or non-randomized clinical trial. Particularly useful when there are many potential confounders

Proportion: The ratio of the number of events of interest to the total number in the sample or population

Proportional hazards assumption: The requirement in a proportional hazards regression model that the relative hazard is constant over time

Proportional hazards regression model (Cox): Used in survival analysis to study the simultaneous effect of a number of explanatory variables on survival

Prospective study: Individuals are followed forward from some point in time

Protocol A full written description of all aspects of a study

Protocol deviations: Patients who enter a clinical trial but do not fulfil the protocol criteria

Pseudo R^2**:** A logistic regression measure, taking a value from 0 to 1, which is similar to R^2 used in multiple regression analysis but it cannot be interpreted in exactly the same way. It is better suited to comparing models than for assessing the goodness of fit of a model

Publication bias: A tendency for journals to publish only papers that contain statistically significant results

Qualitative variable: See categorical variable

Quantitative variable: See numerical variable

Quartiles: Those values that divide the ordered observations into four equal parts

Quota sampling: Non-random sampling in which the investigator chooses sample members to fulfil a specified 'quota'

R^2**:** The proportion of the total variation in the dependent variable in a simple or multiple regression analysis that is explained by the model. It is a subjective measure of goodness of fit

R_I^2**:** An index of goodness of fit of a logistic regression model

Random effect: The effect of a factor whose levels are assumed to represent a random sample from the population

Random effects model: A model, used for the analysis of longitudinal or hierarchical data, containing at least one random effect in addition to the residual. For example, in a two-level structure, level 1 units are nested within level 2 units (clusters), and the model includes a random effect term that varies randomly between clusters to allow for the clustering. See also mixed model and multilevel model

Random error: The differences between the corresponding observed (or measured) and true values of a variable are due to chance

Random intercepts model: A random effects hierarchical model that assumes, for the two-level structure, that the linear relationship between the mean value of the dependent variable and a single covariate for every level 2 unit has the same slope for all level 2 units and an intercept that varies randomly about the mean intercept

Random sampling: Every possible sample of a given size in the population has an equal probability of being chosen

Random slopes model: A random effects hierarchical model that assumes, for the two-level structure, that the linear relationship between the mean value of the dependent variable and a single covariate for each level 2 unit has a slope that varies randomly about the mean slope and an intercept that varies randomly about the mean intercept

Random variable: A quantity that can take any one of a set of mutually exclusive values with a given probability

Random variation: Variability that cannot be attributed to any explained sources

Randomization: Patients are allocated to treatment groups in a random (based on chance) manner. May be *stratified* (controlling for the effect of important factors) or *blocked* (ensuring approximately equally sized treatment groups)

Randomized controlled trial (RCT): A comparative clinical trial in which there is random allocation of patients to treatments

Range: The difference between the smallest and largest observations

Rank correlation coefficient: See Spearman's rank correlation coefficient

Rank methods: See non-parametric tests

Rate: The number of events occurring expressed as a proportion of the total follow-up time of all individuals in the study

RCT: See randomized controlled trial

Recall bias: A systematic distortion of the data resulting from the way in which individuals remember past events

Receiver operating characteristic (ROC) curve: A two-way plot of the sensitivity against one minus the specificity for different cut-off values for a continuous variable. It affords an assessment of the ability of a prognostic score or diagnostic test to discriminate between those with and without a particular condition; may be used to select the optimal cut-off value or to compare procedures. See also *c* statistic and Harrell's *c* statistic

Reference interval: The range of values (usually the central 95%) of a variable that are typically seen in healthy individuals. Also called the normal or reference range

Regression coefficients: The parameters (i.e. the slope and intercept in simple regression) that describe a regression equation

Regression dilution bias: May occur when fitting a regression model to describe the association between an outcome variable and one or more exposure variable(s) if there is substantial measurement error around one of these exposure variables

Regression to the mean: A phenomenon whereby a subset of extreme results is followed by results that are less extreme on average, e.g. tall fathers having shorter (but still tall) sons

Relative frequency: The frequency expressed as a percentage or proportion of the total frequency

Relative hazard: The ratio of two hazards, interpreted in a similar way to the relative risk. Also called the hazard ratio

Relative rate: The ratio of two rates (often the rate of disease in those exposed to a factor divided by the disease rate in those unexposed to the factor)

Relative risk (RR): The ratio of two risks, usually the risk of a disease in a group of individuals exposed to some factor divided by the risk in unexposed individuals

Reliability: A general term that encompasses repeatability, reproducibility and agreement

Repeatability: The extent to which repeated measurements made by the same observer in identical conditions agree

Repeated measures: The variable of interest is measured on the same individual in more than one set of circumstances (e.g. on different occasions)

Repeated measures ANOVA: A special form of analysis of variance used when a numerical variable is measured on each individual more than once (e.g. on different occasions). It is an extension of the paired t-test when there are more than two repeated measures

Replication: The individual has more than one measurement of the variable on a given occasion

Reporting bias: When participants give answers in the direction they perceive are of interest to the researcher or under-report socially unacceptable or embarrassing behaviours or disorders

Reproducibility: The extent to which the same results can be obtained in different circumstances, e.g. by two methods of measurement, or by two observers

Rescaling: See scaling

Residual: The difference between the observed and fitted values of the dependent variable in a regression analysis

Residual variation: The variance of a variable that remains after the variability attributable to factors of interest has been removed. It is the variance unexplained by the model, and is the residual mean square in an ANOVA table. Also called error variation or unexplained variation

Response bias: Caused by differences in characteristics between those who choose or volunteer to participate in a study and those who do not

Response variable: See dependent variable

Retrospective studies: Individuals are selected and factors that have occurred in their past are studied

Right-censored data: Come from patients who were known not to have reached the endpoint of interest when they were last under follow-up

Risk factor: A determinant that affects the incidence of a particular outcome, e.g. a disease

Risk of disease: The probability of developing the disease in the stated time period; it is estimated by the number of new cases of disease in the period divided by the number of individuals disease-free at the start of the period

Risk score: See prognostic score

Robust: A test is robust to violations of its assumptions if its P-value and power and, if relevant, parameter estimates are not appreciably affected by the violations

Robust standard error: Based on the variability in the data rather than on that assumed by the regression model; more robust to violations of the underlying assumptions of the regression model than estimates from ordinary least squares

ROC: See receiver operating characteristic curve

RR: See relative risk

SAMPL guidelines: Provide guidance to authors, journal editors and reviewers on how to optimally report basic statistical methods and results

Sample: A subgroup of the population

Sampling distribution of the mean: The distribution of the sample means obtained after taking repeated samples of a fixed size from the population

Sampling distribution of the proportion: The distribution of the sample proportions obtained after taking repeated samples of a fixed size from the population

Sampling error: The difference, attributed to taking only a sample of values, between a population parameter and its sample estimate

Sampling frame: A list of all the individuals in the population

Saturated model: One in which the number of variables equals or is greater than the number of individuals

Scale parameter: A measure of over- or underdispersion in Poisson (and, sometimes, Binomial) regression. It is equal to one when there is no extra-Poisson dispersion and is used to correct for over or under Poisson dispersion if substantially different from one

Scaling: A process used to improve the interpretation of the parameters in a regression model; achieved by dividing the explanatory variable by a relevant constant. Also called rescaling

Scatter diagram: A two-dimensional plot of one variable against another, with each pair of observations marked by a point

Screening: A process to ascertain which individuals in an apparently healthy population are likely to have (or, sometimes, not have) the disease of interest

SD: See standard deviation

Secondary endpoints: The outcomes in a clinical trial that are not of primary importance

Selection bias: A systematic distortion of the data resulting from the fact that individuals included in the study are not representative of the population from which they were selected

SEM: See standard error of the mean

Sensitivity: The proportion of individuals with the disease who are correctly diagnosed by the test

Sensitivity analysis: Used to assess how robust or sensitive the results of a study or meta-analysis are to the methods and assumptions of the analysis and/or to the data values

Sequential trial: The patients enter the trial serially in time, and the cumulative data are analysed as they become available by performing repeated significance tests. A decision is made after each test on whether to continue sampling or stop the trial by rejecting or not rejecting the null hypothesis

Shapiro–Wilk test: Determines whether data are Normally distributed

Shrinkage: A process used in estimation of parameters in a random effects model to bring each cluster's estimate of the effect of interest closer to the mean effect from all the clusters

Sign test: A non-parametric test that investigates whether differences tend to be positive (or negative); whether observations tend to be greater (or less) than the median; and whether the proportion of observations with a characteristic is greater (or less) than one half

Significance level: The probability, chosen at the outset of an investigation, that will lead us to reject the null hypothesis if our P-value lies below it. It is often chosen as 0.05

Significance test: See hypothesis test

Simple linear regression: The straight-line relationship between a single dependent variable and a single explanatory variable. Also called univariable linear regression

Simpson's (reverse) paradox: Occurs when the direction of a comparison or an association is reversed when data from a single group is split into subgroups

Single-blind: See blinding

Single imputation: A single estimate is derived for each missing value

Skewed distribution: The distribution of the data is asymmetrical; it has a long tail to the right with a few high values (positively skewed) or a long tail to the left with a few low values (negatively skewed)

Slope: The gradient of the regression line, showing the mean change in the dependent variable for a unit change in the explanatory variable

SND: See Standardized Normal Deviate

Spearman's rank correlation coefficient: A non-parametric alternative to the Pearson correlation coefficient; it provides a measure of association between two variables

Specificity: The proportion of individuals without the disease who are correctly identified by a diagnostic test

SPIRIT Statement: Aims to improve the quality of clinical trial protocols by defining an evidence-based set of items to address in a protocol

Standard deviation (SD): A measure of spread equal to the square root of the variance

Standard error of the mean (SEM): A measure of precision of the sample mean. It is the standard deviation of the sampling distribution of the mean

Standard error of the proportion: A measure of precision of the sample proportion. It is the standard deviation of the sampling distribution of the proportion

Standard Normal distribution: A particular Normal distribution with a mean of zero and a variance of one

Standardized difference: A ratio, used in Altman's nomogram and Lehr's formulae, which expresses the clinically important treatment difference as a multiple of the standard deviation

Standardized Normal Deviate (SND): A random variable whose distribution is Normal with zero mean and unit variance

STARD Statement: An initiative to improve the completeness and transparency of reporting of studies of diagnostic accuracy

Statistic: The sample estimate of a population parameter

Statistical heterogeneity: Present in a meta-analysis when there is considerable variation between the separate estimates of the effect of interest

Statistically significant: The result of a hypothesis test is statistically significant at a particular level (say 1%) if we have sufficient evidence to reject the null hypothesis at that level (i.e. when $P < 0.01$)

Statistics: Encompasses the methods of collecting, summarizing, analysing and drawing conclusions from data

Stem-and-leaf plot: A mixture of a diagram and a table used to illustrate the distribution of data. It is similar to a histogram, and is effectively the data values displayed in increasing order of size

Stepwise selection: See automatic model selection

Stratification: Creation of strata where each stratum comprises a group of homogeneous experimental units that share similar characteristics; also called blocking

Stratum: A subgroup of individuals; usually, the individuals within a stratum share similar characteristics. Sometimes called a block

STROBE Statement: Facilitates critical appraisal and interpretation of observational studies by providing guidance, in the form of a checklist, to authors about how to report their studies

Student's *t*-distribution: See *t*-distribution

Subgroup analyses: The data are analysed separately in defined subsets (e.g. sex) which are components of the whole study group

Subjective probability: Personal degree of belief that an event will occur

Superiority trial: Used to demonstrate that two or more treatments are clinically different

Surrogate endpoint: An outcome measure that is highly correlated with the endpoint of interest but which can be measured more easily, quickly or cheaply than that endpoint

Survey: A cross-sectional study that collects detailed information (e.g. opinions, demographic and lifestyle data) from a sample of individuals

Survival analysis: Examines the time taken for an individual to reach an endpoint of interest (e.g. death) when some data are censored

Survivorship bias: Occurs when survival is compared in patients who do or who do not receive a particular intervention where this intervention only becomes available at some point after the start of the study so that patients have to survive long enough to be eligible to receive the intervention

Symmetrical distribution: The data are centred around some midpoint, and the shape of the distribution to the left of the midpoint is a mirror image of that to the right of it

Systematic allocation: Patients in a clinical trial are allocated treatments in a systematized, non-random manner

Systematic error: There is a tendency for the observed (or measured) value to be greater (or less) than the true value of a variable, leading to bias

Systematic review: A formalized and stringent approach to combining the results from all relevant studies of similar investigations of the same health condition

Systematic sampling: The sample is selected from the population using some systematic method rather than that based on chance

t-**distribution:** A continuous distribution, whose shape is similar to the Normal distribution, characterized by its degrees of freedom. It is particularly useful for inferences about the mean. Also called Student's *t*-distribution

Test statistic: A quantity, derived from sample data, used to test a statistical hypothesis; its value is compared with a known probability distribution to obtain a *P*-value

Time-dependent variable: An explanatory variable in a regression analysis (e.g. in Poisson regression or Cox survival analysis) that takes different values for a given individual at various times in the study

Time-varying confounder: A variable that is both a potential confounder for a time-varying exposure variable and also lies on the causal pathway between that exposure and the outcome

Training sample: The first sample used to generate the model (e.g. in logistic regression or discriminant analysis). The results are authenticated by a second (validation) sample

Transformed data: Obtained by taking the same mathematical transformation (e.g. log) of each observation

Transportability: The extent to which a model or prognostic score works in populations other than that used to derive it. Also called generalizability

Treatment effect: The effect of interest (e.g. the difference between means or the relative risk) that affords a treatment comparison

Trend: Values of the variable show a tendency to increase or decrease progressively over time

TRIPOD Statement: An evidence-based minimum set of recommendations for reporting prediction modelling studies, aiding their critical appraisal, interpretation and uptake by potential users

Two-sample *t*-test: See unpaired *t*-test

Two-tailed test: The direction of the effect of interest is not specified in the alternative hypothesis

Type I error: Rejection of the null hypothesis when it is true

Type II error: Non-rejection of the null hypothesis when it is false

Unbiased: Free from bias

Underdispersion: Occurs when the residual variance is less than that expected by the defined regression model (e.g. Binomial, Poisson)

Unexplained variation: See residual variation

Uniform distribution: Has no 'peaks' because each value is equally likely

Unimodal distribution: Has a single 'peak'

Unit of observation: The 'individual' or smallest group of 'individuals' which can be regarded as independent for the purposes of analysis, i.e. its response of interest is unaffected by those of the other units of observation

Univariable regression model: Has one outcome variable and one explanatory variable. Also called simple linear regression

Unpaired (two-sample) *t*-test: Tests the null hypothesis that the means from two independent populations are equal

Validation sample: A second sample, used to authenticate the results from the training sample

Validity: Closeness to the truth

Variable: Any quantity that varies

Variance: A measure of spread equal to the square of the standard deviation

Variance ratio (*F*-) test: Used to compare two population variances by relating the ratio of their sample estimates to the *F*-distribution

Wald test statistic: Used to test the significance of a parameter in a regression model; it follows the Standard Normal distribution and its square follows the Chi-squared distribution

Washout period: The interval between the end of one treatment period and the start of the second treatment period in a cross-over trial. It allows the residual effects of the first treatment to dissipate

Weighted kappa: A refinement of Cohen's kappa, measuring agreement, that takes into account the extent to which two sets of paired ordinal categorical measurements disagree

Weighted mean: A modification of the arithmetic mean, obtained by attaching weights to each value of the variable in the data set

Wilcoxon rank sum (two-sample) test: A non-parametric test comparing the distributions of two independent groups of observations. It produces the same *P*-value as the Mann–Whitney *U* test

Wilcoxon signed ranks test: A non-parametric test comparing paired observations

Appendix F: Chapter numbers with relevant multiple-choice questions and structured questions from *Medical Statistics at a Glance Workbook*

Chapter		Multiple-choice question(s)	Structured question(s)
1.	Types of data	1, 2, 16	1
2.	Data entry	1, 3, 4	1
3.	Error checking and outliers	5, 6	1, 28
4.	Displaying data diagrammatically	7, 8, 9, 37, 50	1, 9
5.	Describing data: the 'average'	1, 10, 11, 12, 13, 19, 39	2, 3, 4, 9
6.	Describing data: the 'spread'	10, 12, 13, 19	2, 3, 4, 16
7.	Theoretical distributions: the Normal distribution	8, 14, 16, 19, 44	–
8.	Theoretical distributions: other distributions	15, 44	–
9.	Transformations	11, 16, 17, 61	3
10.	Sampling and sampling distributions	18, 19	–
11.	Confidence intervals	19, 20, 21, 34, 45	2
12.	Study design I	22, 23, 27, 31, 32, 33, 39	–
13.	Study design II	24, 25, 26, 29, 60	–
14.	Clinical trials	24, 25, 27, 28	5
15.	Cohort studies	20, 22, 29, 30, 31, 48	16
16.	Case–control studies	29, 31, 32, 33	4, 27
17.	Hypothesis testing	16, 24	3
18.	Errors in hypothesis testing	35, 36	6, 28, 29
19.	Numerical data: a single group	37, 38, 40	–
20.	Numerical data: two related groups	35, 39, 40, 41, 42	7, 8
21.	Numerical data: two unrelated groups	40, 41, 42	3, 9, 21, 22
22.	Numerical data: more than two groups	43	10
23.	Categorical data: a single proportion	44, 45	–
24.	Categorical data: two proportions	44, 46, 47, 48, 49	3, 8, 11, 21

continued

Medical Statistics at a Glance, Fourth Edition. Aviva Petrie and Caroline Sabin. © 2020 Aviva Petrie and Caroline Sabin. Published 2020 by John Wiley & Sons Ltd.
Companion Website: www.medstatsaag.com

Chapter		Multiple-choice question(s)	Structured question(s)
25.	Categorical data: more than two categories	48, 49	8, 12
26.	Correlation	50, 51, 74	3, 13, 26
27.	The theory of linear regression	52	13
28.	Performing a linear regression analysis	53, 54	13, 16
29.	Multiple linear regression	33, 55, 56, 57, 81	14
30.	Binary outcomes and logistic regression	33, 46, 57, 58	4, 12, 15
31.	Rates and Poisson regression	59, 60, 61, 62, 63	16, 17, 18, 29
32.	Generalized linear models	64	–
33.	Explanatory variables in statistical models	26, 60, 61, 65	14, 16, 17, 18, 28
34.	Bias and confounding	57, 60, 62, 66	4, 8, 9, 10, 12, 17, 18, 19, 20, 28, 29
35.	Checking assumptions	67, 69	21
36.	Sample size calculations	68, 69	6, 22
37.	Presenting results	70	–
38.	Diagnostic tools	71, 72	23, 24
39.	Assessing agreement	73, 74	25, 26
40.	Evidence-based medicine	75	29
41.	Methods for clustered data	76, 77	20
42.	Regression models for clustered data	78	18, 20
43.	Systematic reviews and meta-analysis	79, 80	27
44.	Survival analysis	81, 82	15, 28, 29
45.	Bayesian methods	83	–
46.	Developing prognostic scores	84, 85	24

Index

Note: Page numbers in *italic* refer to figures
Page numbers in **bold** refer to tables.

Medical Statistics at a Glance, Fourth Edition. Aviva Petrie and Caroline Sabin. © 2020 Aviva Petrie and Caroline Sabin. Published 2020 by John Wiley & Sons Ltd.
Companion Website: www.medstatsaag.com